Perioperative Monitoring

Editors

GABRIELLA IOHOM
GIRISH P. JOSHI

ANESTHESIOLOGY CLINICS

www.anesthesiology.theclinics.com

Consulting Editor
LEE A. FLEISHER

September 2021 • Volume 39 • Number 3

ELSEVIER

1600 John F. Kennedy Boulevard • Suite 1800 • Philadelphia, Pennsylvania, 19103-2899

http://www.theclinics.com

ANESTHESIOLOGY CLINICS Volume 39, Number 3
September 2021 ISSN 1932-2275, ISBN-13: 978-0-323-83526-8

Editor: Joanna Collett
Developmental Editor: Arlene Campos

Anesthesiology Clinics (ISSN 1932-2275) is published quarterly by Elsevier Inc., 360 Park Avenue South, New York, NY 10010-1710. Months of issue are March, June, September, and December. Periodicals postage paid at New York, NY and at additional mailing offices. Subscription prices are $100.00 per year (US student/resident), $368.00 per year (US individuals), $455.00 per year (Canadian individuals), $957.00 per year (US institutions), $1000.00 per year (Canadian institutions), $100.00 per year (Canadian student/resident), $225.00 per year (foreign student/resident), $488.00 per year (foreign individuals), and $1000.00 per year (foreign institutions). To receive student and resident rate, orders must be accompanied by name of affiliated institution, date of term, and the *signature* of program/residency coordinator on institutions letterhead. Orders will be billed at individual rate until proof of status is received. Foreign air speed delivery is included in all *Clinics'* subscription prices. All prices are subject to change without notice. POSTMASTER: Send address changes to *Anesthesiology Clinics,* Elsevier Health Sciences Division, Subscription Customer Service, 3251 Riverport Lane, Maryland Heights, MO 63043. Customer Service (orders, claims, online, change of address): Elsevier Health Sciences Division, Subscription Customer Service, 3251 Riverport Lane, Maryland Heights, MO 63043. **Tel:1-800-654-2452 (U.S. and Canada); 314-447-8871 (outside U.S. and Canada). Fax: 314-447-8029. E-mail: journalscustomerservice-usa@elsevier.com (for print support); journalsonlinesupport-usa@elsevier.com (for online support).**

Reprints. For copies of 100 or more of articles in this publication, please contact the Commercial Reprints Department, Elsevier Inc., 360 Park Avenue South, New York, NY 10010-1710. Tel.: 212-633-3874; Fax: 212-633-3820; E-mail: reprints@elsevier.com.

Anesthesiology Clinics, is also published in Spanish by McGraw-Hill Inter-americana Editores S. A., P.O. Box 5-237, 06500 Mexico D. F., Mexico.

Anesthesiology Clinics, is covered in *MEDLINE/PubMed (Index Medicus), Current Contents/Clinical Medicine, Excerpta Medica, ISI/BIOMED*, and *Chemical Abstracts*.

Contributors

CONSULTING EDITOR

LEE A. FLEISHER, MD, FACC, FAHA
Robert D. Dripps Professor and Chair of Anesthesiology and Critical Care, Professor of Medicine, Perelman School of Medicine, University of Pennsylvania, Philadelphia, Pennsylvania, USA

EDITORS

GABRIELLA IOHOM, MD, PhD
Consultant Anaesthesiologist and Senior Lecturer, Department of Anaesthesiology and Intensive Care Medicine, Cork University Hospital, University College Cork, Cork, Ireland

GIRISH P. JOSHI, MBBS, MD, FFARCSI
Professor of Anesthesiology and Pain Management, The University of Texas Southwestern Medical Center, Dallas, Texas, USA

AUTHORS

FEDERICO BILOTTA, MD, PhD
Department of Anesthesiology, Critical Care and Pain Medicine, Policlinico Umberto I, "Sapienza" University of Rome, Rome, Italy

AMBER BLEDSOE, MD
Department of Anesthesiology, University of Utah, Salt Lake City, Utah, USA

KATHRYN HARTER BRIDGES, MD
Associate Professor, Department of Anesthesia and Perioperative Medicine, Medical University of South Carolina, Charleston, South Carolina, USA

MAXIME CANNESSON, MD, PhD
Department Chair, University of California Los Angeles, David Geffen School of Medicine, Department of Anesthesiology and Perioperative Medicine, Ronald Reagan UCLA Medical Center, Los Angeles, California, USA

ILONKA N. DE KEIJZER, MD
Department of Anesthesiology, University Medical Center Groningen, Groningen, the Netherlands

CIARA FAHY, MD
Specialist Anesthesiology Trainee, Department of Anesthesiology and Intensive Care Medicine, Cork University Hospital, Wilton, Cork, Ireland

CHRISTIAN FENGER-ERIKSEN, MD, PhD
Senior Consultant, Associate Professor, Department of Anaesthesiology, Aarhus University Hospital, Aarhus, Denmark

RALPH GERTLER, MD, PhD
Executive Senior Physician, Department of Anaesthesiology and Intensive Care, HELIOS Klinikum München West, Teaching Hospital of the Ludwig-Maximilians-Universität, München, Germany

GABRIELLA IOHOM, MD, PhD
Consultant Anaesthesiologist and Senior Lecturer, Department of Anaesthesiology and Intensive Care Medicine, Cork University Hospital, University College Cork, Cork, Ireland

GIRISH P. JOSHI, MBBS, MD, FFARCSI
Professor of Anesthesiology and Pain Management, The University of Texas Southwestern Medical Center, Dallas, Texas, USA

CHRISTINE LEE, PhD
Staff Applied Machine Learning Algorithms Engineer, Edwards Lifesciences, Critical Care R&D, Irvine, California, USA

PADRAIG MAHON, MSc, MD, FCARCSI, FJFICMI
Consultant Anaesthesiologist, Department of Anaesthesiology and Critical Care, Cork University Hospital, Honorary Clinical Lecturer, University College Cork, Wilton, Cork, Ireland

JULIE RYAN McSWAIN, MD
Associate Professor, Department of Anesthesia and Perioperative Medicine, Medical University of South Carolina, Charleston, South Carolina, USA

FREDERIC MICHARD, MD, PhD
MiCo, Denens, Switzerland

CORNELIUS O'SULLIVAN, BEng
Senior Clinical Engineer, Biomedical Department, Cork University Hospital, Wilton, Cork, Ireland

MICHAEL RAMSAY, MD, FRCA
Chairman, Department of Anesthesiology, Baylor University Medical Center, Baylor Scott and White Health Care, Dallas, Texas, USA

DAVID ROCHE, BSc, BM, BS, FCAI, FJFICMI
Specialist Registrar Anaesthesiology, Department of Anaesthesiology and Critical Care, Cork University Hospital, Wilton, Cork, Ireland

THOMAS W.L. SCHEEREN, MD, PhD
Professor, Anesthesiologist, Department of Anesthesiology, University Medical Center Groningen, Groningen, the Netherlands

HARSHA SHANTHANNA, MD, FRCPC, PhD
Associate Professor, Department of Anesthesia, Department of Health Research Methods, Evidence and Impact, McMaster University, Hamilton, Ontario, Canada

STEPHAN R. THILEN, MD, MS
Associate Professor, Department of Anesthesiology and Pain Medicine, University of Washington, Seattle, Washington, USA

ALESSIO TRAMONTANA, MD
Department of Anesthesiology, Critical Care and Pain Medicine, Policlinico Umberto I, "Sapienza" University of Rome, Rome, Italy

GEORGIA TSAOUSI, MD, MSc, PhD
Department of Anesthesiology and ICU, School of Medicine, Faculty of Health Sciences, Aristotle University of Thessaloniki, Greece

VISHAL UPPAL, MBBS, FRCA, MSc
Associate Professor, Department of Anesthesia, Dalhousie University, Nova Scotia Health Authority and IWK Health Centre, Halifax, Nova Scotia, Canada

WADE A. WEIGEL, MD
Staff Anesthesiologist, Department of Anesthesiology, Virginia Mason Medical Center, Seattle, Washington, USA

THEODORA WINGERT, MD
Assistant Clinical Professor, University of California Los Angeles, David Geffen School of Medicine, Department of Anesthesiology and Perioperative Medicine, Ronald Reagan UCLA Medical Center, Los Angeles, California, USA

FAROUK YAMANI, MD
Department of Anesthesiology, Critical Care and Pain Medicine, Policlinico Umberto I, "Sapienza" University of Rome, Rome, Italy

JOSH ZIMMERMAN, MD
Department of Anesthesiology, University of Utah, Salt Lake City, Utah, USA

Contents

Since the first public demonstration of general anesthesia in 1846, anesthesiology has seen major advancements as a specialty. These include both important technological improvements and the development and implementation of internationally accepted patient safety standards. Together, these ultimately resulted in the recognition of anesthesiology as the leading medical specialty advocating for patient safety. Modern-day anesthesiology faces a new challenge of automated anesthesia delivery. Despite evidence for a more refined and precise delivery of anesthesia through this platform, there is currently no substitute for the presence of an appropriately trained anesthesia clinician to manage the complex interplay of human factors and patient safety in the perioperative setting.

Ventilation or breathing is vital for life yet is not well monitored in hospital or at home. Respiratory rate is a neglected vital sign and tidal volumes together with breath sounds are checked infrequently in many patients. Medications with the potential to depress ventilation are frequently administered, and may be accentuated by obesity causing airway obstruction in the form of sleep apnea. Sepsis may adversely affect ventilation by causing an increase in respiratory rate, often a very early sign of infection. Changes in ventilation may be early signs of deterioration in the patient.

Today's management of the ventilated patient still relies on the measurement of old parameters such as airway pressures and flow. Graphical presentations reveal the intricacies of patient-ventilator interactions in times of supporting the patient on the ventilator instead of fully ventilating the heavily sedated patient. This opens a new pathway for several bedside technologies based on basic physiologic knowledge; however, it may increase the complexity of measurements. The spread of the COVID-19 infection has confronted the anesthesiologist and intensivist with one of the most severe pulmonary pathologies of the last decades. Optimizing the patient at the bedside is an old and newly required skill for all physicians in the intensive care unit, supported by mobile technologies such as lung ultrasound and electrical impedance tomography. This review summarizes old knowledge and presents a brief insight into extended monitoring options.

Perioperative hemodynamic monitoring is an essential part of anesthetic care. In this review, we aim to give an overview of methods currently used in the clinical routine and experimental methods under development. The technical aspects of the mentioned methods are discussed briefly. This review includes methods to monitor blood pressures, for example, arterial pressure, mean systemic filling pressure and central venous pressure, and volumes, for example, global end-diastolic volume (GEDV) and extravascular lung water. In addition, monitoring blood flow (cardiac output) and fluid responsiveness (preload) will be discussed.

Neuromuscular monitoring is essential for optimal management of neuromuscular blocking drugs. Postoperative residual neuromuscular blockade continues to occur with an unacceptably high incidence and is associated with adverse patient outcomes. Use of a peripheral nerve stimulator and subjective tactile or visual assessment is useful for intraoperative management of neuromuscular blockade, especially when the patient's hand is accessible. Quantitative monitoring is necessary for confirmation of adequate reversal and for identification of patients who have recovered spontaneously and therefore should not receive pharmacologic reversal agents. Guidelines, as well as more user-friendly monitoring equipment, have created momentum toward improving routine perioperative neuromuscular monitoring.

The electroencephalogram (EEG) can be analyzed in its raw form for characteristic drug-induced patterns of change or summarized using mathematical parameters as a processed electroencephalogram (pEEG). In this article we aim to summarize the contemporary literature pertaining to the commonly available pEEG monitors including the effects of commonly used anesthetic drugs on the EEG and pEEG parameters, pEEG monitor pitfalls, and the clinical implications of pEEG monitoring for anesthesia, pediatrics, and intensive care.

Nociception refers to the process of encoding and processing noxious stimuli. Its monitoring can have potential benefits. Under anesthesia, nociceptive signals are continuously generated to cause involuntary effects on the autonomic nervous system, reflex movement, and stress response. Most available systems depend on the identification and measurement of these indirect effects to indicate nociception-antinociception balance. Despite advances in monitoring technology and availability, their limitations presently override their benefits. Hence, their utility and applicability in present-day anesthesia care is uncertain. Future technologies might allow automated closed-loop multimodal anesthesia systems, which includes the components of hypnosis and analgesic balance for a patient.

Accumulating evidence indicates that cerebral desaturation in the perioperative period occurs more frequently than recognized. Combining monitoring modalities that reflect different aspects of cerebral perfusion status, such as near-infrared spectroscopy, jugular bulb saturation, and transcranial Doppler ultrasonography, may provide an extended window for prevention, early detection, and prompt intervention in ongoing hypoxic/ischemic neuronal injury and, thereby, improve neurologic outcome. Such an approach would minimize the impact of limitations of each monitoring modality, while individual components complement each other, enhancing the accuracy of acquired information. Current literature has failed to demonstrate any clear-cut clinical benefit of these modalities on outcome prognosis.

The main goal of perioperative coagulation monitoring is to improve safety of patients undergoing surgical procedures. Various conditions can affect the coagulation system during surgery and bleeding. The value of traditional standard coagulation tests is limited in detecting hemostatic dysfunctions and they are particularly ineffective in diagnosing hyperfibrinolysis. This article reports on key issues and pathophysiologic changes that affect the hemostatic system in the perioperative setting. Values of preoperative coagulation tests are discussed and the basic principles for point-of-care coagulation devices, including platelet analyzers and their clinical use, are evaluated.

 Video content accompanies this article at http://www.anesthesiology. theclinics.com.

Advances in technology have led to more user-friendly ultrasound devices that allow for easy incorporation into daily perioperative practice, with the anesthesiologist serving as the sonographer. With appropriate knowledge and training, bedside ultrasound examinations can be used to better diagnose pathology and guide perioperative strategies. Cardiac ultrasound examination was the initial emphasis in anesthesiology, with now expansion into lung and gastric ultrasound imaging. In this review, the indications,

ANESTHESIOLOGY CLINICS

SERIES OF RELATED INTEREST

Critical Care Clinics

THE CLINICS ARE AVAILABLE ONLINE!
Access your subscription at:
www.theclinics.com

Foreword

Monitoring: Back to the Future

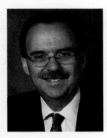

Lee A. Fleisher, MD, FACC, FAHA
Consulting Editor

In 1895, Harvey Cushing and Amory Codman developed the first continuous record for recording pulse and respiration. Over 125 years later, we continue to monitor basic physiology but also have new tools and refinement of old tools to add to our ability to determine the physiologic effects of both surgery and anesthesia. As the editors of the current issue highlight, it is critically important to use technology to provide us with information upon which to make decisions. Therefore, we need to understand that the meaning of this information is critical. Fortunately, our authors have brought together an amazing group of authors to discuss these technologies, including newer modalities like POCUS, wearables, and telemedicine.

In deciding who could assemble a group of experts and provide a vision for this issue, Drs Gabriella Iohom and Girish P. Joshi were clear choices as leaders in anesthesiology. Gabriella Iohom, MD, PhD is Consultant Anaesthesiologist and Senior Lecturer at University College Cork and Cork University Hospital. She is cofounder and codirector of the Cork Regional Anaesthesia Fellowship and Immediate Past Chair and Member, Subcommittee on Regional Anaesthesia of the European Society of Anaesthesiology. Girish P. Joshi, MD, is a professor in the Department of Anesthesiology and Pain Management at UT Southwestern Medical Center. Dr Joshi is an executive section editor for *Anesthesia & Analgesia* and a section editor for UpToDate. He is a past president and current active member of the Society for Ambulatory Anesthesia, the Society of Anesthesia and Sleep Medicine, and the

Anesthesiology Clin 39 (2021) xiii–xiv
https://doi.org/10.1016/j.anclin.2021.06.001
1932-2275/21/© 2021 Published by Elsevier Inc.

anesthesiology.theclinics.com

Texas Society of Anesthesiologists. Together, they have assembled an important issue to ensure we can obtain information from our monitors.

Lee A. Fleisher, MD, FACC, FAHA
Perelman School of Medicine
University of Pennsylvania
3400 Spruce Street, Dulles 680
Philadelphia, PA 19104, USA

E-mail address:
Lee.Fleisher@uphs.upenn.edu

Preface

Monitoring: Back to the Future

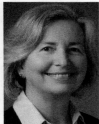
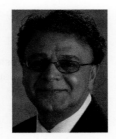

Gabriella Iohom, MD, PhD   Girish P. Joshi, MBBS, MD, FFARCSI
Editors

Monitoring, derived from the Latin *monere* (to warn), meaning continuous measurement of variables over time, is core to the delivery of anesthesia and perioperative care. Currently, the utility of basic standard monitoring is universally accepted as part of a complex man-machine interaction and feedback system aimed at keeping the patient within safe physiologic limits. Perioperative care has always been intimately associated with technological advancements to augment postoperative recovery. Although it may be coincidental, many experts cite improved monitoring as one of the reasons for improved patient safety and perioperative outcomes, as well as enhanced recovery after surgery.

Technological innovation continues to transform perioperative care, and there is much promise for the novel monitors. However, as stated by Albert Einstein (1879-1955): "Not everything that counts can be counted and not everything that can be counted counts." More information is not necessarily always better, but rather the right information must be collected at the right time, interpreted correctly, and acted upon effectively followed by reevaluation. New technology has the potential to become "standard" only if it improves patient outcome in addition to improved patient safety, reliability, and cost-effectiveness.

While the list of topics in this issue of *Anesthesiology Clinics* is far from exhaustive, it provides welcome insights into many exciting innovations in the field without overshadowing embedded standards of monitoring. We are grateful to the authors for their valuable contribution generously delivered amid a global pandemic. We also wish to thank Lee A. Fleisher for the invitation to guest edit this issue, and Elsevier staff, Ms Joanna M. Collett, and Ms Arlene Campos for their support.

Anesthesiology Clin 39 (2021) xv–xvi
https://doi.org/10.1016/j.anclin.2021.04.001
1932-2275/21/© 2021 Published by Elsevier Inc.

We hope you will find this issue enjoyable, informative, and thought provoking.

Gabriella Iohom, MD, PhD
Department of Anaesthesiology and
Intensive Care Medicine
Cork University Hospital
University College Cork
Wilton Road
Cork T12DC4A, Ireland

Girish P. Joshi, MBBS, MD, FFARCSI
Department of Anesthesiology and
Pain Management
University of Texas
Southwestern Medical School
5323 Harry Hines Boulevard
Dallas, TX 75390, USA

E-mail addresses:
giohom@ucc.ie (G. Iohom)
girish.joshi@utsouthwestern.edu (G.P. Joshi)

Clinician Monitoring

Ciara Fahy, MD[a], Cornelius O'Sullivan, BEng[b],
Gabriella Iohom, MD, PhD[c],*

KEYWORDS

- Anesthesia clinician • Clinical monitoring • Monitoring standards
- Clinician presence • History of monitoring

KEY POINTS

- History of monitoring helps appreciate progress made to date.
- Standards of monitoring were formally adopted and subsequently updated by international anesthesia organizations since the late 80s.
- Clinician presence is the first standard of monitoring and a primary determinant of patient safety during all forms of anesthesia and recovery.
- Accurate records of minimum monitoring data must be kept.

HISTORY OF MONITORING

The history of patient monitoring long preceded the first public demonstration of general anesthesia in October 1846 by W.T.G. Morton.[1,2] Before this time, the clinical status of a patient was ascertained by the trained medical gaze of the physician.[1] In 1849, an early British anesthesiologist John Snow published his own set of customary monitoring parameters.[1,3] These included changes in the respiratory rate, patterns, and skin color while undergoing anesthesia.[1,3] The first reported death of a 15-year-old girl, Hannah Greener, under chloroform anesthesia, was a pivotal case in highlighting the importance of patient safety monitoring.[1] Soon after this, early advocacy for patient safety propelled to the forefront of general anesthesia. It began with routine monitoring of respiratory rate, pulse, and skin temperature.[1]

Electrocardiography

Although Willem Einthoven is known as the creator of the electrocardiograph (EKG), the first known EKG recording was obtained in 1887 by Augustus Waller at London's St Mary's Hospital using Lippmann's mercury capillary electrometer.[4] This device had been built on a century's work of electrophysiology, and the discovery of the electrical activity of the heart was done by Köllicker and Müller in 1856.[5] It consisted of a glass

[a] Department of Anesthesiology and Intensive Care Medicine, Cork University Hospital, Wilton, Cork T12 DFK4, Ireland; [b] Biomedical Department, Cork University Hospital, Wilton, Cork T12 DFK4, Ireland; [c] Department of Anesthesiology and Intensive Care Medicine, Cork University Hospital and University College Cork, National University of Ireland, Wilton, Cork T12 DFK4, Ireland
* Corresponding author.
E-mail address: giohom@ucc.ie

Anesthesiology Clin 39 (2021) 389–402
https://doi.org/10.1016/j.anclin.2021.04.002
1932-2275/21/© 2021 Elsevier Inc. All rights reserved.

tube containing mercury. The meniscus of the mercury moved in relation to changes in electrical potentials, which could produce a permanent record by projecting the displacement onto photosensitized paper.[4] It was Waller who demonstrated that, by using this device, the electrical activity of the heart could be recorded externally from the chest wall.[4] He identified two deflections and entitled them V1 and V2.[4] These corresponded to ventricular depolarization (QRS wave) and repolarization (T wave), respectively.[4] Waller presented his findings at the first International Congress of Physiology in 1889, which was attended by Einthoven. Einthoven spent a further 5 years expanding on Waller's discoveries. First, he enhanced the function of the mercury capillary electrometer, which allowed him to further identify five deflections on an EKG tracing, labeled P, Q, R, S, and T.[4] He then developed the string galvanometer, which allowed enhancement of the tracings found on the mercury capillary electrometer to acceptable diagnostic levels.[4] His second article based on his design in 1903 detailed the EKGs he had taken in clinical environments.[6] However, it was not until 1922 that the first prospective study examining the utility of the EKG in monitoring patients under general anesthesia was published.[1]

The effect of anesthesia on cardiac physiology was largely dismissed despite research from Dr J. Clover in 1864.[1] He had observed a link between diminution of pulse, increased pulse irregularities, and death in animals under chloroform anesthesia.[1] Respiratory depression was considered the primary contributing factor to such deaths, and cardiac insult had little part to play. In 1896, Robert Kirk documented the first clinical account of incorporating heart sounds via a stethoscope as part of patient monitoring.[1] Finally, in 1922, the first study advocating the use of continuous cardiac monitoring using a string galvanometer to produce an EKG was reported.[1] It found notable discrepancies between the heart rate recorded via manual pulse palpation and the heart rate recorded by electrocardiography. Interestingly, the EKG trace produced several premature beats that had not been recognized by the anesthesiologist.[1] Unfortunately, various technical issues limited its value in diagnostics and therefore its popularity. This changed in 1952 when Himmelstein and Schneider developed a means by which the EKG could be on continuous display via a cathode-ray screen.[1] With the discovery of lead II mirroring the axis of the heart vector, its reliability in detecting arrhythmias, and the subsequent adaptation of the three-lead configuration, the EKG eventually became of clinical use in the operating theater.

Oxygen Saturation Monitor

The origins of oximetry date back to 1760, with the formulation of Lambert's law by Johann Lambert. The publication of Beer's law soon followed in 1846 by the German physicist August Beer. Together, the Beer-Lambert law demonstrated that the relationship between the amount of light absorbed was related to both the thickness of the material sample and the concentration of the attenuating species.[7] In 1864, the German scientist Felix Hoppe-Seyler used analytical spectroscopy to crystalize the oxygen-carrying pigment in blood.[8] He coined this hemoglobin. He was able to separate it into both iron-rich heme and the protein globin and demonstrated that light was absorbed at wavelengths 540 nm and 560 nm if passed through an oxygenated hemoglobin solution.[8] The British physicist George G. Stokes (1819–1903) expanded on this and showed that hemoglobin exists in two states, oxygenated and deoxygenated.[8] He proved this by observing the changes in the color of blood transitioning from the oxygen-depleted to oxygen-rich envirnonment.[8] Scientists in 1930s Germany applied the Beer-Lambert law to oxyhemoglobin solutions, which absorbed red light. Application of this concept took some time to be incorporated into the development of pulse oximetry. During World War I and II, pilots attempting to fly higher than their enemies were found to be losing consciousness and crashing owing to changing atmospheric pressures that rendered them hypoxic.[1] Primitive oximetry was developed as a warning device for pilots in 1940.[1] This was an invasive procedure requiring blood gas analysis. More than 30 years later, a young Japanese bioengineer, Takuo Aoyagi, while working on the measurement of cardiac output noticed pulsatile variations in dye measurement via light signals with each heart beat or pulse.[8] Using different wavelengths of light, he discovered the isosbestic point for hemoglobin. Eventually, the peripheral pulse oximeter probe came into commercial production in 1977.[8] Yelderman and New published an article in *Anesthesiology* highlighting the importance and utility of continuous pulse oximetry in theaters and in critically ill patients.[9] Soon thereafter, it found its way into the operating room, with the American Society of Anesthesiologists (ASA) incorporating pulse oximetry as a basic standard monitoring device in 1986.[10] The utility of pulse oximetry and its further refinement is discussed in chapters Ventilation monitoring and Cerebral perfusion monitoring-brain oxygen saturation monitoring.

Blood Pressure Monitor

In 1616, the English physician William Harvey proposed that blood was pumped in one direction around the body in a finite amount.[2] The first estimated measurement of blood pressure was performed invasively on animals in the mid-1700s by Stephen Hales.[11] Glass tubes were inserted into the femoral arteries of horses. The height to which blood rose in the glass tubes above the horses' left ventricle was observed.[11] The early 1800s saw the introduction of the mercury hydrodynometer and the millimeter of mercury unit by Jean Léonard Marie Poiseuille (1797–1869).[2] He replaced Hales' long tube for a much smaller column of mercury that connected with an artery.[2,11] Following various advancements, a noninvasive blood pressure monitor finally came about in 1881. The Austrian physician Ritter von Basch (1837–1905) was the first to measure blood pressure noninvasively using a series of sphygmomanometers.[11] His designs, however, were inefficient and unreliable. Scipione Riva Rocci was credited with developing the mercury sphygmomanometer in 1896.[2] At this time, physicians could only measure systolic blood pressures, by palpating the point at which a pulse disappeared on constriction of the artery by the cuff.[1] Normal blood pressure values were unknown, and clinicians therefore followed the changing trends of systolic blood pressure measurement. The basis of current auscultatory blood pressure monitoring is owed to Nikolai Korotkoff.[2] Using Riva Rocci's sphygmomanometer and a stethoscope, he demonstrated certain sounds that could be heard as arteries were decompressed, introducing the concept of diastolic blood pressure.[2] The chapter entitled Hemodynamic monitoring illustrates the sophistication of contemporary methods of monitoring various pressures and flows.

Neuromuscular Monitoring

Muscle relaxants were first introduced into the operating room in 1942.[12] They were used for relaxation of abdominal muscles during surgery.[12] Around the mid-1950s, a higher mortality rate associated with the use of neuromuscular blockade was noticed.[12] This was initially misattributed to neuromuscular blocking agent toxicity, rather than inadequate reversal. By the early 1960s, the notion of toxicity was abolished, and it was agreed that neuromuscular blockade required careful administration and monitoring. The first to describe the neuromuscular monitor was Christie and Churchill-Davidson in the late 1950s.[13] Early monitors measured responses to a single twitch or tetanic stimulation. They were bulky and cumbersome and required an electrical outlet.[13,14] Churchill-Davidson published an article in 1965 outlining the existence of a new portable monitor and the safety value in its implementation during clinical practice.[14] Soon after this, in 1970, the train-of-four ratio was introduced. Initially used to observe treatment responses in patients with myasthenia gravis, it became incorporated into routine clinical practice as a more sensitive index of neuro-muscular blockade reversal.[12,13] Subsequent advances took place with the development of post-tetanic count in 1981 and double burst stimulation in 1989.[13]

Modern neuromuscular monitors have since been developed, which allow objective assessment of the depth of neuromuscular blockade. They differ from peripheral nerve stimulators in that they directly measure the degree of muscle weakness, when stimulated, and display results numerically. Unlike visual and tactile assessments, these quantitative monitors provide a much more accurate assessment of the return of muscle strength after neuromuscular blockade reversal. They are presented in detail in the chapter dedicated to Neuromuscular blockade monitoring.

DEVELOPMENT OF STANDARDS

Patient safety standards have been debated among anesthesiologists since the 1840s.[15] There have been countless peer-reviewed articles published, with a clear focus on training clinicians, a constant drive to develop new enhanced safety equipment, and a growing awareness of risk measurement.[15]

The ASA was founded in 1905. In 1968, the ASA's first set of guidelines was produced.[15] These guidelines defined the role of anesthesiologists, highlighted the importance of preassessment and postoperative care, and described the importance of a universal and expert approach to the deliverance of anesthetic care.[15] However, there were no formal standards of monitoring implemented until a malpractice crisis ensued in the early 1970s. Around this time, it was becoming apparent that a small number of postoperative complications resulted in permanent disability or death due to anesthesia rather than surgery-related incidents.[16] Although these incidents represented only 3% of all claims, they accounted for 11% of projected insurance losses.[17] Sensationalized media depictions of anesthesia-related injury heightened the general public's fear of undergoing general anesthesia. It was now regarded as a high-risk specialty, which saw medical malpractice premiums increase and individual claims reaching multimillion dollar figures.[16] A meeting organized by several hospitals affiliated with Harvard Medical School concluded that adverse outcomes could be reduced by early detection of problems and prompt intervention because the majority of the 1 in 10,000 deaths related to anesthesia were deemed preventable.[16] A risk management committee was formed. This was composed of six affiliated hospitals, six chiefs of anesthesia, and eight other members.[16] They also enlisted Controlled Risk Insurance Company (CRICO), which was formed by Harvard Medical Schools itself to provide medical liability insurance to affiliated hospitals.[17] Together, they investigated all anesthesia-related closed malpractice claims filed between 1976 and 1988.[18] The aim was to identify recurring issues, rather than highlight specific incidents of negligence.[17] CRICO's involvement was to offer recommendations to improve patient safety and therefore lower malpractice premiums.[16] A total of 1,001,000 cases were examined, all of which were ASA grade 1 and 2.[18] Seventy cases of exclusively anesthesia-related injuries were reported; of which, 11 were major intraoperative events, including 5 deaths, four cases of irreversible brain injury, and two cardiac arrests.[18] The committee found that 72% of these adverse events could have been prevented with better monitoring.[19] The main causes included inadequate ventilation (38%), esophageal intubation (18%), and difficult intubation.[20] In addition, the maintenance of any current monitors was found to be substandard.[17] A list of recommendations was formulated including (1) basic monitoring required in both the perioperative and postoperative period, (2) implementation of anesthetic rooms separate to operating rooms, (3) equipment standards, (4) a standard of equipment maintenance, (5) record keeping, and (6) preoperative and postoperative assessments by anesthesiologists.[17]

Adequate patient and anesthetic machine monitoring were the two areas first addressed. This began the formulation of standards such as perioperative and postoperative use of pulse oximetry and capnography.[19,20] Basic or minimal monitoring standards were as follows:[17]

- Continual anesthesiology presence during both general and regional anesthesia
- Blood pressure and heart rate monitoring every 5 minutes
- Auscultation of heart sounds and palpation of pulse
- Continuous electrocardiography
- Ventilation: end-tidal CO_2 in preference to observation of ventilation bag or auscultation of breath sounds
- O_2 analyzer conforming to the requirements of the American National Standards Institute
- Breathing system disconnect alarms
- Temperature monitoring (although not mandatory for every case)

The initial implementation of these standards was met with some resistance. Coinciding with new monitoring devices used in operating rooms, some clinicians felt that these strategies were overriding clinical judgment. Eventually, a compromise was reached in that pulse oximetry and capnography would not be mandatory in all cases and minimal standards would include those already being routinely followed by clinicians until future research was carried out.[16] It was also agreed that the standards established could be overridden by clinical judgment in certain circumstances.[16] These standards were officially adopted as policy on March 25, 1985.[21] After this date, malpractice insurance underwriters lowered the specialty's risk classification, with further incentives of lowered premiums to clinicians who agreed to routinely use pulse oximetry and capnography.[16]

From here, change was beginning to evolve at a national level. Dr Pierce, President of the ASA and an anesthesia chief of Harvard, instigated a closed claim project with aspirations of improving patient safety and expanding patient monitoring standards nationally.[16] Of the 634 claims examined, 69% of the 193 respiratory events were deemed to be preventable if ventilation had been monitored as recommended by the Harvard standards.[16,18] These standards were developed by professionals within anesthesia without any input from regulating bodies. They mandated continuous evaluation of oxygenation, ventilation, and circulation; were approved as ASA National Standards in 1986; and became mandatory in 1987.[16]

The International Task Force on Anesthesia Safety was formed in 1989 with a view to enhance anesthesia safety globally.[22] Comprehensive standard templates and policies were developed over 2 years, looking at monitoring, equipment, and resources available at various geographic locations. This model became known as the International Standards for a Safe Practice of Anesthesia adopted by the World Federation of Societies of Anaesthesiologists (WFSA) in June 1992.[23]

ANESTHESIA CLINICIAN AS THE FIRST STANDARD OF MONITORING

The most important determinant of patient safety during anesthesia is the presence of an appropriately experienced anesthesia practitioner (aka clinician), while monitoring devices supplement clinical observation.[24] Using both clinical skills and monitoring equipment, the anesthesia clinician must care for the patient continuously. In addition, accurate records of the values determined by the monitors must be kept. If handing over patient care under anesthesia becomes necessary, a detailed handover must be delivered to the incoming clinician, and this should also be recorded.

Presence

International anesthesia organizations unanimously agree that the most important monitor is the presence of an anesthesia clinician throughout delivery of anesthesia. Depending on the jurisdiction, this responsibility rests with the consultant anesthesiologist, the attending anesthesiologist, and the anesthesia specialist. It may also be delegated to a suitably trained physician assistant (anesthesia), nurse anesthetist, or anesthesia nurse, supervised or not, in accordance with local guidelines. There is currently no replacement for the expertise, clinical judgment, experience, situational awareness, or the capability of anticipating intraoperative events of an anesthesia practitioner. Absence of an anesthesia clinician has been shown to lead to catastrophic events.

Case 1: Medical Council v Lohan-Mannion: High Court of Ireland, 23rd June 2017

In 2014, Mr FC, a 46-year-old man underwent an elective cervical decompression and discectomy. He sustained a catastrophic, irreversible hypoxic brain injury during the elective procedure. The professional standards of the consultant anesthesiologist were questioned. Seven allegations of professional misconduct and poor professional performance on the part of the anesthesiologist were upheld (https://www.courts.ie/acc/alfresco/2af952ba-54be-4f9d-9973-4a938be0ec61/2017_IEHC_401_1.pdf/pdf#view=fitH).

Allegations were as follows:

1. Failure to appropriately respond to failed, prolonged, or low blood pressure readings.
2. Failure to make note of any of the failed blood pressure readings.
3. Entries of inaccurate blood pressure recordings in the anesthetic chart that were not consistent with readings of the monitor.
4. Failure to record the administration of ephedrine and any responses to the same.
5. Failure to comply with adequate standards of patient safety.
6. Poor professional standards of a consultant anesthesiologist.
7. Absence from the operating theater on two occasions: On one occasion, the anesthesiologist left the patient in the care of an anesthetic nurse while gone for coffee. During this time, the patient had an unrecordable blood pressure. Although the nurse was trained to observe, she was not trained to treat.

Minimal monitoring standards set out by the Association of Anaesthetists state that "The anesthetist must be present and care for the patient throughout the conduct of the anesthetic".[24] This can only be challenged should the anesthetist need to leave for assistance in a lifesaving procedure nearby, when the surgeon must stop what he or she is doing, and the patient must be monitored during this time by a trained anesthetic assistant.[24]

Case 2: Respiratory depression from postoperative analgesia, 2006. Medical Protection Society Report

Mr K was a 37-year-old professional who underwent an elective anterior bowel resection (https://www.medicalprotection.org/world/education-publications/case-reports/case-reports/uk-respiratory-depression-from-postoperative-analgesia). He had an epidural catheter placed by the anesthesiologist for postoperative analgesia, attached to a continuous infusion of bupivacaine and fentanyl. In addition, he had rescue medication prescribed by the same anesthesiologist should his epidural fail. Postoperative care was duly handed over to a nurse and a junior doctor. Epidural analgesia was effective for 24 hours. Unfortunately, it failed to maintain adequate analgesia after this. The junior doctor administered 20 mg of morphine intramuscularly, as prescribed. He also commenced morphine patient-controlled analgesia with a background infusion. The patient received a further 10 mg of morphine intravenously because his pain was deemed uncontrolled. The junior doctor who administered this left soon thereafter without monitoring the patient himself or giving any specific instructions for further monitoring. By this time, the patient had received about 48 mg of morphine within 2 hours. There were no further vital signs recorded until an hour later when the patient was found unresponsive, with an obstructed airway, and his oxygen saturation was recorded at 60%. The junior doctor returned, administered oxygen and naloxone, and called the consultant, who arrived promptly. The patient suffered hypoxic brain injury, which resulted in loss of memory and cognitive function.

It was deemed that this could have been prevented had the patient been adequately monitored and the junior doctor stayed with the patient longer to observe him.

Monitoring

Patient monitoring is a standard of care in anesthesia and is essential for ensuring patient safety.[24] Clinical monitoring using inspection, palpation, and auscultation is augmented by monitoring devices. While these do not replace clinical monitoring, they indisputably offer the anesthesia clinician extended information of the patient's physiologic status, allowing continuous feedback of potentially rapid clinical changes while undergoing surgery under anesthesia.

The anesthesia clinician must ensure that all anesthetic equipment, including relevant monitoring devices, has been checked and alarm limits had been appropriately set before use.[24] If it is absolutely inevitable to continue anesthesia without an essential monitor, the reason should be recorded. However, it is important to acknowledge that the interpretation of numbers on a screen and frequent alarms is not the only type of expertise required of the anesthesiologist. Unlike the machine, anesthesiologists have knowledge of the patient's baseline physiologic status, which must constantly be balanced alongside anticipated physiologic responses to certain surgical interventions. They also have the understanding that monitoring may be disrupted by technical issues, foreign input, or artifact. During regional anesthesia, patient interaction can offer invaluable feedback into the accuracy of any abnormal reading on the monitor, such as extremes of high or low blood pressure. During general anesthesia, clinical skills coupled with cross-checking other monitors are used to investigate any abnormalities. Part of anesthesia training requires formal examination on the fundamental physical principles of monitoring equipment. Interestingly, standard textbooks do not offer statistics of potential issues that may arise with equipment, displaying incorrect vital sign readings with the potential to misrepresent a deteriorating clinical picture, which could assume more importance in less experienced practitioners.[25] The confidence to question and accept deviations from the normal comes with experience and time within the operating room environment.

Electronic monitoring is indispensable and allows continuous assessment of the clinical status of the patient.[26] Subtle changes in clinical signs may precede abnormalities detected by monitoring devices. Anesthesia is not without human error. Equally, monitoring will not prevent all anesthesia-related injuries in the perioperative period.[24]

Record Keeping

Accurate anesthesia record keeping is the responsibility of the anesthesiologist.[27] When John Snow carried out anesthesia in the 1850s, he recorded the events in a notebook.[27] The first official anesthesia record is believed to have been developed in 1894 by two medical students, Cadman and Cushing, who documented observed respiratory rate and palpated pulse rate.[28] Although record keeping has evolved over time, the main aims have remained the same. Record keeping is an integral part to safe patient handover and acts as a source of reference for future anesthetics.

Paper documentation was replaced by automated systems as computers became more available in the 1970s and 1980s.[29] Today's anesthesia record keeping evolved from the Duke Automated Monitoring Equipment (DAME) launched in 1980. This was the first electronic system that could automatically capture physiologic data from a patient monitor. However, the mechanical/semiautomated McKesson Nargraf anesthetic record predated the DAME by over 40 years.[30] The DAME proved initially unreliable and bulky, and user adoption was hampered by a difficult user interface and the size of the system cart.[31] Commercial development improved on the DAME with the launch of Diatek's Arkive (Anesthetic Record Keeper Integrating Voice Recognition) in 1982.[32] This innovation provided an interface to patient monitoring, input via a touchscreen, and audio recording to a diskette. The screen layout was similar to that of paper records, documentation templates were possible, and quick keys were available.

The merits of manual versus automated records are debatable. It has been estimated that about 10% of an anesthesiologist's time can be devoted to manual record keeping during anesthesia.[27] One can argue that this time is inefficient, although it has been suggested that attention to inputting values individually allows for proper assessment of trends. However, when sudden critical events occur, manual record keeping takes a lower priority. A simulated study found that more than 20% of values recorded during such incidents were incorrect by 25% to 200%.[27] Computerized records offer a faithful account of such events during anesthesia. Although they allow clinicians to capture the data and to store and retrieve records when needed, they are far from perfect. Depending on their sophistication, these systems require manual input at the beginning of the case and may be prone to technical errors. Additionally, they are subject to monitoring artifactual input, which may give false readings, misrepresenting the clinical status of the patient. Nonetheless, electronic anesthetic record systems are now the recommended means of record keeping as intuitively, should it be relied on for future reference, it is likely to gain a high standing of evidence over the manual record.[27]

MONITORING THE CLINICIAN

The mandatory requirement for the presence of an appropriately trained and experienced anesthesiologist introduces another facet of patient safety: professional competence. Traditionally, competence encompasses three dimensions: theoretic knowledge, practical skills and attitudes, or nontechnical skills.[33] This has been further expanded within anesthesia to include understanding of work and intuitive expert knowing.[33] The World Health Organization (WHO) and the WFSA published International Standards for a Safe Practice of Anesthesia.[34] They included eight general standards; of which, the first three headings are professional status; professional organizers; and training, certification, and accreditation.[34] Thus, the WHO and WFSA have devised subheadings to ensure that these attributes, or competencies, are measurable and produced as a formal record.

Professional Standards

Professional standards offer a structured set of merits a practitioner must fulfill to ensure fitness to practice. By passing certain examinations set out by accrediting bodies, practitioners should be able to recognize their capabilities and, importantly, the limitations within their field. Professional standards also offer a structure of identifying any gaps in knowledge or capabilities that may require further training or education. By reaching certain standards and levels of competence, a clinician has fulfilled the requirements of the accrediting body and hence obtained certification for safe independent practice.

Accreditation/Professional Organizers

National and international bodies are also accountable for the delivery of safe anesthesia care and must reach certain standards. They must provide a suitable accreditation program, guided by established guidelines, to ensure practitioners are appropriately supervised, trained, and accredited for the same. Appropriate time and facilities must be provided for training of practitioners to ensure these standards are met and maintained.

Continuous Professional Development

The continuous professional development (CPD) is a means of maintaining high quality of patient care. Following basic training, CPD is a lifelong commitment to enhancing knowledge, skills, and up-to-date information. It is a form of regulation that provides assurance of fitness to practice. As anesthesiology is constantly evolving, it is vital to maintain this level of professional growth to ensure safe practice in an environment of rapid technological and scientific advances.

Although CPD serves all generations of anesthesiologists, it has particular importance for the aging anesthesiologist wishing to enhance contemporary competencies. In addition, it plays a role in ensuring clinical fitness for those working close to and beyond the retirement age. As the world's population is aging, there is an increasing demand for healthcare services to cater for it. It is estimated that by 2050, more than a quarter of the European population will be older than 65 years.[35] A third of those born in 2012 in the United Kingdom are expected to survive past 100 years.[36] This puts unprecedented pressure on anesthesia, which already has been reported to have a global shortage.[36] One assumed resolution for alleviating some of this burden is the retention of older anesthesiologists. Although this may sound like a simple solution, it does not come without its own problems. First, as patients age, the proportion of those with complex comorbidities requiring anesthesia increases. This in turn increases the potential for adverse events and outcomes for both the patient and practitioner. Second, as technology is advancing, anesthesia input is being required for more complex interventions outside the standard operating theater, including interventional radiology and cardiology.[37]

Although a highly experienced demographic, it is conceivable that both these workplace challenges impose significant pressure on those who may have completed formalized training thirty or more years ago. Some individual practices may require formal retraining or dedicated teaching to enhance clinical competence. The United States have three formal mechanisms for assessing clinical competency: (1) the Maintenance of Certification in Anesthesiology (MOCA) examinations, performed at 10-year intervals as a means of recertification; (2) the inclusion of anesthesia simulations within these MOCA assessments to observe individual handling of anesthesia emergencies; and (3) requirement of each practitioner to attain a certain amount of Continuing Medical Education (CME) credits for license renewal.[37]

MONITORING THE MONITORS

Provision, maintenance, calibration, and renewal of equipment are the responsibility of the institution in which anesthesia is delivered.

Medical equipment management has traditionally been a risk assessment–based process, often managed by clinical engineers. Preventative maintenance or checks are carried out based on manufacturer guidelines and clinical experience. The combination of equipment complexity and proliferation of devices as well as awareness of safety issues has made management of such risk a broader institutional matter outside the remit of a sole department. Thus, an institution's medical device management policy takes account of relevant standards and guidelines to provide structure and accountability to procurement of devices, training and instruction of users, maintenance/repair procedures and schedules, life cycle assessment, management of medical device alerts and subsequent actions, and disposal of devices.

The International Electrotechnical Commission (IEC) was founded in 1906 and is a worldwide, independent organization for the standardization of matters relating to all electrical, electronic, and information technology fields. The IEC promotes consensus and publishes standards based on international cooperation via national committees.[38] Electrical based medical device standards were first outlined in 1977. The most recent edition serves to ensure that no single point of failure will pose risk to users. Many authorities recognize this standard as the prerequisite for commercialization of electrical medical equipment. Patient monitoring being a multi-parameter device is covered by numerous IEC particular standards.[39]

FUTURE DEVELOPMENTS

Modern-day anesthesia is intrinsically linked to technology with an ever-expanding scope. At first, technology made the practice of anesthesia possible. Then, it made it safe.[40,41] Now, it is at the stage of refining efficiency to improve performance and deliver a more standardized anesthesia care across various healthcare systems and economies. The primary end goal of such developments, however, remains to improve patient safety.

Future of Anesthesia Delivery

Equipment has been described as developing along a continuum of tool to machine to automation.[40] Tools depict devices that have direct user input, and a machine augments that input, while the user still maintains control.[40] Automation implies systems designed to alter function based on a desired user-defined objective without requiring direct user input.[40] Automated anesthesia was first proposed in 1951 by Soltero and colleagues.[42] More recently, closed loop systems have been devised, which rely on a feedback principle.[35]

In general, automated systems were found to be much more efficient in maintaining a desired target range than manual systems.[43] A multicenter analysis found that patients undergoing closed-loop anesthesia delivery system of total intravenous anesthesia had a much tighter control of depth of anesthesia for a longer period of time than those in the traditional manual control group.[44] It has been proposed that this was related to the number of times the system alters settings or the deliverance of medication per unit time, versus the number of adjustments that would be made manually by the anesthesiologist.[45]

Does this mean that automated systems have the potential to take over clinical practice? Even if they do, the extent of such replacement is unclear. Although they have been proven to deliver a more standardized and controlled anesthesia, automated systems do not possess the property of anticipation of events, which is the capability of clinical observation. In addition, there is no perfect system that can counteract intraoperative artifacts. However, it would not be unreasonable to anticipate widespread implementation of automated systems in the coming decade.

This topic is further explored in the chapter entitled Machine learning, deep learning, and closed loop devices – anesthesia delivery.

Future of Monitoring

There is an ever-increasing requirement for anesthesia in remote locations such as MRI departments and interventional radiology.[46] This poses significant ergonomic issues for the anesthesiologist, making the prospect of wireless technology increasingly important. This may be applicable to intensive care units, operating rooms, postanesthesia care units, and transfers of critically ill patients. Wired systems create hazards for all involved as a distraction and tripping hazard for clinicians, a source of potential injury for patients during positioning and transfer, and can lead to dislodged monitors, lines, and ventilation systems when accidently pulled.[47] Wireless infrastructure would require extensive investment and an educated workforce to deal with network failures. This may be difficult to incentivize but remains an exciting area of future development.

Chapters Toward smart monitoring with phones, watches and wearable sensors and Telemedicine for anesthesiologist offer further insights into modern technologies.

Future of Documentation

Anesthesia information management systems (AIMSs) have evolved from electronic anesthesia records into sophisticated software capable of reproducing a patient's entire anesthesia experience. It is composed of either a stand-alone software product or an anesthesia module within a hospital's integrated electronic health record system coupled with hardware components and physiologic device interfaces.[29] This software is installed on the patient's computer workstations and includes preoperative assessment, perioperative events, and postoperative documentation. Clinical decision support systems (CDSSs) within operating theaters have also become possible. Unlike closed loop systems, CDSSs cannot implement any change although they can offer best practice solutions in a given clinical scenario.[32] The ultimate clinical decision-making still lies with the anesthesiologist. Their software requires further refinement. First, the quality of the best practice solutions is dependent on the quality of the input.[48] There is no recognized standard for ensuring quality of input data. Second, there is a risk of this system creating extra workload for the provider because it relies on human attention when it provides notifications and alarms.[48] Alarm fatigue is a well-known phenomenon within anesthesia. Finally, there remains the issue of cost-benefit analysis, with increased workload being required of hospital-based Information Technology (IT) staff, risk of security breaches, and updating hospital networks.[48] Vulnerabilities of contemporary systems to hardware failure can be mitigated, with products installed via virtual servers and the user interface provided on nonspecific terminals. Thus, failure of one component will not impact the operation of the entire system.

The need for committed clinicians to lead installation rollout is seen as key to successful implementation. Benefits to practitioners and institutions are far-reaching ones and include accurately recorded patient data within vastly enhanced documentation, clinical support tools, audit and research repositories, as well as potentials in operation management and cost containment. Enhanced patient safety and quality of information benefits patient outcomes. Importantly, the AIMS has been found to contribute to better risk assessment, thereby offsetting medicolegal costs.[29]

SUMMARY

Anesthesiology has been acknowledged as the leading medical specialty in addressing patient safety.[49] The past 170 years have seen remarkable improvements in patient safety, encompassing new technologies, real-time monitoring, and formulating and defining practice parameters. Anesthesia is on the cusp of new and refined technological advancements. Behavioral science and economics will guide the rate of implementation of these mature technologies. With the Internet era, and more widespread access to online health information, anesthesia will experience new social and economic pressures, which in turn may influence the development of the medical field. "The future is here, and our engagement with innovation will determine our share of its prosperity."[49]

CLINICS CARE POINTS

- The presence of an appropriately trained anesthesia clinician during any form of anesthesia cannot be circumvented.
- The anesthesia clinician must care for the patient continuously using both clinical skills and monitoring equipment.
- Accurate records of the values determined by the monitors must be kept.
- Professional standards represent a structured set of merits a practitioner must fulfill to ensure fitness to practice.
- Provision, maintenance, calibration, and renewal of equipment are the responsibilities of the institution in which anesthesia is delivered.
- Anesthesia clinicians will be faced with a dynamic and challenging interplay between sophisticated technological input and behavioral science.

DISCLOSURE

The authors have nothing to disclose.

REFERENCES

1. Reich DL. The history of anesthesia monitoring and perioperative care. In: Kahn RA, Mittnacht AJC, Leibowitz AB, et al, editors. Monitoring in anesthesia and perioperative care. Cambridge: Cambridge University Press; 2011. p. 1–8.
2. Roguin A. Scipione Riva-Rocci and the men behind the mercury sphygmomanometer. Int J Clin Pract 2006;60:73–9.
3. Snow J. On the fatal cases of the inhalation of chloroform. Edinb Med Surg J 1849;72:75–87.
4. Rivera-Ruiz M, Cajavilca C, Varon J. Einthoven's string galvanometer: the first electrocardiograph. Tex Heart Inst J 2008;35:174–8.
5. Johansson BW. A history of the electrocardiogram. Dan Medicinhist Arbog 2001;163–76.
6. Barold SS. Willem Einthoven and the birth of clinical electrocardiography a hundred years ago. Card Electrophysiol Rev 2003;7:99–104.
7. Al-Shaikh B, Stacey SG. Essentials of equipment in anaesthesia, critical care and peri-operative medicine. 5th edition. Amsterdam: Elsevier; 2018.
8. Van Meter A, Williams U, Zavala A, et al. Beat to beat: a measured look at the history of pulse oximetry. J Anesth Hist 2017;3:24–6.

9. Yelderman M, New W. Evaluation of pulse oximetry. Anesthesiology 1983;59: 349–52.

10. Anesthesiologists ASo. Practice guidelines for preoperative fasting and the use of pharmacologic agents to reduce the risk of pulmonary aspiration: application to healthy patients undergoing elective procedures. Anesthesiology 2017;126: 376–93.

11. Tsyrlin V, Pliss MG, Kuzmenko NV. The history of blood pressure measurement: from Hales to our days. Arterial Hypertens 2016;22:144–52.

12. Loughnan TE, Loughnan AJ. Overview of the introduction of neuromuscular monitoring to clinical anaesthesia. Anaesth Intensive Care 2013;41(Suppl 1):19–24.

13. McGrath CD, Hunter JM. Monitoring of neuromuscular block. Continuing Education in Anaesthesia Critical Care & Pain 2006;6:7–12.

14. Churchill-Davidson HC. A portable peripheral nerve-stimulator. Anesthesiology 1965;26:224–6.

15. Pierce E. The development of anesthesia guidelines and standards. QRB Qual Rev Bull 1990;16:61–4.

16. Pandya AN, Majid SZ, Desai MS. The origins, evolution, and spread of anesthesia monitoring standards: from Boston to across the world. Anaesth Analg 2021;132: 890–8.

17. Eichhorn J, Cooper J, Cullen D, et al. Anesthesia practice standards at Harvard: a review. J Clin Anesth 1988;1:55–65.

18. Eichhorn J. Prevention of intraoperative anesthesia accidents and related severe injury through safety monitoring. Anesthesiology 1989;70:572–7.

19. Tinker JH, Dull DL, Caplan RA, et al. Role of monitoring devices in prevention of anesthetic mishaps: a closed claims analysis. Anesthesiology 1989;71:541–6.

20. Caplan RA, Posner KL, Ward RJ, et al. Adverse respiratory events in anesthesia: a closed claims analysis. Anesthesiology 1990;72:828–33.

21. Eichhorn JH, Cooper JB, Cullen DJ, et al. Standards for patient monitoring during anesthesia at Harvard Medical School. JAMA 1986;256:1017–20.

22. Eichhorn JH. The standards formulation process. Eur J Anaesthesiol Suppl 1993; 7:9–11.

23. Merry A, Cooper J, Soyannwo O, et al. An iterative process of global quality improvement: the International Standards for a Safe Practice of Anesthesia 2010. Can J Anaesth 2010;57:1021–6.

24. Association of Anaesthetists of Great Britain and Ireland. Recommendations for standards of monitoring during anaesthesia and recovery 2015. Anaesthesia 2016;71:85–93.

25. Smith A, Mort M, Goodwin D, et al. Making monitoring 'work': human–machine interaction and patient safety in anaesthesia. Anaesthesia 2003;58:1070–8.

26. Saunders D. On the dangers of monitoring. Or, *Primum non nocere* revisited. Anaesthesia 1997;52:399–400.

27. Peachey T. Anaesthetic records. Anaesth Intensive Care Med 2004;5:402–3.

28. Sundararaman LV, Desai SP. The anesthesia records of Harvey Cushing and Ernest Codman. Anesth Analg 2018;126:322–9.

29. Simpao A, Rehman M. Anesthesia information management systems. Anesth Analg 2018;127:90–4.

30. Madden AP. Clinical systems. Anaesth Intensive Care Med 2004;5:412–4.

31. Block FE. The Diatek Arkive ® patient information management system. Bail Clin Anaesthesiol 1990;4:159–70.

32. Ehrenfeld JM, Rehman MA. Anesthesia information management systems: a review of functionality and installation considerations. J Clin Monit Comput 2011; 25:71–9.

33. Larsson J. Monitoring the anaesthetist in the operating theatre – professional competence and patient safety. Anaesthesia 2017;72:76–83.

34. Merry A, Johnson W, Mets B, et al. The SAFE-T summit and the international standards for a safe practice of anesthesia. APSF Newsl 2019;33:69–104.

35. Redfern N, Gallagher P. The ageing anaesthetist. *Anaesthe*sia 2014;69:1–5.

36. Hutton P, Baker M, Black C, et al. *Age and the Anaesthetist*. AAGBI. Working party report. Anaesth News 2016;3–27.

37. Garfield J, Garfield F. The ageing anaesthetist: lessons from the North American experience. BJA Educ 2021;21:20–5.

38. Bronzino JD. The biomedical engineering handbook. 2nd edition. vol. II. Boca Raton (FL): CRC Press LLC; 2000.

39. TÜV SÜD IEC 60601-1 (EDITION 3.2). Available at: https://www.tuvsud.com/en/industries/healthcare-and-medical-devices/medical-devices-and-ivd/medical-device-testing/physical-testing-of-medical-devices/iec-60601-1.   Accessed February 2, 2021.

40. Seger C, Cannesson M. Recent advances in the technology of anesthesia. F1000Res 2020;18:9.

41. Cannesson M. Innovative technologies applied to anesthesia: how will they impact the way clinicians practice? J Cardiothorac Vasc Anesth 2012;26:711–20.

42. Soltero D, Faulconer A, Bickford R. The clinical application of automatic anesthesia. Anesthesiology 1951;1:574–82.

43. Brogi E, Cyr S, Kazan R, et al. Clinical performance and safety of closed-loop systems: a systematic review and meta-analysis of randomized controlled trials. Anesth Analg 2017;124:446–55.

44. Puri G, Mathew P, Biswas I, et al. A multicenter evaluation of a closed-loop anesthesia delivery system: a randomized controlled trial. Anesth Analg 2016;122: 106–14.

45. Joosten A, Rinehart J, Bardaji A, et al. Anesthetic management using multiple closed-loop systems and delayed neurocognitive recovery: a randomized controlled trial. Anesthesiology 2020;132:253–66.

46. Schubert A, Eckhout G, Ngo A, et al. Status of the anesthesia workforce in 2011: evolution during the last decade and future outlook. Anesth Analg 2012;115: 407–27.

47. Hofer I, Cannesson M. Is wireless the future of monitoring? Anesth Analg 2016; 122:305–6.

48. Freundlich R, Ehrenfeld J. Anesthesia information management. Curr Opin Anaesthesiol 2017;30:705–9.

49. Gaba D. Anaesthesiology as a model for patient safety in healthcare. Br Med J 2000;320:785–8.

Ventilation Monitoring

Michael Ramsay, MD, FRCA

KEYWORDS

- Breath sounds • Respiratory rate • Pulse oximetry • Capnography
- Continuous monitoring • Failure to rescue

KEY POINTS

- Breathing is good.
- Respiratory rate is a vital sign that is neglected.
- Undetected respiratory depression is still common in patients taking opioids.
- Continuous monitoring of ventilation is now available in hospital and at home.

INTRODUCTION

The first medical instrument that the medical student obtains is the stethoscope. This opens the window of physical examination and allows the student to hear the inspiration and expiration of air in to and out from the lungs. Suddenly anatomy and physiology become real, together with the detection of changes that may be early signs of disease. The discovery of the stethoscope by Laennec (1781–1826) in 1816 has brought the importance of ventilation and respiration to the forefront of good health. Listening to breath sounds and counting the respiratory rate has brought forward the importance of monitoring ventilation. Changes in respiratory rate and lung sounds can be early indicators of disease and deterioration in health. Respiratory rate is considered one of the important vital signs in the human because changes from normal values can be an early predictor of deterioration in the patient.[1] Lung sounds also can be good monitors of deterioration in ventilation. Musical sounds such as stridor and wheezing may be indicators of narrowing of the upper or lower airway, respectively.[2] Examples would be vocal cord dysfunction and bronchial constriction caused by asthma. Nonmusical sounds, such as crackles, may indicate pulmonary edema, whereas absent sounds may be caused by pleural effusions, lung collapse, or pneumothorax. Lung auscultation is an important and essential part of monitoring ventilation and the stethoscope is still a very important clinical assessment tool.

The stethoscope has advanced from the wooden tube that Laennec designed and made to digital stethoscopes that deliver computerized recording and analysis of breath sounds. These digital stethoscopes can objectively define the nature of pathologic breath sounds, and the addition of artificial intelligence has improved the

Department of Anesthesiology, Baylor University Medical Center, Baylor Scott and White Health Care, 3500 Gaston Avenue, Dallas, TX 75246, USA
E-mail address: michael.ramsay@bswhealth.org

Anesthesiology Clin 39 (2021) 403–414
https://doi.org/10.1016/j.anclin.2021.03.006
1932-2275/21/© 2021 Elsevier Inc. All rights reserved.
anesthesiology.theclinics.com

diagnostic reliability of these instruments.[3,4] The basic clinical examination of the chest, including auscultation and the monitoring of respiratory rate, are the basis of ventilation monitoring. The monitoring of ventilation in the early days of anesthesia included the continuous use of a monoaural stethoscope attached to the patient's chest where respiratory rate, breath sounds, and heart sounds could be monitored in the anesthetized patient. The clinical importance of respiratory rate has been well documented. It is one of the vital signs, as it is an early detector of serious illness, such as infection, respiratory depression, especially caused by opioids or sedatives, and respiratory failure, yet it has been reported as the "neglected vital sign," probably because in many situations it has to be counted manually.[5]

The latest technology now allows continuous monitoring of ventilation noninvasively. As this becomes more available, the early detection of deterioration in patients becomes possible so that early interventions can be made, preventing "failure to rescue" events in our hospitals. This technology is now becoming available for home monitoring with signals transmitted to the smart phone of a caregiver. This will allow patients to spend less time in the hospital, and illness maybe detected earlier, especially in those with specific risks factors. The current Covid-19 pandemic is still affecting populations across the globe, and with remote monitoring, early hypoxemia could be detected sooner, and interventions made.[6]

PULSE OXIMETRY

The goal of ventilation is to get oxygen to the mitochondria to allow respiration to occur and remove the carbon dioxide that is produced as a result of the metabolism of glucose to carbon dioxide and water with the formation of energy. This relies not only on oxygenation but on the circulation and the red cells to carry the oxygen to the tissues. Normally, approximately 1000 mL of oxygen is delivered to the tissues each minute. This oxygen delivery (DO_2) is dependent on the circulation, which is driven by the cardiac output and the circulation volume status, and the hemoglobin (Hgb) concentration.

The amount of oxygen carried in 100 mL of blood (CaO_2) depends on the Hgb concentration, the O_2 saturation (SaO_2) and the partial pressure of O_2 (Pao_2) and is calculated with the following formula: $CaO_2 = Hgb \times 1.39 \times SaO_2 + (Pao_2 \times 0.0032)$. The pulse oximeter allows a continuous monitoring of the oxygen saturation in arterial blood (SpO_2).

The institution of continuous pulse oximetry surveillance on rescue events, and intensive care unit (ICU) transfers, on postoperative patients at risk for unrecognized respiratory depression has demonstrated a significant reduction in the need for patient rescue and ICU admissions.[7] The concern about pulse oximetry is that when the patient is receiving supplemental oxygen, the SpO_2 can remain in the normal range even though the carbon dioxide level ($Paco_2$) maybe dangerously high.[8] Lynn and Curry examined the clinical patterns of different types of "in-hospital" unexpected deaths and also the number and reasons for rapid response team calls.[9] They found that many patients fit into 3 different clinical pattern types. The first was hyperventilation compensated respiratory distress; usually this was a result of sepsis, congestive heart failure, or pulmonary embolism. The pattern presented was stable SpO_2, with progressively falling $Paco_2$ as respiratory rate increased with the sepsis and fever, followed by a steep decline in SpO_2 when the metabolic acidosis became severe. This was then followed by a code (**Fig. 1**). The next 2 clinical patterns raise concern, as they are often avoidable or preventable situations if the correct care and monitoring of ventilation had been applied. The second pattern was a progressive unidirectional hypoventilation

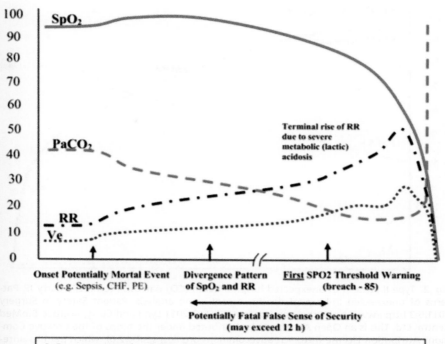

Fig. 1. Type 1: Hyperventilation in response to sepsis. (Lynn LA, Curry JP. Patterns of unexpected in-hospital deaths: a root cause analysis. Patient Safety in Surgery 2011;5:3 http://www.pssjournal.com/content/5/1/3. © 2011 Lynn and Curry; licensee BioMed Central Ltd. This is an Open Access article distributed under the terms of the Creative Commons Attribution License (http://creativecommons.org/licenses/by/2.0), which permits unrestricted use, distribution, and reproduction in any medium, provided the original work is properly cited.)

with the development of CO_2 narcosis. This is caused by increasing respiratory depression, possibly due to overprescribing of narcotics and/or sedatives. There is a rise in $Paco_2$ and a fall in SpO_2, but this may be masked by the addition of supplemental O_2, which allows the $Paco_2$ to reach very high levels before there is a decline in oxygenation, which may occur suddenly (**Fig. 2**). These patients may be better monitored with capnography, respiratory rate, and a sedation scale. When the $Paco_2$ reaches 80 mm Hg, most patients become unresponsive, so placing a sedation score next to a pain score may assist in detecting opioid-induced respiratory depression, especially in patients receiving supplemental oxygen.[10,11] A further study testing the rapidity of oxygen desaturation once the decline started demonstrated no difference between patients on supplemental oxygen or on room air.[12] The third pattern of ventilation failure is the patient with sleep apnea, which if it goes undetected and no intervention is made, could lead to a code situation. There is a state of "arousal-dependent survival" where patients, when asleep, frequently obstruct and become hypoxic but then wake themselves up and relieve the obstruction. When opioids or sedatives are administered postoperatively, this arousal mechanism may be obtunded, and

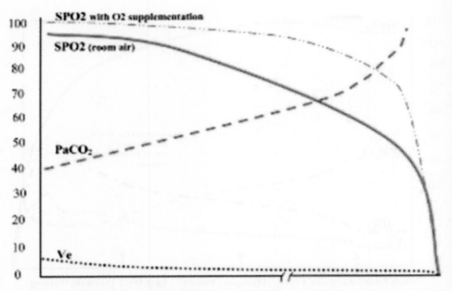

Fig. 2. Type II pattern of unexpected hospital death (CO_2 narcosis). (Lynn LA, Curry JP. Patterns of unexpected in-hospital deaths: a root cause analysis. Patient Safety in Surgery 2011;5:3 http://www.pssjournal.com/content/5/1/3. © 2011 Lynn and Curry; licensee BioMed Central Ltd. This is an Open Access article distributed under the terms of the Creative Commons Attribution License (http://creativecommons.org/licenses/by/2.0), which permits unrestricted use, distribution, and reproduction in any medium, provided the original work is properly cited.)

the patient may not be aroused and stays obstructed and a hypoxic arrest will follow (**Fig. 3**).

Multiwavelength pulse oximetry can provide trend values for hemoglobin and pleth variability indices for volume status that can help to determine the oxygen delivery DO_2 to the mitochondria.[13,14] The multiwave pulse oximeters can also provide an estimation of venous oxygen saturation displayed as an index, the Oxygen Reserve Index. This is a unitless index from 0.00 to 1.00. At 1.00 the venous blood is approximately 80% saturated and the Pao_2 is approximately 100 to 200 mm Hg and the patient may be hyperoxic. When the Oxygen Reserve Index is 0.00 then the SpO_2 is about to decline and this can be an early warning that the patient on supplemental O_2 is not ventilating adequately and is potentially about to desaturate. The low index may also be an early sign of fever or low cardiac output. The Oxygen Reserve Index is not equivalent to Pao_2 but is complementary to SpO_2 for monitoring patients receiving supplementary oxygen.[15]

MONITORING VENTILATION WITH CAPNOGRAPHY

Carbon dioxide (CO_2), one of the end-products of respiration, is transported in the bloodstream to the lungs where it enters the alveoli and is ventilated out of the lungs during expiration. The measurement of expired CO_2 provides information on metabolism, cardiac output, and ventilation. Capnography, the measurement of exhaled CO_2 (or End-Tidal CO_2), is the standard of care for monitoring the adequacy of ventilation for patients under general anesthesia. It is a major patient safety technology that monitors the adequacy of ventilation in patients supported by mechanical ventilation

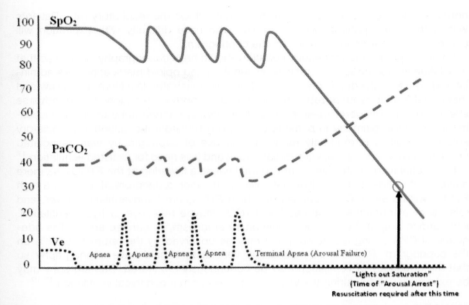

Fig. 3. Type III pattern of unexpected hospital death (sleep apnea with arousal failure). (Lynn LA, Curry JP. Patterns of unexpected in-hospital deaths: a root cause analysis. Patient Safety in Surgery 2011;5:3 http://www.pssjournal.com/content/5/1/3. © 2011 Lynn and Curry; licensee BioMed Central Ltd. This is an Open Access article distributed under the terms of the Creative Commons Attribution License (http://creativecommons.org/licenses/by/2.0), which permits unrestricted use, distribution, and reproduction in any medium, provided the original work is properly cited.)

and in those receiving sedation or anesthesia medications that can depress ventilation. The presence and the amount of $ETCO_2$ may be used to assess not only adequacy of ventilation but the effectiveness of resuscitation in creating an adequate return of circulation.[16]

Devices used to detect and monitor CO_2 include colorimetric detectors in the form of disposable discs that change color when exposed to exhaled CO_2. These are useful for confirming tracheal intubation in an emergency situation or confirming the adequacy of cardiopulmonary resuscitation (CPR) during a code. The discs are pH sensitive and the amount of color change reflects the CO_2 concentration in the expired gas. They are not for long-term use and are disposable. The other devices used to measure CO_2 may be "Mainstream" or "Side-stream," depending on whether the sensor is placed directly in the gas flow pathway in the airway or a gas sample is aspirated from the breathing circuit. The side-stream devices use an infrared monitor located away from the patient, whereas the mainstream devices are limited to intubated patients as the infrared practice device is sited in the connector to the endotracheal tube.

Capnography is the graphic display of the concentration of exhaled and inhaled CO_2 plotted against time. It is used whenever a patient is intubated to monitor the adequacy of ventilation and more importantly to confirm that the endotracheal tube is in the trachea and not the esophagus. The $ETCO_2$ value in normal lungs is approximately 2 to 5 mm Hg less than the $Paco_2$. If the lungs are diseased with chronic obstructive pulmonary disease, this difference may be much greater, as there is a ventilation perfusion (V/Q) mismatch in the lungs. The normal capnogram for a patient with normal lungs is a nearly square waveform that follows the respiratory rate. Patients with asthma and patients with bronchitis who have difficulty with expiration will demonstrate a flattened upstroke on the capnogram.

Patients undergoing procedural sedation should have capnography applied so that ventilation is monitored continuously as sedation and opioid medications are administered. The efficacy of this practice has been demonstrated in a literature review and meta-analysis of randomized controlled trials reporting sedation-related adverse events. The incidence of these events when adding capnography to visual assessment and pulse oximetry in patients undergoing procedural sedation in ambulatory surgery hospitals is markedly reduced. The use of capnography was associated with less mild and severe oxygen desaturation and less need for assisted ventilation.[17]

Hypoventilation or shallow breathing may cause a lowering of the $ETCO_2$, as there maybe just dead-space ventilation if severe, but when a deep breath occurs, a high $ETCO_2$ will be seen. Other causes of a high $ETCO_2$ are hypoventilation, fever, and release of a tourniquet, whereas low $ETCO_2$ maybe reflective of hyperventilation, low cardiac output, hypotension, pulmonary embolism, or cardiac arrest. The adequacy of CPR during a cardiac arrest may be observed by the return of $ETCO_2$ on the capnogram. Patients on mechanical ventilation should have capnography so that the adequacy of ventilation may be continuously monitored. Capnography may be extremely helpful during the weaning process from mechanical ventilation.[18,19]

RESPIRATORY RATE MONITORS

As reported earlier, respiratory rate is an important vital sign that is frequently not recorded, as it often must be counted manually; however, continuous monitoring does exist. Everyday electrocardiogram monitors can record respiratory rate by changes in the bioimpedance across the chest wall with each chest excursion moving the electrocardiogram pads. The problem with this technology is that it counts chest movement, not respiratory volume, thus obstructed breathing will not be recognized. This problem has been resolved by the respiratory volume monitor, which is described later, and is able to monitor minute volume and respiratory rate accurately. Respiratory rate also may be monitored by acoustic sensors applied to the neck. These sensors detect air movement, and this is displayed as a waveform. The noisier the sound of breathing, the larger the amplitude of the wave generated. Therefore, snoring would be depicted as very large waves and quiet nonlabored breathing would have small amplitude waves. In one study in the recovery room after surgery, the acoustic monitor compared well with capnography.[20]

A new contactless sensor system using an Ultra-Wideband radio transceiver capable of detecting chest wall rise has been developed. It is currently undergoing clinical trial to determine if it can measure respiratory rate from a distance.[21]

MONITORING INVASIVE MECHANICAL VENTILATION

Invasive mechanical ventilation is used frequently during major surgery and in the ICU. The invasion component is attributed to the presence of an endotracheal tube or tracheostomy, compared with noninvasive ventilation, which implies the presence of a facemask or helmet.

Mechanical ventilators may control and measure volume, pressure, rate, and flow so that a predetermined tidal volume and minute volume are delivered and monitored. The delivery may be volume controlled or pressure controlled, and within these parameters assist control, synchronized intermittent mandatory ventilation, and pressure-regulated volume control may be added. The respiratory rate may be set by time or may be patient triggered by inspiratory effort or both, and positive end-expiratory pressure (PEEP) may be set as well as inspired oxygen. All these parameters are continuously monitored as is airway pressure.[22] To assist in ensuring adequate ventilation, capnography and pulse oximetry should be used continuously to monitor ventilation.

Lung protective ventilation was found to improve outcomes in patients with acute respiratory distress syndrome. This protection consists of low-tidal volumes and low pressures, compensated with high respiratory rate and PEEP. This has now been shown to reduce acute lung injury in surgical patients.[23–25]

Mechanical ventilation may have adverse effects on the diaphragm as well as the lung. The lung injury occurs from the excessive mechanical stress and strain; the diaphragm, however, becomes atrophied because of little respiratory effort. Now strategies are being developed to provide both lung and diaphragm protection when a patient is being mechanically ventilated. The focus of lung protective ventilation is to reduce lung stress by keeping a low driving pressure, and reduce strain from over-distension, repetitive tidal volume recruitment, and collapse. The lung injury may be inflicted by the ventilator or by the patient's own breathing efforts. The weight of the chest wall in obese patients results in a high intrathoracic pressure that maybe measured as transpulmonary pressure.

Diaphragm protective ventilation endeavors to reduce the impact of unloading the work of this respiratory muscle pump as we assist breathing by mechanical ventilation. After 24 hours of mechanical ventilation, 64% of patients have diaphragm weakness. Poor diaphragm effort as a result of paralysis or sedation will result in atrophy, whereas too much diaphragm muscle work may lead to load-induced injury. The key to diaphragm muscle protection is to titrate ventilation and sedation to restore early diaphragm activity without excessive work[26] (**Fig. 4**).

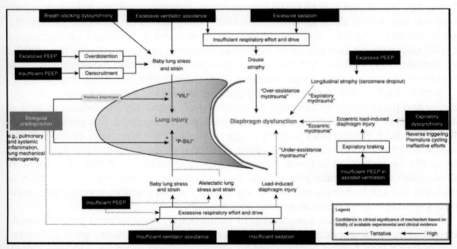

Fig. 4. Mechanisms of injury to the lung and diaphragm during mechanical ventilation. P-SILI, patient self-inflicted lung injury. VILI, ventilator-induced lung injury. (*From* Goligher EC, Dres M, Patel BK et al. Lung and diaphragm protective ventilation. Am J Respir Crit Care Med 2020;202:950-61. Reprinted with permission of the American Thoracic Society. Copyright © 2021 American Thoracic Society. All rights reserved. The American Journal of Respiratory and Critical Care Medicine is an official journal of the American Thoracic Society.)

Monitoring strategies to provide lung and diaphragm protective strategies include tidal volume, airway driving pressure, airway pressure and flow wave forms, airway occlusion pressure, airway pressure swing during a whole breath occlusion, esophageal pressure and transpulmonary pressure, transdiaphragmatic pressure swing, and gastric pressure swing.[27]

Monitoring ventilation and the end result, respiration, includes gas exchange effects that are reflected by continuous pulse oximetry and capnography. Arterial blood gas analysis and the Pao_2/Fio_2 ratio, in particular, is used to assess the severity of respiratory failure, whereas $Paco_2$ reflects the degree of ventilatory depression. The monitoring of respiratory mechanics, compliance and resistance, are essential for the comprehension of the work of breathing.[28] Esophageal pressure measured from an air-filled balloon placed in the esophagus permits accurate monitoring of controlled and assisted mechanical ventilation to allow personalized protective settings of the ventilator. It can also detect patient-ventilator asynchrony and allows bedside monitoring of ventilation, especially transpulmonary pressure, in patients with acute respiratory failure.[29]

POSTOPERATIVE OPIOID-INDUCED RESPIRATORY DEPRESSION

A major cause of preventable hospital mortality and brain damage is postoperative opioid-induced respiratory depression. An analysis of the Anesthesia Closed Claims Project database between 1990 and 2009 revealed 92 claims that met the criteria for inclusion, and of these 77% resulted in severe brain damage or death.[30] Most occurred within 24 hours of surgery and 97% were judged as preventable with better monitoring and response to signals. Confounding factors were multiple prescribers, and the addition of nonopioid sedatives. The time from the last nursing assessment and the finding of the patient with severe respiratory depression was 42% within 2 hours and 16% within 15 minutes. This brings home the difficulty of recognizing respiratory depression with the naked eye and the need for appropriate continuous monitoring equipment. Another study examined risk factors and noted the following: elderly women, obstructive sleep apnea, chronic obstructive pulmonary disease, cardiac disease, diabetes, hypertension, neurologic and renal disease, 2 or more comorbidities, opioid dependance, use of patient-controlled analgesia pump, and finally the addition of sedatives. This list was virtually uniformly inclusive. Enhanced monitoring of sedation level, respiratory rate, pulse oximetry, and capnography were recommended.[31]

Another multicenter study monitoring patients on opioids with continuous capnography and pulse oximetry detected an incidence of respiratory depression in 46% of 1335 patients on the general floor. The investigators derived a risk prediction tool that included 5 independent variables: age older than 60 years, sex, opioid naivety, sleep disorders, and chronic heart failure.[32] They identified multiple risk factors that basically mean that all patients taking parenteral opioids are at risk of respiratory depression in the hospital and should be continuously monitored. The addition of sedative therapy to opioids resulted in significantly higher cardiopulmonary and respiratory arrests in both medical and surgical patients.[33]

A real-time quantitative assessment of ventilation in nonintubated patients would detect early respiratory compromise before pulse oximetry or capnography. Oxygen desaturation lags behind hypoventilation when breathing room air and very significantly if supplemental O_2 is being administered. Capnography is a measure of respiratory rate as well as ventilation, but it still lacks the sensitivity in demonstrating a decrease in ventilation, when compared with a sensitive respiratory volume monitor. A recently designed impedance-based noninvasive respiratory volume monitor has been demonstrated to measure continuously minute ventilation, tidal volume, and respiratory rate accurately. In a 48-subject study, changes were seen more rapidly and to a greater degree in minute ventilation when compared with capnography. This could result in earlier detection and enable earlier intervention if respiratory depression occurred.[34] Another study examined the close correlation of the respiratory volume monitor with those of a mechanical ventilator when used on intubated patients. This demonstrated good accuracy and a similar accuracy was maintained after extubation.[35]

DETECTING PATIENT DETERIORATION WITH CONTINUOUS MONITORING

The early detection of the deteriorating patient is key to reducing the number of "failure to rescue" events and the number of rapid response team calls that occur in hospital patients. The implementation of continuous surveillance monitoring is now being applied in some centers. An early implementation using pulse oximetry formed a good template as a data source and enabled the impact of adding more monitors to be explored.[36] Postoperative patients receiving opioids are at particular risk for preventable respiratory depression.[37] Intermittent sampling of vital signs is insufficient to detect physiologic deterioration and this leads to a failure of adequate intervention in a timely fashion.[38]

A pulse oximeter surveillance system with pager notification of nursing staff when alarm thresholds were reached resulted in a 65% reduction in rapid response team calls and a reduction in unplanned ICU transfers of more than 40%. Significant cost savings were calculated within the first year of use.[39]

Patients with chronic hypercapnic respiratory failure maybe treated at home with noninvasive mechanical ventilation. Ventilation monitoring has been developed that can evaluate the effectiveness of the ventilation and provide data on compliance, leaks, and respiratory parameters. Telemonitoring now allows the potential of adjusting ventilator settings remotely.[40]

Continuous monitoring of a patient's respiratory status often includes $ETCO_2$, respiratory rate, SpO_2, and pulse rate. Interpreting these data for nonanesthesiologists or intensivists may be challenging, so an algorithm has been designed to integrate these parameters to make an overall assessment of the patients' respiratory status. This is called the Integrated Pulmonary Index and prospective studies are being performed to evaluate its usefulness in the clinical setting.[41]

The Covid pandemic has resulted in many patients requiring mechanical ventilation, and this has created a shortage of ventilators, and therefore anesthesia machine ventilators are being converted into remote monitoring and intensive care ventilators.[42] The future of smart phones or similar devices to be remote monitors of ventilation, vital signs, and overall well-being is here. Failure to rescue should become a rare event, as early deterioration will be detected and interventions made.

CLINICS CARE POINTS

- The pulse oximeter may be a delayed indicator of respiratory depression if supplemental oxygen is being delivered to the patient.
- Respiratory rate is an early detector of clinical deterioration in a patient. It may increase with sepsis or decrease with sedation but is rarely accurately documented, as it is usually measured manually, and this should take a minute to do.
- Capnography should be applied to all patients undergoing procedural sedation to monitor the adequacy of ventilation. However, if the patient is severely hypoventilating, the capnogram may exhibit a low number for several breaths as only "dead-space" air may be expired until a deep breath occurs and exhibits a high value.

- The adequacy of CPR may be assessed by the return of carbon dioxide on the capnogram
- Continuous monitoring of ventilation is an early detector of patient deterioration and should lead to early intervention and drastically decrease patients on the general wards being found "dead in bed."

DISCLOSURE

The author has received Research Grants from Masimo Corp, Irvine, California.

REFERENCES

1. Loughlin PC, Sebat F, Kellett JG. Respiratory rate : the forgotten vital sign – make it count! Joint Comm J Qual Patient Saf 2018;44:494–9.
2. Bohadana A, Izbicki G, Kraman SS. Fundamentals of lung auscultation. N Engl J Med 2014;370:744–51.
3. Kevat AC, Kalirajah A, Roseby R. Digital stethoscopes compared to standard auscultation for detecting abnormal paediatric breath sounds. Eur J Pediatr 2017;176:989–92.
4. Kevat AC, Kalirajah A, Roseby R. Artificial intelligence accuracy in detecting pathological breath sounds in children using digital stethoscopes. Respir Res 2020;21:253.
5. Cretikos MA, Bellomo R, Hillman K, et al. Respiratory rate: the neglected vital sign. Med J Aust 2008;188:657–9.
6. Tobin MJ, Laghi F, Jubran A. Why Covid-19 silent hypoxemia is baffling to physicians. Am J Respir Crit Care Med 2020;202:356–60.
7. Taenzer AH, Pyke JB, McGrath SP, et al. Impact of pulse oximetry surveillance on rescue events and intensive care unit transfers. a before and after concurrence study. Anesthesiology 2010;112:282–7.
8. Fu ES, Downs JB, Schweiger JW, et al. Supplemental oxygen impairs the detection of hypoventilation by pulse oximetry. Chest 2004;126:1552–8.
9. Lynn LA, Curry JP. Patterns of unexpected in-hospital deaths: a root cause analysis. Patient Saf Surg 2011;5:3. Available at: http://www.pssjournal.com/content/5/1/3.
10. Kelley SD, Ramsay MA. Respiratory rate monitoring: characterizing performance for emerging technologies. Anesth Analg 2014;119:1246–8.
11. Lam T, Nagappa M, Wong J, et al. Continuous pulse oximetry and capnography monitoring for postoperative respiratory depression and adverse events: a systematic review and meta-analysis. Anesth Analg 2017;125:2019–29.
12. Taenzer AH, Perreard IM, MacKenzie T, et al. Characteristics of desaturation and respiratory rate in postoperative patients breathing room air versus supplemental oxygen: are they different? Anesth Analg 2018;126:826–32.
13. Barker SJ, Shander A, Ramsay MA. Continuous noninvasive hemoglobin monitoring: a measured response to a critical review. Anesth Analg 2016;122:565–72.
14. Chu H, Wang Y, Sun Y, et al. Accuracy of pleth variability index to predict fluid responsiveness in mechanically ventilated patients: a systematic review and meta-analysis. J Clin Monit Comput 2016;30:265–74.
15. Scheeren TWL, Belda FJ, Perel A. The oxygen reserve index (ORI): a new tool to monitor oxygen therapy. J Clin Monit Comput 2018;32:379–89.
16. Whitaker DK. Time for capnography everywhere. Anaesthesia 2011;66:544–9.
17. Saunders R, Struys MRF, Pollock RF, et al. Patient safety during procedural sedation using capnography monitoring: a systematic review and meta-analysis. BML Open 2017;7:e013402.

18. Ortega R, Connor C, Kim S, et al. Monitoring ventilation with capnography. N Engl J Med 2012;367:19.

19. Siobal MS. Monitoring exhaled carbon dioxide. Respir Care 2016;61:1397–416.

20. Ramsay MA, Usman M, Lagow E, et al. The accuracy, precision and reliability of measuring ventilatory rate and detecting ventilatory pause by rainbow acoustic monitoring and capnometry. Anesth Analg 2013;117:69–75.

21. Goldfine CE, Oshim FT, Carreiro SP, et al. Respiratory rate monitoring in clinical environments with a contactless ultra-wideband impulse radar-based sensor system. Proc Annu Hawaii Int Conf Syst Sci 2020;2020:3366–75.

22. Walter J, Corbridge TC, Singer BD. Invasive mechanical ventilation. South Med J 2018;111:746–53.

23. Acute Respiratory Distress Syndrome Network, Brower RG, Matthay MA, Morris A, et al. Ventilation with lower tidal volumes as compared to traditional tidal volumes for acute lung injury and the acute respiratory distress syndrome. N Engl J Med 2000;342:1301–8.

24. Neto AS, Hemmes SNT, Barbas CSV, et al. Association between driving pressure and development of postoperative pulmonary complications in patients undergoing mechanical ventilation for general anesthesia: a meta-analysis of individual patient data. Lancet Resp Med 2016;4:272–80.

25. Futier E, Constantin JM, Paugam-Burtz C, et al. IMPROVE Study Group: A trial of intraoperative low-tidal-volume ventilation in abdominal surgery. N Engl J Med 2013;369:428–37.

26. Goligher EC, Dres M, Patel BK, et al. Lung and diaphragm protective ventilation. Am J Respir Crit Care Med 2020;202:950–61.

27. Gologher EC, Jonkman AH, Dianti J, et al. Clinical strategies for implementing lung and diaphragm protective ventilation: avoiding insufficient and excessive effort. Intensive Care Med 2020;46:2314–26.

28. Brochard L, Martin GS, BlanchL, et al. Clinical Review: respiratory monitoring in the ICU – a consensus of 16. Crit Care 2012;16:219. Available at: http://ccforum.com/content/16/2/219.

29. Mauri T, Yoshida T, Bellani G, et al. Esophageal and transpulmonary pressure in the clinical setting: meaning, usefulness and perspectives. Intensive Care Med 2016;42:1360–73.

30. Lee LA, Caplan RA, Stephens LS, et al. Postoperative opioid-induced respiratory depression; a closed claims analysis. Anesthesiology 2015;122:659–65.

31. Gupta K, Prasad A, Nagappa M, et al. Risk factors for opioid-induced respiratory depression and failure to rescue: a review. Curr Opin Anesthesiol 2018;31:110–9.

32. Khanna AK, Bergese SD, Jungquist CR, et al. Prediction of opioid-induced respiratory depression on inpatient wards using continuous capnography and oximetry: an international prospective observational trial. Anesth Analg 2020;131:1012–24.

33. Izrailtyan I, Qiu J, Overdyk FJ, et al. Risk factors for cardiopulmonary and respiratory arrest in medical and surgical hospital patients on opioid analgesics and sedatives. PLoS One 2018;13:e0194553.

34. Williams GW, George CA, Harvey BC, et al. A comparison of measurement of change in respiratory status in spontaneously breathing volunteers by the Ex-Spiron Noninvasive respiratory volume monitor versus the Capnostream capnometer. Anesth Analg 2017;124:120–6.

35. Voscopoulos CJ, MacNabb CM, Brayanov J, et al. The evaluation of a noninvasive respiratory volume monitor in surgical patients undergoing elective surgery with general anesthesia. L Clin Monit Comput 2015;29:223–30.

36. Pyke J, Taenzer AH, Renaud CE, et al. Developing a continuous monitoring infrastructure for detection of inpatient deterioration. Jt Comm J Qual Patient Saf 2012; 38:428–31.
37. Overdyk FJ, Carter R, Maddox RR, et al. Continuous oximetry/capnometry monitoring reveals frequent desaturation and bradypnea during patient-controlled analgesia. Anesth Analg 2007;105:412–8.
38. Taenzer AH, Pyke J, Herrick MD, et al. A comparison of oxygen saturation data in inpatients with low oxygen saturation using automated continuous monitoring and intermittent manual charting. Anesth Analg 2014;118:326–31.
39. Taenzer AH, Spence BC. The afferent limb of rapid response systems: continuous monitoring on general care units. Crit Care Clin 2018;34:189–98.
40. Borel JC, Palot A, Patout M. Technological advances in home non-invasive ventilation monitoring: reliability of data and effect on patient outcomes. Respirology 2019;24:1143–51.
41. Ronen R, Weissbrod R, Overdyk FJ, et al. Smart respiratory monitoring: clinical development and validation of the IPI^{tm} algorithm. J Clin Monit Comput 2017; 31:435–42.
42. Connor CW, Palmer LJ. Remote control and monitoring of GE Aisys anesthesia machines repurposed as intensive care unit ventilators. Anesthesiology 2020; 133(2):477–9.

Respiratory Mechanics

Ralph Gertler, MD, PhD

KEYWORDS

- Respiratory mechanics • Mechanical ventilation • Monitoring

KEY POINTS

- Measurement of respiratory mechanics is still the mainstay of bedside monitoring of mechanical ventilation.
- Ideally, the energy applied to the lung is optimized based on the equation of mechanical power.
- Setting the ventilator considers multiple aspects of energy transfer and protection against ventilator-associated injury.
- Newer technologies appear promising; particularly, electrical impedance tomography and lung ultrasound in combination with conventional monitoring are currently the direction for the future.

INTRODUCTION

Mechanical ventilation can harm lung tissue through barotrauma, volutrauma, atelectrauma, oxytrauma, and biotrauma. These 5 mechanisms have their own specific pathophysiological features but share similarities in their pathways of injuring the lungs (ventilator-induced lung injury [VILI]).[1] All these mechanisms together may result in inflammation through local production and release of inflammatory mediators, which is known as biotrauma. The so-called lung-protective ventilation strategies aim to minimize the occurrence of the pathophysiological features of VILI. To prevent VILI, the amount of energy transferred from the mechanical ventilator to the patient should be limited to a bare minimum. To do so, tidal volume (VT) and inspiratory pressures should be kept low to minimize the risk of barotrauma and volutrauma. This review provides a brief overview on the measurement of respiratory (also referred to as pulmonary) mechanics and current developments in the field to achieve this goal.

WHAT ARE RESPIRATORY MECHANICS?

Respiratory mechanics refer to the expression of lung function through measures of pressure and flow. From these, a variety of derived indices can be determined, such as flow, pressure, volume, compliance, resistance, and work of breathing (WOB). These factors directly affect lung volumes and therefore functional residual

Department of Anaesthesiology and Intensive Care, HELIOS Klinikum München West, Teaching Hospital of the Ludwig-Maximilians-Universität, Steinerweg 5, München 85241, Germany
E-mail address: Ralph.Gertler@gmail.com

Anesthesiology Clin 39 (2021) 415–440
https://doi.org/10.1016/j.anclin.2021.04.003
1932-2275/21/© 2021 Elsevier Inc. All rights reserved.

capacity (FRC) and gas exchange. Waveforms are derived when one of the parameters of respiratory mechanics is plotted as a function of time or as a function of one of the other parameters. This produces scalar tracings of pressure-time, flow-time, and volume-time graphics, as well as flow-volume (V̇-V) and pressure-volume (P-V) loops. All current-generation positive-pressure ventilators—including those in the operating room—provide some monitoring of pulmonary mechanics at the bedside. Additionally, advanced respiratory mechanics monitoring modalities, such as esophageal pressure and electrical activity of the diaphragm, are available to provide sophisticated analysis of breathing efforts and diaphragmatic function. They will only be touched upon briefly because they are beyond the scope of this article. Lung ultrasound has improved the diagnostic accuracy of these modalities and nowadays is the second mainstay of ventilator management at the bedside.

WHY MEASURE RESPIRATORY MECHANICS?

Artificial ventilation is a temporary measure to replace or augment the function of the inspiratory muscles, providing the necessary energy to ensure a flow of gas into the alveoli during inspiration. When this support is removed, gas is exhaled passively as the lung and chest wall recoil to their original volume. An understanding of respiratory mechanics is vital to patient assessment during mechanical ventilation in order to match the available technology to the patient's needs. The goals are optimizing the patient's pulmonary physiology, providing effective gas exchange, maintaining alveolar recruitment, reducing injury potential, and ensuring hemodynamic stability. Analyzing and incorporating measurements of respiratory mechanics during your assessment will provide the information required for optimal intraoperative mechanical ventilation. Optimizing settings requires that the physician understands the intricacies of patient-ventilator interactions, particularly in terms of the measured variables as they are displayed by ventilator graphics. They represent the interaction between the ventilator and the patient's respiratory mechanics described by the equation of motion and therefore the power applied to the lung.

PHYSIOLOGY OF CHEST MECHANICS

The respiratory system can be simplified using a linear one-compartment model, which comprises a tube representing the airways and a balloon representing the alveoli and the chest wall.

The impedance to ventilation has numerous origins, the most important of which are the following:

- Elastic resistance of lung tissue and the chest wall
- Resistance from surface forces at the alveolar gas-liquid interface
- Frictional resistance to gas flow through the airways
- Frictional resistance from deformation of thoracic tissues (viscoelastic tissue resistance)
- Inertia associated with movement of gas and tissue (negligible at normal respiratory rates)

The first two forms of impedance may be grouped together as elastic resistance. These are measured when gas is not flowing within the lung and represent the total compliance of the lung and chest wall:

- Compliance $C_{rs} = \Delta$ volume$/\Delta$ pressure
- Elastance $EL_{rs} = \Delta$ pressure$/\Delta$ volume $= 1/C$

The last three forms may be grouped together as nonelastic resistance or respiratory system resistance. They occur while gas is flowing within the airways, and work performed in overcoming this frictional resistance is dissipated as heat and lost. Impedance to flow represents resistance of the airways:

- Resistance R = Δ pressure/flow

Note that the linear one-compartment model does not take into account the fact that resistance and compliance are not constant in the case of lung and chest wall disease; instead, they exhibit a flow and volume dependency. Work performed in overcoming elastic resistance is stored as potential energy, and elastic deformation during inspiration is the usual source of energy for expiration during both spontaneous and artificial breathing.

CONCEPT OF MECHANICAL POWER

In the past, adjusting the ventilator often only considered the variables positive end-expiratory pressure (PEEP), tidal volume (VT), P_{Plat}, and ΔP.[2] Other components such as flow and respiratory rate were neglected. The problem is that any alterations of one component changes another and makes it even more difficult to understand the relationship of the variables, blurring the overall picture. With this in mind, Gattinoni and colleagues[3] proposed the concept of mechanical power (MP) in 2016. The equation for MP is the product of ventilating frequency and the inflation energy of the tidal cycle. The latter consists of three components: (1) the power required to overcome tissue and airways resistance during gas movement (flow-resistive work), (2) the power required to inflate the lung and chest wall from their shared initial position (VT-associated work), and (3) the (nonrecurring) power required to overcome PEEP-related recoil of the lung and respiratory system. Ultimately, in the expression for MP, every component is subsumed:

$$P_{APPL} = P_{VENT} + P_{MUS} = V_T/C + \dot{V} \times R$$

where P_{appl} is the applied power to the lung and P_{vent} and P_{Mus} are the pressures applied by the ventilator and the muscles, respectively.

Elastance (E) relates P to V, and resistance relates P to ($\dot{V}$), so the equation of motion can be modified to explain how the pressure at the airway opening (P_{aw}) can be partitioned into a resistive and an elastic pressure component.

$$P_{AW(t)} = P_0 + E(V)_{(t)} + R\left(\dot{V}\right)_{(t)}$$

Here, P_0 is the starting pressure, either zero end expiratory pressure or PEEP.

Written differently, these components can be divided into the following more familiar variables, which can be measured easily at the bedside:

$$Power_{rs} = RR \cdot \left\{ \Delta V^2 \cdot \left[\frac{1}{2} \cdot EL_{rs} + RR \cdot \frac{(1+I:E)}{60 \cdot I:E} \cdot R_{aw} \right] + \Delta V \cdot PEEP \right\}$$

where ΔV marks VT, EL_{rs} is the elastance of the respiratory system (the reciprocal of compliance), RR is the respiratory rate, and I:E is the time ratio of inspiration and expiration. To begin inflation, the lung requires an energy input greater than the potential energy stored in the system by PEEP at end-exhalation. The term Δ V · PEEP is the energy required to equilibrate the potential energy stored in the system at the PEEP level (ie, PEEP-related MP, when related to time).

Recruitment diminishes and distention increases as airway pressure rises. Therefore, although its mechanical effects on atelectrauma may be, on balance, lung protective over its lower range, rising PEEP is unquestionably a component of MP and, as such, favors VILI by increasing lung stress and strain. MP can be calculated using the P-V curve. The power is defined as the area between the inspiratory limb of the Δ-transpulmonary pressure (x)-volume curve, and the volume axis (y) and is measured in joules.[4]

Following this basic idea, Collino and colleagues[5] carried out a set of animal experiments in which the MP was modified by changing the PEEP. The total MP remained unchanged, with a PEEP between 0 and 7 cmH_2O. The components of energy changed, however. While the PEEP-associated energy increases, the energy decreases owing to the components of the driving pressure (ΔP) and the flow resistance, with a PEEP level up to 7 cmH_2O. If the PEEP is raised further (up to 11–18 cmH_2O), all components of MP as well as the total energy are steadily increasing. VT, driving pressure, and inspiratory flow exponentially increased MP by a factor of 2. A 1.4 exponential increase in MP was registered with frequency, whereas a linear increase was observed with PEEP. The same MP may produce different effects in healthy or injured lungs. A power of 12 J/min may be a meaningful upper threshold of VILI and may be a predictor of survival. MP normalized to predicted body weight was a good ventilator variable in predicting mortality in patients with adult respiratory distress syndrome (ARDS).[6]

STRESS

Stress is a force applied to an area, such as pressure applied to the lung parenchyma. Force applied at an angle generates shear stress. In clinical terms, lung stress refers to the distending pressure within the lung, and the counterforce (external load) is the chest wall. The best indicator of the amount of stress applied to the lungs is the transpulmonary pressure, which is difficult to measure in routine practice, but can be estimated with transpulmonary pressure measurements (eg, with an esophageal balloon, see the following information). At the bedside, plateau pressure is often used as a surrogate, although this comes with limitations. Plateau pressure does not represent the actual force on the lung fibers but the pressure needed to expand the lungs and the chest wall consisting of the rib cage and the diaphragm. Patients with a stiff chest wall, for example, during pneumoperitoneum, will have a high plateau pressure that cannot automatically be translated into lung overdistension.[7] Maintaining a plateau pressure less than 25 cmH_2O in most patients (<30 cmH_2O in patients with ARDS) would limit lung strain to less than 2 cmH_2O (considered detrimental) and lung stress to 22 to 24 cmH_2O (considered the upper limit of stress).[8]

STRESS INDEX

The index is used to assess the shape of the pressure-time curve during constant V̇-V control ventilation.[9] A linear increase in pressure (constant compliance, index 1) suggests adequate alveolar recruitment without overdistention. If compliance worsens as the lungs are inflated (progressive decrease in compliance, upward concavity, index >1), this suggests overdistention, and the recommendation is to decrease the PEEP, VT, or both. If compliance improves as the lungs are inflated (progressive increase in compliance, downward concavity, index <1), this suggests tidal recruitment and potential for additional recruitment, and the recommendation is to increase PEEP (**Fig. 1**).

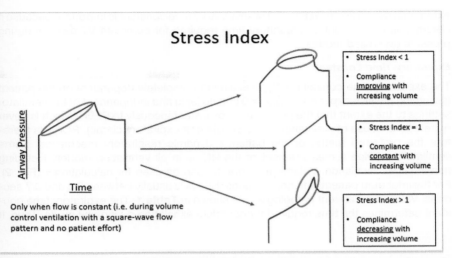

Fig. 1. Stress Index. (*Courtesy of* Willard Applefeld MD, Clinical Fellow in Critical Care Medicine, The National Institutes of Health, Bethesda, Maryland.)

STRAIN

Strain refers to the deformation, or change, in the shape of a structure compared with its resting condition. Lung strain is directly related to lung stress: stress = k × strain, where k is the specific lung elastance (13.5 cmH$_2$O in humans).[8] For the calculation of lung strain, values of FRC are obtained at zero end-expiratory pressure: lung strain = ΔV/FRC, where ΔV refers to the change in volume during inspiration. It is possible to measure strain and then calculate stress if the end-expiratory lung volume (EELV) is measured at FRC without PEEP. However, the concept of lung strain becomes complicated and less intuitive with the application of PEEP.[8,10,11]

TIME CONSTANT

When a step change in pressure is applied to the respiratory system, the change in volume (and flow and alveolar pressure) follows an exponential curve. The speed of the volume change is described by the time constant (τ) (seconds). The time constant determines the rate of change in the volume of a lung unit that is passively inflated or deflated. It is expressed by the following relationship:

$$V_t = V_i \times e^{-t/T},$$

where V_t is the volume of a lung unit at time t, V_i is the initial volume of the lung unit, e is the base of the natural logarithm, and τ is the time constant.

The time constant can be calculated during inspiration or expiration. Mathematically, one time constant is equal to the product of resistance and compliance and describes the time needed to increase or decrease the volume by 63% of the total volume change: $τ = R * C$. Lung units with a higher resistance and/or compliance will have a longer time constant and require more time to fill and to empty.

Inspiratory Time Constant

Because the time constant represents the response to a step change (ie, a square pressure waveform), the inspiratory time constant (RC$_{INSP}$) will be inaccurate to the extent that rise time is never zero. The inspiratory time constant is important because it determines the amount of inspiratory time required for complete VT delivery during pressure controlled modes.

Expiratory Time Constant

The expiratory time constant (RC_{EXP}) is almost completely dependent on the patient (assuming passive expiration, $P_{MUS} = 0$ and no leak) and independent of the ventilator settings to the extent that the pressure drops instantaneously to PEEP (which is never quite true because of resistance in the ventilator's expiratory circuit). RC_{EXP} is therefore the preferred metric of the patient's dynamic respiratory mechanics. Some ventilators provide a measurement of the RC_{EXP} in all ventilation modes, including non-invasive ventilation. Volume-time graphs can be used for calculating τ (**Fig. 2**). For the intubated patient with normal lungs, RC_{EXP} is usually between 0.5 and 0.7 seconds. Values for different pathologies are shown in **Table 1**. The expiratory time constant determines the time required for complete exhalation during any mode. Thus, if

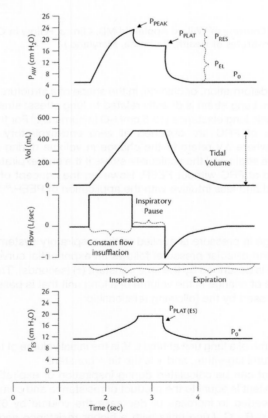

Fig. 2. Ventilator screen image representing changes in airway pressure (P_{AW}), flow, volume, and esophageal pressure (P_{ES}) versus time. PPEAK, inspiratory peak pressure; PPLAT, plateau airway pressure; PPLAT(ES), plateau esophageal pressure; P0, total PEEP at the airway pressure waveform; P0*, total PEEP at the esophageal pressure waveform; VT, tidal volume. (In: Cordioli, R and Brochard, L, Respiratory system compliance and resistance in the critically ill, Oxford Textbook of Critical Care, ISBN: 9780198855439.)

Table 1
Overview of the static lung compliance (Cstat), inspiratory resistance (Rins) and expiratory
time constant (Rexp) for different lung pathologies

	Normal Lung	ARDS	COPD
C_{stat} (ml/cmH$_2$O)	50–70	<40	> 50
R_{ins} (cm HsO s/L)	<10	10–15	15–40
RC_{EXP} (s)	0.5–0.7	< 0.5	> 0.7

expiratory time is set less than five time constants, gas trapping with intrinsic PEEP will occur (auto-PEEP >0).

PERIOPERATIVE MEASUREMENTS

In general, modern ventilators are all able to measure airway pressure and flow. Volume is derived from the flow measurement. Apart from airway pressure displayed on the mechanical ventilator, additional sources of pressure measurements (eg, tracheal pressure, gastric pressure, and esophageal pressure) are useful for separating the effects of airway resistance and chest wall elastance on the lung mechanics.

Pressure Measurements

Airway pressure is measured universally during mechanical ventilation using a pressure transducer that converts pressure into an electrical signal (see **Fig. 2**). Pressure is ideally measured at the proximal airway, for example, at the tip of the endotracheal tube. The ventilator can approximate proximal airway pressures by measuring airway pressures proximal to the inspiratory and expiratory valve during zero-flow condition in the alternating limb of the ventilator circuit. Inspiratory pressure is measured proximal to the expiratory valve during inspiration and vice versa. Airway pressure is typically displayed on the ventilator screen as a function of time and can be predicted mathematically by the equation of motion.

Peak airway pressure

Peak airway pressure (P$_{aw}$) is the maximum pressure recorded during inspiration. Inspiratory P$_{aw}$ is divided into two components, (1) resistive pressure to generate airflow through the airways and (2) alveolar pressure to distend the alveoli and chest wall. Peak P$_{aw}$ includes both resistive and alveolar components, but because there is no flow at end-inspiration (by brief inspiratory occlusion), plateau pressure can purely reflect alveolar pressure to distend the alveoli and chest wall.[12] As per the equation of motion, P$_{PEAK}$ depends on PEEP$_{TOT}$, flow, inspiratory resistance, VT, and respiratory system compliance (assuming muscle activity [P$_{MUS}$ = 0]). Therefore, any worsening of respiratory mechanics is associated with an increase in P$_{PEAK}$. To distinguish between increased resistance and decreased compliance, the first step is to perform an end-inspiratory occlusion to measure plateau pressure (P$_{PLAT}$). If P$_{PLAT}$ has not changed, the increase in P$_{PEAK}$ was due to an increase in resistance. If P$_{PLAT}$ is higher, the change in P$_{PLAT}$ resulted either from an increase in total PEEP or a decrease in compliance. Subsequently, an end-expiratory occlusion should be performed to measure total PEEP and detect occult or intrinsic PEEP.

End-inspiratory plateau pressure

Plateau pressure (P$_{PLAT}$) is measured during mechanical ventilation by applying an end-inspiratory breath-hold for a short period of time, usually 0.5 to 2 seconds, or intermittently by manually performing an end-inspiratory occlusion. During the hold, pressure equilibrates throughout the system to approximate the proximal airway pressure P_{alv}. As per the equation of motion, P_{PLAT} depends on $PEEP_{TOT}$, V_T, and respiratory system compliance. P_{plat} is determined by V_T and C_{RS} during full ventilatory support: $P_{plat} = VT/C_{RS}$. Measurement of P_{plat} is valid only during passive inflation of the lungs, but not during active breathing. During pressure control ventilation, the flow might decrease to zero at the end of the inspiratory phase; in this case, peak inspiratory pressure (PIP) and P_{plat} are equal.

The pressure drop between P_{PEAK} and P_{PLAT} is called transairway pressure and represents the resistive pressure. Owing to the airway resistance (R_{aw}), proximal airway pressure will always be greater than alveolar pressure (P_{alv}) during inspiration if flow is present. If the inspiratory flow is still positive at the end of inspiratory time, plateau pressure will be lower than the preset inspiratory pressure. In such a case, an end-inspiratory occlusion is required to measure plateau pressure. P_{plat} should ideally be kept at less than 30 cmH_2O, or even lower in patients with ARDS. This assumes that chest wall compliance (C_{CW}) is normal, whereas higher P_{plat} may be safe if C_{CW} is decreased.

End-inspiratory occlusion pressure
In patients with normal lungs, an end-inspiratory occlusion of at least 0.5 seconds allows for an accurate measurement of P_{PLAT}. However, in patients with associated lung inhomogeneity, a longer end-inspiratory occlusion of up to 5 seconds is required to reach a plateau. This long end-inspiratory occlusion must be performed manually. An end-inspiratory occlusion produces an immediate drop in peak airway pressure (P_{PEAK}) down to a lower initial pressure (P1). Then, pressure continues to decline gradually—even after the ventilator valves are closed—to reach a plateau after 3 to 5 seconds (P_{PLAT}) depending on lung mechanics. Maximum resistance, ($P_{PEAK}-P_{PLAT}$)/flow, is then partitioned into minimum resistance, ($P_{PEAK}-P1$)/flow, and additional resistance, ($P1-P_{PLAT}$)/flow. Minimum resistance represents the flow resistance of the airways and the endotracheal tube. Additional resistance represents the viscoelastic behavior or stress relaxation of the pulmonary tissues and decay of flow (pendelluft) among lung units with different time constants. Newer concepts use the expiratory time constant (τ_E) to provide real-time determinations of P_{plat} without the need for an end-inspiratory pause maneuver. This is helpful if expiration is not fully passive as in the awake patient.[13]

Mean airway pressure
The mean airway pressure is the average pressure over the whole ventilatory cycle. Graphically, it is represented by the area below the pressure time curve divided by the ventilatory period (inspiratory time plus expiratory time). During pressure control ventilation, the inspiratory pressure waveform is rectangular, and mean P_{AW} can be estimated as follows:

Mean P_{AW} = (PIP - PEEP) × (Ti/Ttot) + PEEP

Using a volume mode, the waveform is triangular, therefore cutting the aforementioned value in half:

Mean P_{AW} = 0.5 (PIP - PEEP) × (Ti/Ttot) + PEEP

Many current microprocessor ventilators display mean P_{AW} from integration of the P_{AW} waveform as the average of samples taken over the ventilatory period (eg, every

20 milliseconds). Mean airway pressure is clinically important because P_aO_2 is proportional to mean airway pressure. On the other hand, cardiac output may be inversely proportional to mean airway pressure. Typical mean P_{AW} values for fully ventilated patients are 5 to 10 cmH$_2$O for patients with normal lungs, 10 to 20 cmH$_2$O for patients with airflow obstruction, and 15 to 30 cmH$_2$O for patients with ARDS. Anything that increases airway pressure or the I:E ratio by increasing inspiratory time or decreasing expiratory time increases mean airway pressure.

End-expiratory pressure and auto-positive end-expiratory pressure

It is generally preferable that expiratory flow should reach zero before the end of expiration (**Fig. 3**). Incomplete emptying of the lungs occurs if the expiratory phase is terminated prematurely. The pressure produced by this trapped gas is called auto-PEEP, intrinsic PEEP, or occult PEEP. Auto-PEEP increases EELV and causes dynamic hyperinflation.[14,15] Auto-PEEP is measured by applying an end-expiratory pause for 0.5 to 2 seconds or longer. The pressure measured at the end of this maneuver in excess of the PEEP set on the ventilator is defined as auto-PEEP. For a valid measurement, the patient must be relaxed and breathing in synchrony with the ventilator because active breathing during exhalation invalidates the measurement. The end-expiratory pause method can underestimate auto-PEEP when some airways close during exhalation, as may occur during ventilation of the lungs of patients with severe asthma (airway closure). Auto-PEEP reduces VT during PC ventilation and may contribute to ineffective trigger efforts and dyssynchrony. In spontaneously breathing patients, measurement of esophageal pressure (P_{es}) can be used to determine auto-PEEP (see the following information). Auto-PEEP can be decreased by decreasing

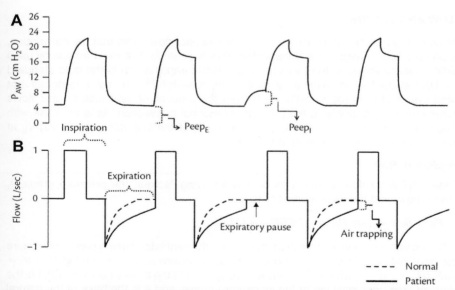

Fig. 3. The occurrence of intrinsic PEEP can be observed on the screen of the ventilator from a patient with obstructive lung disease. (A) Airway pressure waveform with an expiratory pause showing the existence of PEEPI (or auto-PEEP). (B) Flow curve demonstrating the failure to exhale all gas during the expiratory time and, consequently, formation of gas trapping. (In: Cordioli, R and Brochard, L, Respiratory system compliance and resistance in the critically ill, Oxford Textbook of Critical Care, ISBN: 9780198855439.)

minute ventilation (rate or VT), increasing expiratory time T_E (decreasing rate or T_I), or decreasing R_{aw} (eg, bronchodilator administration). The pressure curve during expiration also reflects the status of the exhalation valve. If the exhalation valve demonstrates significant airflow resistance, the pressure drop at the beginning of expiration will be smooth. If the exhalation valve is leaking, the expiratory pressure will be lower than the set PEEP.

Driving pressure

Driving pressure (ΔP) (more accurately, tidal pressure) is the pressure required to overcome elastic forces during tidal inflation of the respiratory system. Driving pressure is calculated as follows:

$$\Delta P = E_{RS} \times V_T = V_T / C_{STAT} = P_{PLAT} - PEEP_{TOT}$$

Driving pressure is one metric of the strain applied to the respiratory system and represents the risk of volutrauma. In retrospective studies on patients with ARDS, there is a clear association between driving pressure (ΔP) and mortality. This clinical observation confirms the assumption that ΔP is a measure of detrimental energy to the lung. The higher the ΔP, the more the MP is applied to the lung. ΔP represents an attractive shortcut to the equation of motion because it combines the variables P_{Plat} and PEEP. P_{Plat} represents total inspiratory forces, and PEEP represents the expiratory one. Increased P_{Plat} is associated with overdistention and an insufficient amount of PEEP with atelectasis and atelectrauma. This is further complicated by the fact that changes in PEEP necessarily increase P_{plat}. It was shown that survival does not depend on the position of ΔP on the P-V graph, but rather on the absolute value of ΔP.[16,17]

FLOW AND VOLUME

All current-generation critical care ventilators monitor flow. Note that, by convention, expiratory flow is negative and inspiratory flow is positive. The most frequently used airflow measurement is the Fleisch pneumotachograph, which is the gold standard for flow evaluation in respiratory mechanics research.[18] Thermal cooling (or hot wire) pneumotachographs estimate V from the amount of heat loss as gas flows across the device, applying the principle of thermal convection. As is the case with P_{AW} measurements, most ventilators measure $\dot{V}_I$ at the inspiratory valve and $\dot{V}_E$ at the expiratory valve rather than at the airway.

Inspiratory Flow

Peak inspiratory flow $\dot{V}_I$ depends on the following factors: the pressure gradient, driving flow, and the inspiratory resistance.

$$Peak\ flow = (set\ P_{PEAK} - PEEP_{TOT}) / R_{INSP}$$

During volume control ventilation, $\dot{V}_I$ is set on the ventilator. During passive pressure control ventilation, flow is the pressure applied to the airway, R_{aw}, and τ (Fig. 13) : $\dot{V}_I = (\Delta P / R_{aw}) \times e^{-t/T}$, where P is the pressure applied to the airway above PEEP, t is the elapsed time after initiation of the inspiratory phase, and e is the base of the natural logarithm.

Expiratory Flow

Expiratory flow (V_E) is normally passive and is determined by Palv, R_{aw}, the elapsed time since initiation of exhalation, and τ : $\dot{V} = -(P_{alv} / R_{aw}) \times e^{-t/T}$.

End-expiratory flow is present if R_{aw} is high and expiratory time T_E is not sufficient, indicating the presence of air trapping (auto-PEEP). It may be of value to determine whether auto-PEEP is due to flow limitation. If pushing on the abdomen results in no additional expiratory flow, flow limitation is present. The presence of missed triggers and flow limitation suggests that PEEP might effectively counterbalance auto-PEEP. Notching in the expiratory flow waveform suggests the presence of missed trigger efforts.[19]

Tidal Volume

Most ventilators do not measure volume directly but derive this from the integration of flow. Because flow is usually not measured directly at the proximal airway, volume output from the ventilator is less than the volume delivered to the patient. Modern ventilators correct volume for circuit compression, which can be as much as 0.5 to 1.5 mL/ cmH_2O.

DERIVED MEASUREMENTS

For an easy assessment, the ventilator is set in the volume-controlled mode with a constant inspiratory flow pattern. Care must be paid to minimize the patient's own respiratory efforts, which would invalidate or complicate these measurements. The relationship between respiratory mechanics and lung volume/volume-derived indices critically depends on the presence of aeration loss from predicted FRC: C_{RS} reflects end-expiratory aerated volume, DP roughly measures dynamic strain, and PEEP-induced alveolar recruitment can be detected at the bedside by changes in these two parameters only if aerated lung volume is lower than the individual predicted FRC.[20]

Measurement of Compliance

Compliance measurements are key to ventilator management in patients with and without lung disease. Respiratory system static compliance (C_{rs}) is the pressure burden exerted on the lung for any volume change. It is calculated as change in volume over the change in pressure as follows:

$$C_{rs} = \Delta V/\Delta P = VT/\text{Plateau Pressure (Pplat)} - PEEP.$$

The normal respiratory compliance is in the range of 50 to 70 mL/cmH_2O.
Static compliance is relatively simple to measure, but it has some limitations: Most importantly, it does not distinguish between the lung and chest wall.

$$1/C_{rs} = 1/C_{lung} + 1/C_{chest\ wall}$$

Next, it is measured at just one VT and assumes the respiratory system to be a single compartment, which may underestimate the complexity of regional compliances in clinical situations with great inhomogeneity, for example, ARDS. The distinction between the two requires measuring the intrathoracic (or pleural) pressure. Even in the absence of a direct measurement, a significant contribution of the chest wall to a low C_{RS} can be suspected in the presence of morbid obesity, abdominal distention, tight chest bandages, and large pleural effusions.[21]

Dynamic compliance (DyC_{rs}) is similar; however, it incorporates airway resistance (R_{aw}) within the calculated value. For the single-compartment model of the respiratory system, $C_{STAT} = C_{DYN}$ and is independent of the respiratory rate. For a multiple-compartment model of the lungs, as the distribution of resistance and compliance becomes less homogeneous, C_{STAT} becomes greater than C_{DYN} because flow persists among lung units with different mechanical properties (pendelluft), and this flow increases ΔP for the same ΔV. In this case, C decreases as the respiratory rate increases. Optimal compliance demonstrates ideal distending pressures, alveolar recruitment, V/Q matching, homogeneity, and therefore prevention of VILI. Static compliance values are relative to each patient and circumstance, often between 40 and 80 mL/cmH$_2$O. The crucial factor is ensuring each patient's best and optimal compliance. Recruited open lungs are compliant, whereas atelectatic or overinflated lungs are not. Plateau pressure may also be trended as a surrogate of compliance when calculations are not expedient. It is determined by the compliance of the lungs and chest wall.

Chest Wall Compliance

To calculate C$_{CW}$, changes in P$_{es}$ (P$_{pl}$) are used during passive inflation: C$_{CW}$ =V/P= VT/P$_{es}$.

The normal C$_{CW}$ is 200 mL/cmH$_2$O and is decreased in morbid obesity, abdominal compartment syndrome, chest wall edema, chest wall burns, and thoracic deformities (eg, kyphoscoliosis). C$_{CW}$ is also decreased with an increase in muscle tone (eg, a patient who is asynchronous with the ventilator). C$_{CW}$ is increased with flail chest and paralysis.

Lung Compliance

To calculate lung compliance (C$_L$), the change in P$_L$ when the lungs are inflated is used:

$$C_L = V/P = V_T/P_L.$$

The normal C$_L$ is 150 to 200 mL/cmH$_2$O.[22] The variability of C$_L$ may be related to the surface tension of alveoli and the viscosity of lung tissue. C$_L$ is decreased with ARDS, cardiogenic pulmonary edema, pneumothorax, consolidation, atelectasis, pulmonary fibrosis, pneumonectomy, bronchial intubation, and overdistention. C$_L$ is increased with emphysema.

AIRWAY RESISTANCE

R$_{aw}$ reflects the resistance to ventilation imposed by the airways as well as by the endotracheal tube. However, the resistance of endotracheal tubes is known, and one can use this knowledge[23] and clinical judgment (presence of secretions within the tube as seen in the flow curve) in estimating the airway-versus-equipment contribution onto R$_{aw}$. The resistance imposed by the ventilator circuit (generally minimal) is not part of this measurement. R$_{aw}$ is affected by flow, lung volume, and the phase of respiration. Resistance forces disappear before reaching the deep lung and are not present in alveoli, therefore not contributing to the risk of VILI.

During volume control ventilation, R$_I$ can be estimated from the PIP, P$_{plat}$, and end-inspiratory flow:

$$R_I = (PIP - P_{plat})/ V_I$$

R$_E$ can be estimated from the V$_{EXH}$ and the difference between P$_{plat}$ and PEEP:[24]

$$R_E = (P_{plat} - PEEP)/ V_{EXH}$$

Common causes of increased R$_{aw}$ are bronchospasm, secretions, and a small inner diameter endotracheal tube. For intubated and mechanically ventilated patients, R$_I$

should be less than 10 cmH$_2$O/L/s. Inspiratory R$_{aw}$ is typically lower than expiratory R$_{aw}$ owing to the increased diameter of the airways during inspiration, particularly in patients with chronic obstructive respiratory disease (COPD) and dynamic hyperinflation.[25]

The PIP-P$_{plat}$ differential can offer a surrogate indicator of inspiratory R$_{aw}$ during rapid assessment. R$_{aw}$ can also be estimated from the time constant ($\tau = R \times C$) of the respiratory system. This method permits to calculate both inspiratory and expiratory R$_{aw}$. R$_{aw}$ cannot be determined when using variable flow modes such as pressure control ventilation. Flow/time, volume/time, and pressure/time waveforms may demonstrate a failure to reach baseline, indicating high expiratory R$_{aw}$, air trapping, dynamic hyperinflation, and/or auto-PEEP. The lowest R$_{aw}$ will often coincide with optimal compliance and PEEP. In the heterogeneous obstructive lung, optimal PEEP will splint airways, improve the distribution of ventilation, diminish air trapping, prevent auto-PEEP, and yield the lowest expiratory R$_{aw}$.[15,26] Removing externally set PEEP to decrease air trapping in obstructive lung disease is an erroneous technique not in-line with current empiric data. R$_{aw}$ may be minimized through optimal PEEP, treating airway abnormalities such as secretions or bronchospasm, and ensuring a patent airway.

MEASUREMENT OF DEAD SPACE

Approximately 33% of each breath does not participate in gas exchange, termed dead space (V$_{DS}$) and averaging 2 mL/kg of ideal body weight. Dead space is divided into 2 categories: anatomic and alveolar. Together, the two encompass the physiologic (total) dead space and are measured in ratio to the V$_T$ (V$_{DS}$/V$_T$). Applying the Enghoff modification of the Bohr equation, V$_{DS}$/V$_T$ =P$_a$CO$_2$ – PeCO$_2$/Paco$_2$, values for dead space fraction may be estimated. Although not technically equivalent, the end-tidal carbon dioxide (ETCO$_2$) may act as a surrogate for PeCO$_2$. C$_{RS}$ and alveolar dead space have been previously proposed to optimize the PEEP setting during surgery.[27] Trending V$_{DS}$/V$_T$ allows ventilation titration for the best possible V/Q matching and gas exchange. Intrapulmonary shunt measurements can offer additional data on oxygenation and V/Q mismatch, but shunt calculation is complex. Alveolar-to-arterial gradients from a blood gas analysis can act as a substitute (A/a gradient = P$_{AO_2}$ – Pao$_2$). Confirming optimal C$_{rs}$, DyC$_{rs}$, R$_{aw}$, V$_{DS}$/V$_T$, and gas exchange is the key facet in providing optimal mechanical ventilation, which in turn minimizes the risk of postoperative pulmonary complications (PPCs) and VILI.

EXTENDED MONITORING

Airway flow and pressure curves display the complex interaction between the ventilator settings and the patient's respiratory mechanics. Pressure, volume, and flow curves displayed by the ventilator are nothing more than graphical representations of the equation of motion.

P-V Loops

The P-V relation as displayed by the P-V loop is linear in a normal lung that is fully aerated at the beginning of the maneuver. This means that the compliance remains constant throughout inflation. The slope of the P-V curve is C$_{RS}$. Deflation is also linear. There is a small degree of physiologic hysteresis (area between the inflation and deflation limbs of the P-V loop) that occurs owing to the viscoelastic property of tissues. In a patient with early-onset ARDS, the shape of the P-V loop may differ compared with that of a patient with normal lungs (see **Fig. 4**). The inflation and deflation limbs demonstrate a change in slope, which means that the respiratory system compliance varies at different levels of pressure. In addition, hysteresis is greater than in patients with normal lungs owing to recruitment occurring during inflation and derecruitment occurring during deflation. Recruitment occurs at a higher pressure than derecruitment. Therefore, a quasi-static P-V loop can be used to assess the potential for recruitment and predict the effect of a recruitment maneuver. The larger the volume difference between inflation and deflation, the higher the potential for recruitment. Hysteresis is quite awkward to calculate but can easily be estimated using the volume difference between inflation and deflation measured at 20 cmH$_2$O of pressure. If the volume difference is higher than 500 mL, it means there is high potential for recruitment. A number of issues preclude routine use of P-V curves to set the ventilator in patients with ARDS.[28] Correct interpretation of the P-V curve during nonconstant flow ventilation (eg, pressure control ventilation) and with higher V_I is problematic. Measurement of the P-V curve requires deep sedation, and often paralysis, to correctly make the measurement. Chest wall mechanics potentially affect the shape of the P-V curve, necessitating P_{es} measurement to separate lung from chest wall effects. As with most measures of respiratory mechanics, the P-V curve treats the lungs as a single compartment, disregarding the inhomogeneity of the lungs of patients with ARDS. Performing subsequent P-V curves and measuring lung volume corresponding to different PEEP levels can be used to assess PEEP-induced lung recruitment.[29,30] Lung recruitment at a given airway pressure is observed as the difference in lung volume between P-V curves starting at different lung volumes corresponding to different levels of PEEP (**Fig. 4**).

$\dot{V}$-V Loops

$\dot{V}$-V loops are displayed with flow as a function of volume. Analysis of the $\dot{V}$-V loop may be helpful for identifying flow limitation during expiration and bronchodilator response.[31] The inability to reach zero flow indicates that exhalation ends at a lung volume higher than FRC, which exerts an auto-PEEP (PEEP$_i$). The $\dot{V}$-V curve can provide an indication of excessive secretions more reliably than clinical examination, with the presence of excessive secretions in the airways producing a sawtooth pattern on both the inspiratory and expiratory $\dot{V}$-V curves[32] $\dot{V}$-V loops are also useful in the detection of air leaks that cause a loss of volume with each breath, as well as a difference between the delivered and the exhaled VT. Air leaks can occur all the way from within the

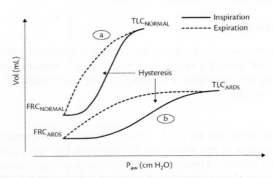

Fig. 4. Pressure-volume curve (P/V) and its hysteresis. (a) P/V curve from a normal patient. (b) P/V curve from a patient with ARDS. (In: Cordioli, R and Brochard, L, Respiratory system compliance and resistance in the critically ill, Oxford Textbook of Critical Care, ISBN: 9780198855439.)

ventilator system, between the ventilator and the patient and within the patient, for example, when a bronchopleural fistula is present. Regardless of their location, air leaks cause a characteristic failure of the V-V loop to close at the end of expiration because a portion of the inspired VT does not return to the site of measurement on the expiration side (**Fig. 5**).

BEST POSITIVE END-EXPIRATORY PRESSURE VENTILATION

An optimal PEEP is a pressure at end-expiration, which should be set to an end-expiratory pressure that prevents injurious energy expenditure to the lung. Providing PEEP levels sufficient to maintain alveolar recruitment is instrumental in protective ventilation. All other parameters and settings rely on appropriate levels of PEEP to ensure adequate ventilation, FRC, and recruitment. If PEEP exceeds the level required to stabilize the lungs, overdistension may result, despite the use of low VT. Thus, moderate levels of PEEP in noninjured lungs may represent a compromise between cyclic overdistension and closing/reopening of lung units. The optimal PEEP to apply remains debated. Ventilation with higher PEEP (10–12 cmH$_2$O) may be without clinical benefit because studies so far have shown no protection against development of PPCs, suggesting that the optimal setting has a wide intersubject variability. This might be attributable to its two-edged nature: PEEP generates overinflation with lung injury in already open alveoli (ie, static strain) but lowers dynamic strain when it is effective in recruiting new compartments.[20] There are arguments against use of higher PEEP owing to its effect on circulation and the need for intraoperative administration of vasoactive drugs.[7]

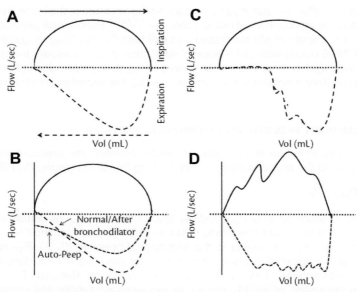

Fig. 5. Flow-volume curves in different situations. (*A*) Normal patient; (*B*) patient with COPD and dynamic hyperinflation and auto-PEEP and after bronchodilator treatment; (*C*) sudden interruption of exhalation flow representing an important gas leak from the patient (bronchopleural fistulae) or from the ventilator circuit; (*D*) a sawtooth pattern is observed in both inspiratory and expiratory limbs and indicates the presence of secretions in the airways. (In: Cordioli, R and Brochard, L, Respiratory system compliance and resistance in the critically ill, Oxford Textbook of Critical Care, ISBN: 9780198855439.)

WHAT IS THE OPTIMAL POSITIVE END-EXPIRATORY PRESSURE AND HOW IS IT DETERMINED?

PEEP must be individually determined for each patient. The lowest sum of collapse and overdistension will be the optimal PEEP, which will lead to the least lung injury. Basic PEEP trial methods involve monitoring compliance and/or its surrogates (PIP, P_{plat}) with progressive changes in PEEP. During PEEP trials, DyC_{rs} has proved to be a particularly valuable indicator, accounting for changes in R_{aw} in addition to C_{rs}. Alveolar-to-arterial gradient, oxygenation, and V_{DS}/V_T will generally improve in conjunction with compliance and resistance, indicating optimal settings. Suter and colleagues[33] discovered that the best C_{rs} coincided with maximum oxygen transport and the lowest V_{DS}/V_T. An increase in PIP/P_{plat} greater than the change in PEEP would indicate a drop in compliance, overdistention, and increased risk of VILI. For patients being ventilated with pressure control ventilation, the anesthesia provider may use a similar extrapolation in DyC_{rs} or C_{rs}, noting changes in the delivered V_T for a set PIP and/or ΔP. Because pressure is fixed, V_T changes are indicative of changes in compliance, recruitment, and FRC in contrast to PIP/P_{plat} changes during volume ventilation. Optimal PEEP promotes these goals without compromising hemodynamics; otherwise, oxygen delivery would be curtailed.

The most relevant clinical consequence of these considerations is that C_{RS} and DP are the best available bedside tools to monitor aeration loss, dynamic strain, and PEEP-induced recruitment.

INTRATHORACIC OR PLEURAL PRESSURE

Pleural pressure (P_{PL}) is estimated by measuring the pressure in the lower third of the esophagus using an esophageal balloon catheter.[11,34–36] Esophageal pressure (P_{ESO}) is used as a surrogate of pleural pressure to estimate C_L and C_{CW}, to quantify auto-PEEP and WOB during assisted modes of ventilation, and to evaluate the degree of diaphragmatic dysfunction. The measurement of P_{PL} is of great value in the assessment of respiratory mechanics and can be used by the experienced clinician at the bedside.[11]

TRANSPULMONARY PRESSURE AND ESOPHAGEAL PRESSURE

Transpulmonary Pressure (P_{TP}) is the difference between the pressure inside the alveoli (P_{ALV}) and the pressure surrounding the lung (pleural pressure, P_{PL}) (**Fig. 6**):

$$P_{TP} = P_{ALV} - P_{PL}$$

As in vivo measurements of P_{ALV} and P_{PL} are not feasible, P_{ALV} is usually assumed to be approximately equal to the static pressure at the airway opening (P_{PLAT}, PEEP) and P_{PL} is assumed to be equal to the esophageal pressure (P_{ESO}). P_{TP} is usually described as the distending pressure of the lungs because it best describes the sum of the interactions of P_{PL} and P_{ALV} across the lungs. Because P_{ESO} can be elevated in the setting of ARDS, obesity, or increased intraabdominal pressure, the use of P_{TP} allows the titration of positive pressure based on the actual pressure applied to the lung. To allow optimal recruitment, PEEP could be increased until P_{TP} becomes positive at end-expiration, to keep airways and alveoli open during the tidal cycle.[36] End-inspiratory P_{TP} is evaluated by calculating the $P_{PLAT} - P_{ESO}$ difference during an inspiratory hold. It is useful in the assessment of safety pressure thresholds: an end-inspiratory P_{TP} lower than 20 cmH_2O is generally considered safe.[36]

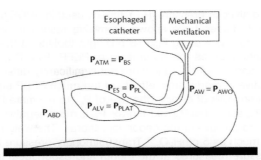

Fig. 6. The main different pressures involved in pulmonary mechanics. (In: Cordioli, R and Brochard, L, Respiratory system compliance and resistance in the critically ill, Oxford Text-book of Critical Care, ISBN: 9780198855439.)

For the lung, only transpulmonary pressure ($P_L = P_{pl} - P_{alv}$, with P_{pl} being the intra-pleural pressure) determines alveolar distention. Intrapleural pressure is not easily accessible, besides being unequally distributed throughout the lung. As a surrogate, esophageal pressure (P_{es}) can be used as an estimate of mean P_{pl}.[37] This minimally invasive approach can be used to estimate P_L, which is particularly advantageous in cases of a decreased extrathoracic compliance such as obesity or an elevated intra-obdominal pressure. In the supine position, the weight of the mediastinum and abdominal pressure both increase P_{es}. Some studies have pointed out that P_{es} is higher than P_{pl} by about 5 cmH$_2$O owing to the effects of body position and medias-tinum.[38] P_{es} can represent the average level of P_{pl}, and P_{es} and P_{pl} have a good cor-relation. For making sure P_{es} reflects P_{pl} accurately, the technical aspects of P_{es} measurement are important. It usually includes the characteristics of the esophageal manometers, placement position, balloon inflating volume, and data interpretation. In order to ensure the accuracy of P_{es}, its positioning needs to be tested by an occlusion test. In some cases, such as obesity, thoracic, or abdominal disease, P_{aw} cannot reflect actual pressure gradient over the lung because the higher percentage of P_{aw} is used to overcome the elastance of the chest wall. The monitoring of pleural pressure (P_{pl}) or esophageal pressure (P_{es}) may help to distinguish the pressure gradients acting on the lung and chest wall. On the other hand, when the patient makes spon-taneous breathing efforts, the inspiratory muscles and the ventilator both participate in breathing activity during assisting ventilation mode. The pressure inflating the lung comes from the pressure generated by the ventilator and the patient's inspiratory muscles. However, excessive breathing effort also can induce spontaneous patient self-inflicted lung injury.[39] Therefore, it is very important to monitor spontaneous breathing efforts and to balance the relationship between mechanical ventilation and spontaneous breathing effort during assisted ventilation. The Monitoring of P_{es}, intragastric pressure (P_{ga}), and a series of parameters derived from P_{es} and P_{ga} can be used to quantitatively assess spontaneous breathing efforts.

CHOICE OF POSITIVE END-EXPIRATORY PRESSURE USING ESOPHAGEAL PRESSURE

For the choice of PEEP levels, airway pressure P_{aw} is primarily chosen. This, however, rather represents pressure at the artificial airway or the ventilator, respectively. P_{aw} is easily displayed and measures the mechanical properties of the whole respiratory sys-tem including the artificial airway. Therefore, only during zero-flow conditions (end-inspiratory pause, end of expiration, or during occlusion) is P_{aw} equal to tracheal pressure (P_{trach}) and alveolar pressure (P_{alv}). Initially used in ARDS to choose the right PEEP value, several studies have shown promising results in terms of improved oxygenation and compliance using P_{es}. Surprisingly, looking at the results, mortality and other end points such as measurements of PEEP, P_{TP}, P_{aw}, driving pressure ($\Delta P = P_{Plat}$-PEEP), and P_aO_2/FiO$_2$ ratio were not significantly different.[36,40] This may be due to the negative hemodynamic effects of too much PEEP on oxygen delivery. There are potential sources of error in the use of P_{es} to estimate P_{pl}. It is important to appreciate that P_{es} estimates P_{pl} mid-thorax. P_{pl} is more negative in the nondependent thorax and more positive in the dependent thorax. The weight of the heart can bias the P_{es} by as much as 5 cmH$_2$O.[41] Transpulmonary pressure (P_{TP}) is the difference between pressure measured at the mouth and esophageal (pleural) pressure. During no flow (inspiratory or expiratory pause maneuvers), P_{TP} becomes the alveolar distending pressure. In this article, the assumption is that P_{TP} is measured under static conditions and thus represents alveolar distending pressure. The ventilator should be set to avoid a negative P_{TP} during exhalation (contributing to cyclical opening and closing injury) and to avoid excessive P_{TP} at the end of inspiration (overdistention).

COMPLIANCE OF LUNGS AND CHEST WALL

P_{es} is required to separate C_L and C_{CW}. Measurement of end-inspiratory P_{ESO} ($P_{ESO,i}$) and end-expiratory P_{ESO} ($P_{ESO,e}$) allows to distinguish the two components of C_{RS}: C_{CW} and C_L.

$$1/C_{RS} = 1/C_{CW} + 1/C_L$$

$$C_{CW} = V_T / (P_{ESO,i} - P_{ESO,c})$$

$$C_L = V_T / [(P_{PLAT} - P_{ESO,i}) - (PEEP - P_{ESO,i})]$$

or

$$C_L = V_T / (P_{TP,i} - P_{TP,c})$$

The partitioning of the elastic properties of the respiratory system is useful to understand whether a low C_{RS} as a whole might be due to low C_L, low C_{CW}, or both. Impairment of the elastic properties of the chest wall, as in morbid obesity, pneumoperitoneum, or increased intra-abdominal pressure, gives us an indication that additional pressure needs to be applied to the lung and transmitted to the pleural space in order to achieve adequate thoracic inflation.[29] As the chest wall becomes stiffer, the proportion of P_{AW} that is spent for lung distention becomes smaller. The degree of stiffness of the chest wall (low C_{CW}) must be taken into account when titrating P_{AW} to recruit the lung of ARDS patients because higher P_{AW} levels might be needed to achieve the desired recruitment, without the same risk of injuring the lung. Using P_{TP} rather than P_{PLAT} as a target of P_{AW} titration has been shown to be safe and effective.[30]

FUNCTIONAL RESIDUAL CAPACITY AND END-EXPIRATORY LUNG VOLUME

FRC represents the unstressed volume at the end of lung expiration. In critically ill patients receiving mechanical ventilation and different levels of PEEP, it is better to speak of the EELV. Calculation of EELV is based on a step change in F_iO_2 and the assumption that N_2 is the balance gas. Baseline determination is made of end-tidal N2 (FET$_{N2}$). It is assumed that oxygen consumption and carbon dioxide

(CO_2) production remain constant throughout the measurement. A 20% step change in F_iO_2 then occurs, and the EELV is calculated as follows: V_{N2}/FET_{N2}, where FET_{N2} is the change following the step change in F_iO_2. The breath-to-breath changes are calculated over 20 breaths. The EELV measurement is implemented in some modern ventilators. For this application, nitrogen concentration in inhaled and exhaled gas is not directly measured but estimated from the end-tidal concentrations of oxygen and CO_2.[42–44]

WHY MEASURE LUNG VOLUMES DURING INVASIVE VENTILATION?

The use of EELV during PEEP titration would seem attractive. An increase in PEEP will always increase EELV, and respiratory system compliance can predict the amount of volume it would increase. A PEEP-induced increase in EELV might be the result of recruitment, or it might be the result of overdistention of already open alveoli. Therefore, both PEEP and EELV might contribute to lung strain, and EELV by itself might not be useful to assess PEEP response.

ELECTRICAL IMPEDANCE TOMOGRAPHY

Electrical impedance tomography (EIT) is a noninvasive and radiation-free imaging technique that uses a minimum of 16 to 32 leads positioned around the thorax. EIT provides breath-by-breath dynamic imaging of regional ventilation distribution through measuring impedance changes across lung regions; such information cannot be obtained by global monitoring (eg, airway pressure, flow monitoring). EIT can detect the changes in lung impedance associated with a recruitment maneuver and an incremental or decremental PEEP trial, enabling the identification of the PEEP level at which tidal ventilation is most homogeneous.[45,46] EIT combined with lung mechanics can avoid hyperinflation because of excessive PEEP, which may be reached if PEEP is titrated on the basis of gas exchange alone.[47] Indeed, high impedance associated with reduced compliance is the hallmark of changes suggestive of hyperinflation, whereas low impedance associated with reduced compliance is suggestive of collapse.[48–50] In patients with severe ARDS, EIT-guided PEEP titration has been associated with improved oxygenation, compliance, driving pressure, and weaning success rate.[51]

MECHANICAL VENTILATION IN SPECIAL SUBSETS OF PATIENTS
Spontaneously Breathing Patient

In spontaneously breathing patients, the pressure generated by the patient's muscle (PMUS) is added to the pressure applied by the ventilator:

$$P_{AW} + (P_{MUS} - PEEP_{TOT}) = (tidal\ volume\ /\ compliance) + (flow \times resistance)$$

There are two implications of this equation:

- First is that for PC modes, increasing P_{MUS} does not affect P_{AW} (because this is preset), but it increases volume and flow (ie, it deforms the volume and flow curves). For volume controlled modes, increasing P_{MUS} decreases P_{AW} (ie, it deforms the pressure curve), but it does not affect volume or flow (because they are preset).
- Second, it follows that P_{MUS} must exceed $PEEP_{TOT}$ in order for P_{AW} to drop (or flow to increase) enough to trigger inspiration. Otherwise a patient-ventilator asynchrony occurs, which is known as an ineffective trigger effort.

Increased Abdominal Pressure

Intra-abdominal pressure is the steady-state pressure in the abdominal cavity.[52] The normal intra-abdominal pressure is 5 mm Hg; it increases during inhalation with diaphragmatic contraction. Direct measurement of intraperitoneal pressure is not practical, so the bladder method is thus most commonly used for intermittent intra-abdominal pressure measurement.[53] Intra-abdominal pressure should be measured at the end of exhalation in the supine position, ensuring that abdominal muscle contractions are absent. In mechanically ventilated patients, an increase in intraabdominal pressure results in decreased C_{RS} with flattening and a rightward shift of the P-V curve of the respiratory system. These changes are due to decreased C_{CW}, whereas C_L remains unchanged. In deeply sedated patients with ARDS, the diaphragm behaves as a passive structure, and thus moves upward in the rib cage, transmitting increased intra-abdominal pressure to the lower lobes of the lung, where it causes compression atelectasis. Surgical abdominal decompression recruits lung volume and increases $Pa_{O_2}/F_{i_{O_2}}$. Upright positioning increases intra-abdominal pressure and decreases C_{RS}, suggesting that this position might result in a deterioration of respiratory function in patients with intra-abdominal hypertension.[54]

Pneumoperitoneum

Insufflation of CO_2 into the abdomen in the context of minimally invasive surgery leads to significant changes to the mechanical characteristics of the respiratory system. On the one hand, thoracic compliance changes with cranial shift of the diaphragm; on the other hand, compressive atelectasis leads to a reduction in EELV. Conventional monitoring, for example, of parameters relating to respiratory mechanics as provided by the mechanical ventilator (plateau and peak pressures, compliance), is not suitable for quantifying these two (lung/thorax) mechanical components. As such, faced with an increase in plateau pressure during otherwise unchanged volume-controlled ventilation, the anesthesiologist will be unable to discern whether this is solely the result of CO_2 insufflation into the abdomen with a subsequent change in thoracic compliance or whether it instead represents an actual mismatch between VT and EELV, causing increased strain and potentially lung damage. Strict limitation of those pressures cannot as a concept simply be applied to the setting of minimally invasive surgery. One option to estimate pressure acting directly on the lungs is to measure transpulmonary pressure (see the aforementioned information). To date, however, there is no evidence that adjusting ventilation parameters, and especially PEEP, in accordance with transpulmonary pressure measurements can avoid PPCs. The increase in arterial CO_2 caused by transperitoneal resorption of insufflated gas can require a significantly increased respiratory minute volume. Increasing alveolar ventilation primarily by increasing VTs may cause VILI. Increasing the respiratory rate is a useful measure but may, in the context of increased airway resistance in the setting of pneumoperitoneum, limit expiratory flow. Higher peak airway pressures do not necessarily reflect the pressure at the level of the alveoli and may instead be primarily associated with higher airway resistance in the face of increased flow. The aggressivity with which these respiratory measures are pursued can be tempered, however, if moderate hypercapnia based on pH is tolerated.

Chronic Obstructive Respiratory Disease/Asthma

Patients with obstructive lung disease cannot generate a normal expiratory flow. Normally, lung volume returns to the relaxed volume at the end of passive expiration. This relaxed lung volume is defined as FRC during spontaneous breathing. Dynamic hyperinflation occurs whenever the respiratory system cannot generate the necessary expiratory flow near FRC. In patients with increased expiratory resistance due to airflow obstruction, the EELV may increase higher than the predicted FRC. Along with the increase in EELV, end-expiratory alveolar pressure increases, which is called intrinsic PEEP.[55] Mechanical causes of dynamic hyperinflation include an increased expiratory resistance resulting in a longer time constant and a reduced lung elastance which results in a decreased expiratory driving pressure. Expiratory flow limitation is defined as the inability of augmentation of expiratory flow regardless of an increased expiratory driving pressure.[56] The consequences of hyperinflation and intrinsic PEEP are an increased inspiratory threshold during assisted mechanical ventilation. Patients have to generate an additional pleural pressure to counterbalance the intrinsic PEEP to be able to trigger the ventilator. This can be considered wasted energy cost of breathing because inspiratory muscle contraction to counterbalance intrinsic PEEP does not generate inspiratory flow. The increased inspiratory muscle load results in muscle fatigue and patient-ventilator asynchrony[57–60] and leads to an increasing pulmonary vascular resistance and right ventricular failure.

By conducting end-expiratory occlusion, static intrinsic PEEP can be measured. In combination with end-inspiratory occlusion, the static compliance of the respiratory system can be obtained. In patients with dynamic hyperinflation and intrinsic PEEP, the calculation of static compliance should be calibrated by intrinsic PEEP; otherwise, the true compliance will be underestimated.[61] Dynamic hyperinflation-induced elevation of EELV can be measured at the bedside using release and prolonged expiration maneuver.[62] No matter what ventilation model is selected, monitoring of expiration should be performed periodically to allow lung emptying. For patients with severe asthma, a relatively small VT and a higher inspiratory flow have been recommended to preserve expiratory time and minimize dynamic hyperinflation. To counterbalance intrinsic PEEP during ventilator triggering, PEEP may be applied in patients with COPD. The PEEP level is usually set as 80% of baseline intrinsic PEEP, which has been explained by the waterfall analogy.[55]

Adult Respiratory Distress Syndrome

In a heterogeneous lung in patients with ARDS, the local strain (lung tissue deformation or volume change) and the transpulmonary pressure (airway pressure-pleural pressure) are different in different locations.[8,63] In patients with ARDS, high inspiratory and expiratory resistance as well as low compliances of the baby lung are the leading pathologies. Assuming that all alveoli are open, plateau pressure (P_{plat}) reflects end-inspiratory alveolar pressure.[64] A short end-inspiratory occlusion (0.3 seconds) is sufficient to estimate injurious pressure applied to the alveoli, especially in passive breathing. Nowadays, maintaining P_{plat} at or lower than 25 cmH_2O as used in a large trial seems to be a reasonable and safe threshold. At end-inspiration, P_{TP} as derived by the insertion of an esophageal balloon is a more reliable measurement of the distending pressure of the lung because P_{plat} also depends on pleural pressure (P_{pl}). In some patients, C_{cw} is responsible for almost 50% of the C_{RS}, whereas in other cases, it is only about 15% to 20%.[65] Separation of these two factors improves ventilator settings and outcomes. P_{TP} at end-expiration ($P_{TP,ee}$) is the pressure distending the lungs at end-expiration. Negative $P_{TP,ee}$ values are common in ARDS, potentially favoring cyclic reopening and closing of alveoli during ventilation and atelectrauma.[37] Setting PEEP to a positive $P_{TP,ee}$ was associated with improved physiologic parameters.[36] A ΔP value higher than 14 to 15 cmH_2O was independently associated with higher mortality.[16] An optimal PEEP is essential in ARDS and has been discussed previously. Excluding lung imaging methods, the most common methods for the PEEP setting is the use of respiratory mechanics. Best compliance methods or the ARDS PEEP table are commonly used. Airway closure at end-expiration is another feature of ARDS, and close attention needs to be paid to the end-expiratory flow curve as well as esophageal pressures for the detection of airway closure. With the development of newer technologies, EIT has been used to select the optimal PEEP and may actually be the simplest and most promising way at the bedside. This method can be used to calculate the percentage of overdistention and collapse.

SUMMARY

Contemporary management of the ventilated patient still relies on the measurement of old parameters such as airway pressures and flows. Graphical presentations—in particular of the pressure and flow curves at different locations—reveal the intricacies of patient-ventilator interactions. This increases the complexity of measurements and opens a new pathway for several bedside technologies based on basic physiologic knowledge. The spread of COVID-19 has confronted the anesthesiologist and intensivist with one of the most severe pulmonary pathologies of the last decades. Optimizing the patient's respiratory mechanics at the bedside is a valuable skill for the physician in the ICU, which is further refined and supported by mobile technologies such as lung ultrasound and electrical impedance tomography.

CLINICS CARE POINTS

- Always evaluate the pressure-time and flow-time curves of the patient in combination with your clinical assessment.
- Use additional imaging modalities such as radiological tests, ultrasound, and EIT.
- Pressure-volume curves provide insight into compliance and recruitability.
- Keep safe airway pressures in mind: ideally P_{plat} less than 30 cmH_2O, or even lower in patients with ARDS, and driving pressure less than 15 cmH_2O.
- ΔP is a measure of detrimental energy to the lung and represents an attractive shortcut to the equation of motion because it combines the variables P_{Plat} (inspiratory forces) and PEEP (expiratory forces). Survival does not depend on the position of ΔP on the pressure-volume graph, but rather on the absolute value of ΔP.
- Mean airway pressure is clinically important because P_aO_2 is proportional to mean airway pressure and inversely proportional to cardiac output. Typical mean P_{AW} values for fully ventilated patients are 5 to 10 cmH_2O for patients with normal lungs, 10 to 20 cmH_2O for patients with airflow obstruction, and 15 to 30 cmH_2O for patients with ARDS.
- Optimal compliance demonstrates ideal distending pressures, alveolar recruitment, V/Q matching, and homogeneity and therefore prevents VILI.

DISCLOSURE

The author has nothing to disclose.

REFERENCES

1. Slutsky AS, Ranieri VM. Ventilator-induced lung injury. N Engl J Med 2013; 369(22):2126–36.
2. Tonetti T, Vasques F, Rapetti F, et al. Driving pressure and mechanical power: new targets for VILI prevention. Ann Transl Med 2017;5(14):286.

3. Gattinoni L, Tonetti T, Cressoni M, et al. Ventilator-related causes of lung injury: the mechanical power. Intensive Care Med 2016;42(10):1567–75.

4. Cressoni M, Gotti M, Chiurazzi C, et al. Mechanical power and development of ventilator-induced lung injury. Anesthesiology 2016;124(5):1100–8.

5. Collino F, Rapetti F, Vasques F, et al. Positive end-expiratory pressure and mechanical power. Anesthesiology 2019;130(1):119–30.

6. Zhang Z, Zheng B, Liu N, et al. Mechanical power normalized to predicted body weight as a predictor of mortality in patients with acute respiratory distress syndrome. Intensive Care Med 2019;45(6):856–64.

7. Hol L, Nijbroek S, Schultz MJ. Perioperative lung protection: clinical implications. Anesth Analg 2020;131(6):1721–9.

8. Chiumello D, Carlesso E, Cadringher P, et al. Lung stress and strain during mechanical ventilation for acute respiratory distress syndrome. Am J Respir Crit Care Med 2008;178(4):346–55.

9. Grasso S, Stripoli T, De Michele M, et al. ARDSnet ventilatory protocol and alveolar hyperinflation: role of positive end-expiratory pressure. Am J Respir Crit Care Med 2007;176(8):761–7.

10. Terragni PP, Rosboch G, Tealdi A, et al. Tidal hyperinflation during low tidal volume ventilation in acute respiratory distress syndrome. Am J Respir Crit Care Med 2007;175(2):160–6.

11. Benditt JO. Esophageal and gastric pressure measurements. Respir Care Jan 2005;50(1):68–75 [discussion 75-7].

12. Carvalho AR, Spieth PM, Pelosi P, et al. Ability of dynamic airway pressure curve profile and elastance for positive end-expiratory pressure titration. Intensive Care Med 2008;34(12):2291–9.

13. Al-Rawas N, Banner MJ, Euliano NR, et al. Expiratory time constant for determinations of plateau pressure, respiratory system compliance, and total resistance. Crit Care 2013;17(1):R23.

14. Marini JJ. Dynamic hyperinflation and auto-positive end-expiratory pressure: lessons learned over 30 years. Am J Respir Crit Care Med 2011;184(7):756–62.

15. Blanch L, Bernabe F, Lucangelo U. Measurement of air trapping, intrinsic positive end-expiratory pressure, and dynamic hyperinflation in mechanically ventilated patients. Respir Care 2005;50(1):110–23 [discussion 123-4].

16. Amato MB, Meade MO, Slutsky AS, et al. Driving pressure and survival in the acute respiratory distress syndrome. N Engl J Med 2015;372(8):747–55.

17. Bellani G, Laffey JG, Pham T, et al. The LUNG SAFE study: a presentation of the prevalence of ARDS according to the Berlin Definition! Crit Care 2016;20:268.

18. Giannella-Neto A, Bellido C, Barbosa RB, et al. Design and calibration of unicapillary pneumotachographs. J Appl Physiol (1985) 1998;84(1):335–43.

19. Ninane V, Leduc D, Kafi SA, et al. Detection of expiratory flow limitation by manual compression of the abdominal wall. Am J Respir Crit Care Med 2001;163(6):1326–30.

20. Fernandez-Bustamante A, Vidal Melo MF. Bedside assessment of lung aeration and stretch. Br J Anaesth 2018;121(5):1001–4.

21. Ranieri VM, Giuliani R, Mascia L, et al. Chest wall and lung contribution to the elastic properties of the respiratory system in patients with chronic obstructive pulmonary disease. Eur Respir J 1996;9(6):1232–9.

22. Faffe DS, Zin WA. Lung parenchymal mechanics in health and disease. Physiol Rev 2009;89(3):759–75.

23. Rossi A, Gottfried SB, Higgs BD, et al. Respiratory mechanics in mechanically ventilated patients with respiratory failure. J Appl Physiol (1985) 1985;58(6): 1849–58.
24. Hess D, Tabor T. Comparison of six methods to calculate airway resistance during mechanical ventilation in adults. J Clin Monit 1993;9(4):275–82.
25. Smith TC, Marini JJ. Impact of PEEP on lung mechanics and work of breathing in severe airflow obstruction. J Appl Physiol (1985) 1988;65(4):1488–99.
26. Ranieri VM, Grasso S, Fiore T, et al. Auto-positive end-expiratory pressure and dynamic hyperinflation. Clin Chest Med 1996;17(3):379–94.
27. Maisch S, Reissmann H, Fuellekrug B, et al. Compliance and dead space fraction indicate an optimal level of positive end-expiratory pressure after recruitment in anesthetized patients. Anesth Analg 2008;106(1):175–81, table of contents.
28. Gattinoni L, Vagginelli F, Chiumello D, et al. Physiologic rationale for ventilator setting in acute lung injury/acute respiratory distress syndrome patients. Crit Care Med 2003;31(4 Suppl):S300–4.
29. Gattinoni L, Chiumello D, Carlesso E, et al. Bench-to-bedside review: chest wall elastance in acute lung injury/acute respiratory distress syndrome patients. Crit Care 2004;8(5):350–5.
30. Sarge T, Talmor D. Targeting transpulmonary pressure to prevent ventilator induced lung injury. Minerva Anestesiol 2009;75(5):293–9.
31. Dhand R. Ventilator graphics and respiratory mechanics in the patient with obstructive lung disease. Respir Care Feb 2005;50(2):246–61 [discussion 259-61].
32. Jubran A, Tobin MJ. Use of flow-volume curves in detecting secretions in ventilator-dependent patients. Am J Respir Crit Care Med 1994;150(3):766–9.
33. Suter PM, Fairley B, Isenberg MD. Optimum end-expiratory airway pressure in patients with acute pulmonary failure. N Engl J Med 1975;292(6):284–9.
34. Petit JM, Milic-Emili G. Measurement of endoesophageal pressure. J Appl Physiol 1958;13(3):481–5.
35. Walterspacher S, Isaak L, Guttmann J, et al. Assessing respiratory function depends on mechanical characteristics of balloon catheters. Respir Care 2014; 59(9):1345–52.
36. Talmor D, Sarge T, Malhotra A, et al. Mechanical ventilation guided by esophageal pressure in acute lung injury. N Engl J Med 2008;359(20):2095–104.
37. Talmor D, Sarge T, O'Donnell CR, et al. Esophageal and transpulmonary pressures in acute respiratory failure. Crit Care Med 2006;34(5):1389–94.
38. Terragni P, Mascia L, Fanelli V, et al. Accuracy of esophageal pressure to assess transpulmonary pressure during mechanical ventilation. Intensive Care Med 2017;43(1):142–3.
39. Brochard L, Slutsky A, Pesenti A. Mechanical ventilation to minimize progression of lung injury in acute respiratory failure. Am J Respir Crit Care Med 2017;195(4): 438–42.
40. Beitler JR, Sarge T, Banner-Goodspeed VM, et al. Effect of Titrating Positive End-Expiratory Pressure (PEEP) with an esophageal pressure-guided strategy vs an empirical high PEEP-Fio2 strategy on death and days free from mechanical ventilation among patients with acute respiratory distress syndrome: a randomized clinical trial. JAMA 2019;321(9):846–57.
41. Loring SH, O'Donnell CR, Behazin N, et al. Esophageal pressures in acute lung injury: do they represent artifact or useful information about transpulmonary pressure, chest wall mechanics, and lung stress? J Appl Physiol (1985) 2010;108(3): 515–22.

42. Olegard C, Sondergaard S, Houltz E, et al. Estimation of functional residual capacity at the bedside using standard monitoring equipment: a modified nitrogen washout/washin technique requiring a small change of the inspired oxygen fraction. *Anesth Analg* Jul 2005;101(1):206–12, table of contents.

43. Chiumello D, Cressoni M, Chierichetti M, et al. Nitrogen washout/washin, helium dilution and computed tomography in the assessment of end expiratory lung volume. Crit Care 2008;12(6):R150.

44. Dellamonica J, Lerolle N, Sargentini C, et al. PEEP-induced changes in lung volume in acute respiratory distress syndrome. Two methods to estimate alveolar recruitment. Intensive Care Med 2011;37(10):1595–604.

45. Blankman P, Hasan D, van Mourik MS, et al. Ventilation distribution measured with EIT at varying levels of pressure support and Neurally Adjusted Ventilatory Assist in patients with ALI. Intensive Care Med 2013;39(6):1057–62.

46. Dargaville PA, Rimensberger PC, Frerichs I. Regional tidal ventilation and compliance during a stepwise vital capacity manoeuvre. Intensive Care Med 2010; 36(11):1953–61.

47. Yoshida T, Piraino T, Lima CAS, et al. Regional ventilation displayed by electrical impedance tomography as an incentive to decrease positive end-expiratory pressure. Am J Respir Crit Care Med 2019;200(7):933–7.

48. Hinz J, Hahn G, Neumann P, et al. End-expiratory lung impedance change enables bedside monitoring of end-expiratory lung volume change. Intensive Care Med 2003;29(1):37–43.

49. Meier T, Luepschen H, Karsten J, et al. Assessment of regional lung recruitment and derecruitment during a PEEP trial based on electrical impedance tomography. Intensive Care Med 2008;34(3):543–50.

50. Spadaro S, Mauri T, Bohm SH, et al. Variation of poorly ventilated lung units (silent spaces) measured by electrical impedance tomography to dynamically assess recruitment. Crit Care 2018;22(1):26.

51. Zhao Z, Chang MY, Chang MY, et al. Positive end-expiratory pressure titration with electrical impedance tomography and pressure-volume curve in severe acute respiratory distress syndrome. Ann Intensive Care 2019;9(1):7.

52. Malbrain ML, Deeren D, De Potter TJ. Intra-abdominal hypertension in the critically ill: it is time to pay attention. Curr Opin Crit Care 2005;11(2):156–71.

53. Malbrain ML. Different techniques to measure intra-abdominal pressure (IAP): time for a critical re-appraisal. Intensive Care Med 2004;30(3):357–71.

54. Cheatham ML, De Waele JJ, De Laet I, et al. The impact of body position on intra-abdominal pressure measurement: a multicenter analysis. Crit Care Med 2009; 37(7):2187–90.

55. Tobin MJ, Lodato RF. PEEP, auto-PEEP, and waterfalls. Chest 1989;96(3):449–51.

56. Koutsoukou A, Pecchiari M. Expiratory flow-limitation in mechanically ventilated patients: a risk for ventilator-induced lung injury? World J Crit Care Med 2019; 8(1):1–8.

57. Fernandez R, Benito S, Blanch L, et al. Intrinsic PEEP: a cause of inspiratory muscle ineffectivity. Intensive Care Med 1988;15(1):51–2.

58. Nava S, Bruschi C, Fracchia C, et al. Patient-ventilator interaction and inspiratory effort during pressure support ventilation in patients with different pathologies. Eur Respir J 1997;10(1):177–83.

59. Young IH, Bye PT. Gas exchange in disease: asthma, chronic obstructive pulmonary disease, cystic fibrosis, and interstitial lung disease. Compr Physiol 2011; 1(2):663–97.

60. MacDonald MI, Shafuddin E, King PT, et al. Cardiac dysfunction during exacerbations of chronic obstructive pulmonary disease. Lancet Respir Med 2016; 4(2):138–48.
61. Rossi A, Polese G, Brandi G, et al. Intrinsic positive end-expiratory pressure (PEEPi). Intensive Care Med 1995;21(6):522–36.
62. Patroniti N, Bellani G, Cortinovis B, et al. Role of absolute lung volume to assess alveolar recruitment in acute respiratory distress syndrome patients. Crit Care Med 2010;38(5):1300–7.
63. Perchiazzi G, Rylander C, Derosa S, et al. Regional distribution of lung compliance by image analysis of computed tomograms. Respir Physiol Neurobiol 2014;201:60–70.
64. Loring SH, Topulos GP, Hubmayr RD. Transpulmonary pressure: the importance of precise definitions and limiting assumptions. Am J Respir Crit Care Med 2016; 194(12):1452–7.
65. Gattinoni L, Pelosi P, Suter PM, et al. Acute respiratory distress syndrome caused by pulmonary and extrapulmonary disease. Different syndromes? Am J Respir Crit Care Med 1998;158(1):3–11.

Perioperative Hemodynamic Monitoring
An Overview of Current Methods

Ilonka N. de Keijzer, MD*, Thomas W.L. Scheeren, MD, PhD

KEYWORDS

- Hemodynamic monitoring • Blood pressure • Mean systemic filling pressure
- Central venous pressure • Cardiac output monitoring • Fluid responsiveness
- Volume monitoring

KEY POINTS

- The aim of hemodynamic management is to optimize the amount of oxygen delivered to tissues.
- Because direct monitoring of the amount of oxygen delivered remains difficult, hemodynamic variables are monitored instead.
- Hemodynamic monitoring itself does not improve patient outcomes and needs to be combined with treatment protocols.
- Pressures, from arterial blood pressure through pulmonary artery occlusion pressure, can be measured using invasive catheters, but are subject to artifacts (e.g. over- and under-damping, patient movements) and should be zeroed correctly before adequate measurements can be obtained.
- Flow, that is cardiac output, is mostly obtained by indicator dilution techniques or pulse wave analysis. The evidence for using other noninvasive techniques, for example pulse wave transit time, bioimpedance and bioreactance, is limited.

INTRODUCTION

The word "hemodynamic" is derived from the Greek words *haima* and *dunamiko´s*. Hemodynamic monitoring, therefore, freely translates into observing the motion of blood. As the word itself, hemodynamic monitoring originates from ancient times: Feeling the pulse was first described in 2600 BCE in the myth of a Mesopotamian king whose friend had died, and by "touching" his heart, he realized that it did not beat any more,[1] demonstrating that at that time mankind understood the heart was beating and that its pulsations could be felt. Two thousand years later, Hippocrates described

Department of Anesthesiology, University Medical Center Groningen, Hanzeplein 1, PO Box 30.
001, 9700 RB Groningen, The Netherlands
* Corresponding author.
E-mail address: i.n.de.keijzer@umcg.nl

Anesthesiology Clin 39 (2021) 441–456
https://doi.org/10.1016/j.anclin.2021.03.007   **anesthesiology.theclinics.com**
1932-2275/21/© 2021 The Authors. Published by Elsevier Inc. This is an open access article under
the CC BY license (http://creativecommons.org/licenses/by/4.0/).

pulse characteristics during different states of disease, while Praxagoras (born around 340 BCE) was the first one to use the pulse for indication of disease.[2] The actual circulation was first described by William Harvey in the seventeenth century, and this was considered one of the greatest contributions to the field of cardiovascular science.[3] Further development of measuring hemodynamic variables took until 1733, when Stephen Hales pioneered measuring intra-arterial pressure in horses[4] and this discovery was followed by the development of the "Stromuhr" in 1867 by Carl Ludwig, a device able to quantify blood flow through perfused organs.[5] From there on forward, important discoveries followed more rapidly, including the first noninvasive systolic blood pressure measuring device using a cuff-based version of the mercury sphygmograph by Riva Rocci in 1896.[6] In 1905, Nicolai Korotkoff described the sounds auscultating the brachial artery while deflating the cuff.[7] This way, it became possible to also determine diastolic blood pressure. Around the same time, in 1901, Willem Einthoven invented the electrocardiograph for which he later (1924) received the Nobel Prize.[8,9] The foundation for modern hemodynamic monitoring was laid.

PRESSURE MONITORING
Arterial Blood Pressure

Arterial blood pressure was one of the first hemodynamic variables that could be measured.[7] Currently, different techniques are available for continuous and intermittent arterial blood pressure monitoring in the perioperative period. Arterial catheterization is the gold standard for measuring blood pressure continuously.[10] A catheter is placed into a superficial artery (mostly radial artery) and is connected via a fluid filled tube to a pressure transducer and a pressurized bag of fluids which creates counterpressure for the arterial pressure.[11] The pressure transducer transforms mechanical pressure into an electrical signal, which is used to depict the arterial pressure waveform on a monitor. The arterial pressure waveform is the result of the interaction between the left ventricle and the systemic arteries. The pressure sensor should be placed at right atrium level and zeroed against atmospheric pressure to obtain reliable measurements. Over- and underdamping can underestimate or overestimate arterial blood pressure.[11] Additionally, blood pressure measurements can be influenced by movement of the patient's arm or a kink in the pressure system.[10,11] The use of invasive blood pressure monitoring is limited owing to the risk of complications and costs associated with arterial catheterization.[12,13] Frequently used alternative techniques for invasive blood pressure monitoring are noninvasive intermittent oscillometry and the continuous volume clamp method.[14] The most widely used method of measuring arterial blood pressure noninvasively is oscillometry. Usually, a brachial cuff is inflated and instead of Korotkoff sounds, oscillations of the blood pressure signal are detected.[15] The pressure which causes maximum oscillations is closest to the mean arterial pressure (MAP), and systolic and diastolic blood pressures are mathematically derived from this mean value.[16] The noninvasive volume clamp method uses a plethysmograph and an inflatable finger cuff. The plethysmograph detects the blood volume in the digital arteries and subsequently the pressure from the inflatable finger cuff is adjusted with high frequency to keep the blood volume in the digital arteries constant (volume clamp). Subsequently, the arterial pressure waveform can be constructed from the amount of pressure in the finger cuff needed to ensure constant volume.[17–19] Calibration is periodically performed by applying a constant pressure, to determine MAP and subsequently calibrate the plethysmography signal.[14] The use of the volume clamp method has also been validated in obese patients[20] and in patients with atrial fibrillation[21]; however, the use is limited in patients with impaired peripheral perfusion, for example in patients receiving high doses of vasopressors or during peripheral hypothermia or edema.[14,21] Other methods for measuring blood pressure noninvasively include applanation tonometry, hydraulic coupling, pulse wave transit time, and pulse decomposition. The evidence for the accuracy of these methods is limited and therefore these are not (yet) widely used in daily clinical routine.[10]

Central Venous Pressure

The central venous pressure (CVP) is the pressure measured in the vena cava near the right atrium, and is commonly obtained by placing a central venous catheter in the superior vena cava via the internal jugular vein or the subclavian vein.[22] The catheter is then connected to a pressure transducer via a fluid filled line. The CVP is determined by cardiac function and venous return to the heart,[23,24] and has traditionally been used to estimate preload and volume status,[23,25] and also to guide fluid therapy.[26] It was assumed that, because obtaining ventricular end-diastolic volume was not suitable in many clinical settings, the CVP would be a surrogate measure of preload.[25] However er the use of the CVP as a surrogate for end-diastolic volume was questioned owing to the poor correlation with the volume status of the patient[25,27–29] and should no longer be used to assess fluid responsiveness.[29,30] Nonetheless, the CVP is still measured frequently and might be used instead as an indication to stop fluid resuscitation.[31] Although the CVP is not able to predict fluid responsiveness, it can be used to assess right ventricular function, for example, in pulmonary embolism, right ventricular failure, or after heart transplantation.[29] Another advantage from using a central venous catheter is the possibility of taking blood gas samples for measuring the central venous oxygen saturation.[32]

Pulmonary Artery Pressures

Pulmonary artery pressures include the systolic and diastolic pressures and the pulmonary artery occlusion pressure (PAOP) and can be assessed by a pulmonary artery catheter (PAC).[33,34] A PAC is inserted via the internal jugular vein, subclavian vein, or femoral vein through the right atrium and right ventricle until its tip is positioned in the pulmonary artery.[34] The catheter is then connected via a tubing to a pressure transducer to obtain pressure measurements. These pressure measurements can be used during insertion to assess the position of the tip. The catheter contains 2 or more ports; the distal port is located at the tip and the other port is located more proximal and can be used to measure the CVP.[34] A PAC contains a balloon close to the tip, which can be inflated to float the catheter into the pulmonary artery and to determine PAOP.[33] The PAOP reflects the pressure in the pulmonary veins and left atrium.[33,35] In analogy to the CVP for the right ventricle, the PAOP was used as a predictor of left ventricular preload, but turned out to be unreliable for this purpose as well.[25] The use of a PAC can be associated with several (severe) complications,[33] and treatment benefits of using a PAC have not been clearly established in critically ill patients.[36,37] Therefore, the evidence for using a PAC has been questioned. The use of a PAC should always be combined with a specific treatment protocol to improve patient outcomes.[38] The PAC is still frequently used worldwide, particularly in cardiac surgery, in patients with pulmonary arterial hypertension (suspected or known), severe cardiogenic shock, unknown volume status in shock, or other severe cardiopulmonary disease.[39–41] It has been suggested that clinicians use the PAC to gain a clear understanding of the pathophysiology.[42] Similar to the central venous catheter, a PAC can be used to obtain blood samples for measuring mixed venous oxygen saturation, a marker of the global relation between oxygen delivery and consumption or the ability of the tissues to extract oxygen from the blood.

Mean Systemic Filling Pressure

The mean systemic filling pressure (P_{msf}) is the pressure that equilibrates in the systemic circulation when the heart stops pumping and all blood is distributed equally throughout the systemic circulation.[43] The value of the P_{msf} is therefore between MAP and CVP (closer to the latter owing to the size of the venous blood reservoir). The P_{msf} does not include the pressures in the pulmonary circulation and cardiac chambers (mean cardiopulmonary filling pressure). The P_{msf} and mean cardiopulmonary filling pressure combined are the mean circulatory filling pressure.[43] The P_{msf} resembles the stressed blood volume, that is, the amount of blood that exerts pressure against the vascular walls. The unstressed blood volume in turn is the amount of blood, which can be held within the vascular system without creating pressure.[43] The P_{msf} can be measured in different ways: (1) by the inspiratory hold method, (2) by the arm stop-flow method, or (3) through a calculated model.[44,45] The inspiratory hold method uses inspiratory holds of several seconds at plateau pressure to briefly increase the CVP. When the CVP increases, the venous return decreases and consequently the cardiac output (CO) decreases as well. Multiple inspiratory hold maneuvers at different plateau pressure levels are performed to derive pairs of CO and CVP measurements, which are then correlated and extrapolated to zero CO (which resembles a no flow state) and the pressure that remains is the estimated P_{msf} **(Fig. 1)**. For this method, a central venous catheter and CO monitoring are required.[46] However, the P_{msf} might be overestimated by this method because high airway pressures may redistribute blood from the pulmonary to the systemic circulation.[47] The arm stop-flow method is performed using a rapidly inflating arm cuff, which occludes

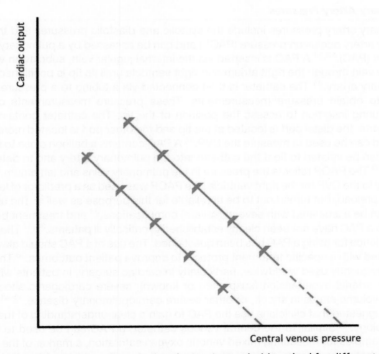

Fig. 1. Venous return curves plotted using the inspiratory hold method for different volume states. The right/upper curve is the higher volume state. Inspiratory hold maneuver.

the arteries in the arm creating a status of zero flow. The intravascular pressure will equilibrate between the venous and arterial compartment after approximately 30 seconds. The equilibration pressure is an estimation of the P_{msf}. For this method, only an arterial catheter is required.[44] The last method uses a mathematical model to estimate the P_{msf}. The P_{msf} comprises of the arterial and venous compartment and resistance to flow, resulting in the following formula: $P_{msf} = aRAP + bMAP + cCO$, in which RAP is right atrial pressure, MAP is mean arterial pressure, and CO is cardiac output[48], a and b are both dimensionless constants (often $a = 0.96$, $b = 0.04$), reflecting the contribution of venous and arterial blood, and c is a constant determined by age, height, and weight, resembling resistance.[48] The P_{msf} can be used to accurately assess volume status, although it is quite difficult to measure and thus of limited clinical use. Additionally, the P_{msf} minus the right atrial pressure is the driving force for venous return.[49] An overview of all pressure monitoring methods can be found in **Table 1**.

Table 1 Overview of pressure monitoring methods			
Arterial Blood Pressure	**Central Venous Pressure**	**Pulmonary Artery Pressures**	P_{msf}
Arterial catheter	Central venous catheter	Pulmonary artery catheter	Inspiratory hold method
Volume clamp method			Arm stop-flow method
Intermittent oscillometry			Calculated model

FLOW MONITORING
Cardiac Output

Invasive cardiac output monitoring

The CO is the product of stroke volume and heart rate and is the primary determinant of oxygen delivery to organs and peripheral tissues, therefore being one of the most clinically relevant hemodynamic variables. Invasive methods of determining CO include pulmonary artery thermodilution (PATD), transpulmonary thermodilution (TPTD), and lithium dilution.[50] All of these techniques use modified versions of the Stewart Hamilton equation to determine CO.[51] The Stewart Hamilton equation is based on the fact that, if the volume and temperature or concentration of an injected indicator are known, then the change in temperature or indicator concentration downstream is related to the flow, that is CO, and can be calculated as follows:

$$CO = \frac{Temperature\ of\ indicator}{Area\ under\ the\ temperature\ curve}$$

PATD requires a PAC, through which a cold fluid bolus can be injected to the right atrium and downstream temperature changes can be measured at the tip thermistor. Because the tip of the PAC is located in the pulmonary artery, this method actually measures right ventricular output.[50,51] Newer generation PACs incorporate electric heating elements to continuously assess temperature differences downstream and, thus, CO.[52] TPTD requires a central venous catheter and an arterial catheter placed in a systemic artery in proximity to the heart.[51] Using this technique, a cold fluid bolus is injected in the central venous circulation and the blood temperature difference is measured in the systemic circulation, therefore measuring the global CO. Unlike PATD, TPTD is not influenced by the ventilatory cycle.[52] The use of both methods is limited in patients with intracardiac shunts, low-flow states, or tricuspid regurgitation.[52] For lithium dilution, a bolus of lithium chloride solution is injected in a peripheral or central vein, and the systemic lithium concentration is detected downstream by an electrode sensor implanted in the arterial catheter. The lithium dilution method for assessing CO is limited in patients treated with lithium and is contraindicated in the first trimester of pregnancy. Additionally, lithium boluses cannot be given frequently, because of lithium accumulation.[52] All these indicator dilution techniques are primarily used in patients undergoing cardiac surgery.[50]

Minimally invasive cardiac output monitoring

Minimally invasive CO measurement methods use a peripheral arterial catheter to obtain the arterial pressure waveform. By analyzing this waveform an estimation of the stroke volume and, thus, the CO can be made.[50] There are calibrated and uncalibrated minimally invasive methods to estimate CO. Calibrated methods need an externally derived CO value, that is one obtained by PATD or TPTD, to adjust the estimated CO. Uncalibrated methods estimate CO solely based on characteristics of the arterial pressure waveform[53,54] in combination with demographic factors. Pulse wave analysis is indicated in high-risk patients or in patients who are planned to undergo a high-risk procedure.[50] Calibrated methods are preferred in patients with low systemic vascular resistance, such as liver disease and sepsis.[55] The use of pulse wave analysis is limited in patients with frequent and fast changes in vascular tone and in patients with cardiac arrhythmias.[50] Naturally, the quality of the arterial pressure waveform signal is of crucial importance to the reliability of the derived CO estimates.[50]

Noninvasive cardiac output monitoring

Multiple methods are available for assessing CO noninvasively including volume clamp method, electrical bioimpedance, thoracic bioreactance, and pulse wave transit time.[56] As explained elsewhere in this article, the volume clamp method obtains the arterial pressure waveform noninvasively from which the stroke volume and thus CO can be derived. Electrical bioimpedance is based on the assumption that resistance to electrical current (impedance) changes during the cardiac cycle owing to the fluctuating blood volume in the thorax. These changes can be quantified by measuring the changes in voltages from the applied and detected current via surface electrodes to estimate CO. In the majority of studies it has been shown that the CO estimates by electrical bioimpedance lack accuracy and precision.[56–59] Additionally, the use of bioimpedance is limited in patients with cardiac arrhythmias,[60] pathologic accumulation of fluid in the thorax,[61] and during electrical interference (such as electrocautery). A new device was developed that used electrodes attached to an endotracheal tube to obtain the bioimpedance signal closer to the source, that is, the ascending aorta.[62] Thoracic bioreactance is a newer technology also based on the principle of bioimpedance. However, bioreactance focuses on the phase shift of the bioimpedance signal. The phase shift occurs owing to pulsatile flow, primarily coming from the aorta. Because only pulsatile flow is accounted for, pathologic fluid collections in the thorax do not affect these measurements.[63] However, thoracic bioreactance is also disturbed by electrical interference, and the agreement between bioreactance and reference methods was poor.[56] The pulse wave transit time is defined as the time that the stroke volume travels from the heart to the periphery, and can be measured as the time difference between the R top in the electrocardiogram and the start of the plethysmographic waveform obtained by pulse oximetry.[56] The pulse wave transit time is inversely correlated with stroke volume and thus the CO; that is it decreases when stroke volume and CO increase. Evidence for the use of the pulse wave transit time method is limited. Currently, the volume clamp method is the most studied one of the methods described in this paragraph.[18] An overview of all CO monitoring methods can be found in **Table 2**.

VOLUME MONITORING

Besides measuring blood pressure and blood flow, and in contrast with measuring total blood volume, which is highly complex, several compartmental volumes with clinical relevance can be measured with sufficient accuracy. These include GEDV and extravascular lung water (EVLW).

Global End-Diastolic Volume

The GEDV is the amount of blood volume present in all heart chambers at the end of the diastole. During diastole the heart is passively filled with blood and thus the GEDV resembles cardiac preload.[27] TPTD can be used to calculate the GEDV[51] as the difference between the intrathoracic thermal volume (ie, total intrathoracic volume) and the pulmonary thermal volume (ie, pulmonary volume and volume of the pulmonary circulation) (**Fig. 2**). Intrathoracic thermal volume is calculated by multiplying CO with the mean transit time, that is the time from injection of the indicator until one-half of the indicator passes the detection point. The pulmonary thermal volume is calculated as the CO multiplied by the downslope time of the natural log-transformed blood temperature curve measured in a systemic artery.[51] Because the GEDV is a static variable, it is known to be a less reliable predictor of fluid responsiveness compared with dynamic indices (as discussed elsewhere in this article).[64] However, the GEDV can be used to assess whether the cardiac preload adequately increases during volume loading.

Extravascular Lung Water

Fluid accumulated in the extravascular space within the lungs, that is in the interstitial space and alveoli, is called the EVLW. Fluid can leak from the capillaries owing to increased hydrostatic pressure (fluid overload) or increased lung permeability (acute respiratory distress syndrome).[65] TPTD can be used to estimate the EVLW by subtracting the intrathoracic blood volume from the intrathoracic thermal volume.[51] The intrathoracic blood volume can be estimated by multiplying the GEDV by 1.25.[66] EVLW can aid in the diagnosis and severity assessment of pulmonary edema and acute respiratory distress syndrome and has been shown to predict adverse outcome.[66] The estimation of EVLW by TPTD is compromised by major pulmonary embolism, in patients with a partial lung resection, and in patients with significant pleural effusion.[51] **Fig. 2** gives a graphical display of all volumetric calculations.

FLUID RESPONSIVENESS

Fluid responsiveness is mostly defined as an increase in stroke volume or CO of 10% to 15% after the administration of a fluid bolus.[67] Because poor outcomes are

Table 2 Overview of CO monitoring methods		
Invasive Methods	**Minimally Invasive Methods**	**Noninvasive Methods**
PATD	Pulse wave analysis	Volume clamp method
TPTD	(calibrated and uncalibrated)	Electrical bioimpedance
Lithium dilution		Thoracic bioreactance
		Pulse wave transit time

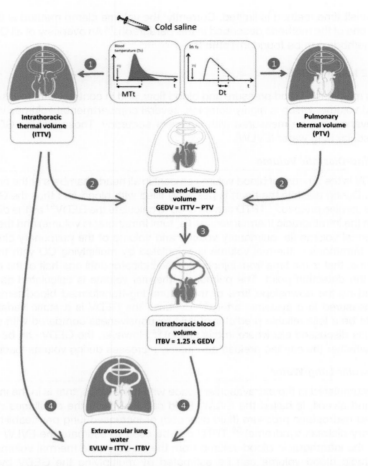

Fig. 2. Example of a volume estimation of intrathoracic compartments using TPTD. (Reproduced with permission from Monnet and Teboul Critical Care (2017) 21:147.)

associated with both hypovolemia and fluid overload, efforts have been made to find reliable predictors of fluid responsiveness, so that fluids can be administered only if an increase in CO is expected. In the past, filling pressures (CPV or PAOP) and volumetric variables (GEDV or intrathoracic blood volume) were used to estimate fluid responsiveness. However, studies have shown that those (static) indicators cannot reliably predict fluid responsiveness.[68–72] Instead, there is increasing evidence that dynamic variables such as stroke volume variation and pulse pressure variation, which are based on the heart–lung interaction during mechanical ventilation, reliably predict fluid responsiveness. Dynamic variables are based on the changes in cardiac preload during different phases of the respiratory cycle, resulting in variations of stroke volume and pulse pressure.[64,68,73–76] When intrathoracic pressure decreases during the ventilatory cycle, venous return increases, causing an increase in the stroke volume. In contrast, stroke volume decreases with the subsequent increase in intrathoracic pressure. Stroke volume variation is the maximum difference in stroke volume during a ventilatory cycle divided by the mean stroke volume. The pressure between the systolic and diastolic blood pressures is the pulse pressure. Pulse pressure variation is the maximum difference in pulse pressure during a ventilatory cycle divided by the mean pulse pressure. Patients who are fluid the responsive are on the steep part of the Frank–Starling curve and have high variations in stroke volume and pulse pressure during the ventilatory cycle (**Fig. 3**).

Minimally Invasive Methods

Stroke volume variation and pulse pressure variation are probably the most well-known dynamic indices for predicting fluid responsiveness in mechanically ventilated patients. Both the stroke volume variation and the pulse pressure variation can be obtained with minimally invasive methods using an arterial catheter and monitor for pulse wave analysis[64,68,73–76] or noninvasively using the volume clamp method.[77] The use of stroke volume variation and pulse pressure variation is limited in several situations, including irregular heartbeats, spontaneously breathing patients or mechanical ventilation with low tidal volumes, open thorax, increased abdominal pressure, and a low heart rate to respiratory rate ratio.[78] Previously, the variation of the systolic pressure during 1 mechanical respiratory cycle had been shown to predict hypovolemia and is calculated as the systolic arterial pressure during inspiration minus the systolic arterial pressure during expiration.[79,80] The systolic pressure variation is not used in clinical routine anymore.

Noninvasive Methods

Noninvasive methods of assessing fluid responsiveness include noninvasively obtained stroke volume variation and pulse pressure variation using the volume clamp

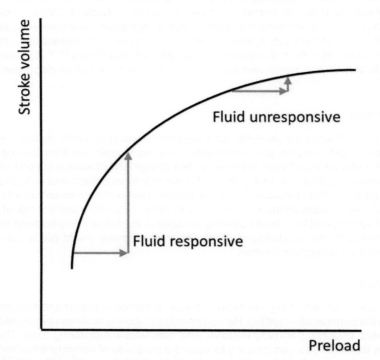

Fig. 3. Display of the fluid-responsive and fluid-unresponsive states of the left ventricle on the Frank–Starling curve.

Table 3
Overview of dynamic indices calculations

Dynamic Variable	Calculation
Stroke volume variation	$SVV = \dfrac{SVV_{max} - SVV_{min}}{SVV_{mean}}$
Pulse pressure variation	$PPV = \dfrac{PPV_{max} - PPV_{min}}{PPV_{mean}}$
Systolic pressure variation	$SPV = SAP_{insp} - SAP_{exp}$
Respiratory variations in ΔPOP	$\Delta POP = \dfrac{POP_{max} - POP_{min}}{POP_{mean}}$
PVI	$PVI = \dfrac{PI_{max} - PI_{min}}{PI_{max}} \times 100$

method, respiratory variations in pulse oximetry plethysmographic waveform amplitude (ΔPOP), and automated pleth variability index (PVI).[68,77,81] The volume clamp method was explained previously. Noninvasively obtained stroke volume variations and pulse pressure variations are acceptable predictors of fluid responsiveness.[77] The ΔPOP is strongly correlated with the pulse pressure variation in mechanically ventilated patients[82–84] and is able to predict fluid responsiveness in the operating room.[81,84] The PVI is based on a commercial algorithm, which continuously assesses the ΔPOP using the perfusion index[85] and has been shown to predict fluid responsiveness accurately.[86,87] The use of ΔPOP and PVI might be limited during severe vasoconstriction[88] and in patients with a low perfusion index.[89] An overview of the calculations used for the dynamic indices are given in **Table 3**. Other methods of assessing fluid responsiveness include echocardiographic measurements, such as the peak aortic flow velocity variation or vena cava collapsibility/distensibility, the passive leg raising test, the end-expiratory occlusion test, and others.[68,90] Because these methods can only be performed intermittently, they are not further discussed in this review.

DISCUSSION

Many different tools are available for perioperative hemodynamic monitoring, both noninvasive and invasive, and a multitude of hemodynamic variables can be monitored. A profound knowledge of the methods and their limitations is required to choose the most appropriate monitoring device for the individual patient and indication. The type of perioperative hemodynamic monitoring should be chosen based on a thorough risk and benefit assessment, including the risk of the procedure and the risk of the individual patient, and this should be weighed against the risk of complications from the invasiveness of the monitoring method. The current review might guide the user in choosing the appropriate method.

SUMMARY

In this review, we aimed to provide an overview of hemodynamic monitoring methods used in the perioperative setting. Hemodynamic monitoring tools can be divided into 3 categories: invasive, minimally invasive, and noninvasive monitoring tools. The most invasive tool, the PAC, can be used to assess a multitude of hemodynamic variables, for example, CO, pulmonary artery pressures, systemic vascular resistance, pulmonary vascular resistance, right ventricle end-diastolic volume or ejection fraction, and so on. However, owing to the risks associated with its invasiveness, the use of PAC is limited to select patient populations and procedures (mainly cardiac surgery). It remains unclear if PAC based treatment algorithms improve clinical outcomes. Slightly less invasive is the TPTD technique, which can be used to obtain the CO, GEDV, and EVLW. For arterial blood pressure monitoring, an arterial catheter remains the gold standard and pulse wave analysis can be used to estimate CO, stroke volume, and dynamic indices (stroke volume variation and pulse pressure variation) for predicting fluid responsiveness. Pulse waves can also be derived and analyzed from the noninvasive continuous volume clamp method, which can provide the same hemodynamic variables. The CVP has been used for a long time for assessing fluid responsiveness; however, it has been shown to correlate poorly with the volume status of the patients, and therefore it has been proposed to use dynamic indices instead, obtained either invasively or noninvasively. Besides stroke volume variation and pulse pressure variation, the ΔPOP and PVI can be used to predict fluid responsiveness in the operating room. The P_{msf} can be used to accurately assess a patient's volume status, although it is quite difficult to measure and, thus, is of limited clinical use.

CLINICS CARE POINTS

- The CVP should not be used to assess preload or fluid responsiveness; dynamic variables should be used instead.
- The P_{msf}, although difficult to measure, can be used to accurately assess a patient's volume status.
- CO can be monitored using different methods with different levels of invasiveness and risks of complications. The best suited type of monitoring should be determined for every individual patient and procedure.

DISCLOSURE

I.N. de Keijzer has nothing to disclose. T.W.L. Scheeren received research grants and honoraria from Edwards Lifesciences (Irvine, California, USA) and Masimo (Irvine, CA) for consulting and lecturing and from Pulsion Medical Systems SE (Feldkirchen, Germany) for lecturing.

REFERENCES

1. Dalley S. Myths from Mesopotamia: creation, the flood, Gilgamesh and others. Oxford (England, UK): Oxford University Press; 1989.
2. Ghasemzadeh N, Zafari AM. A brief journey into the history of the arterial pulse. Cardiol Res Pract 2011;2011:164832.
3. Bolli R. William Harvey and the Discovery of the Circulation of the Blood. Circ Res 2019;124:1169–71.
4. Esunge PM. From blood pressure to hypertension: the history of research. J R Soc Med 1991;84:621.
5. Neil E. Carl Ludwig and His Pupils. Circ Res 1961;IX:971–8.
6. Roguin A. Scipione Riva-Rocci and the men behind the mercury sphygmomanometer. Int J Clin Pract 2006;60:73–9.
7. Wesseling K. A century of non-invasive arterial pressure measurement: form Marey to Peñáz and Finapres. Homeost Heal Dis 1995;36:50–66.

8. Einthoven W. Un nouveau galvanomètre. Arch Neerl Sc Ex Nat 1901;6:625–33.

9. Burnett J. The origins of the electrocardiograph as a clinical instrument. Med Hist 1985;(Supplement 5):53–76.

10. Saugel B, Sessler DI. Perioperative Blood Pressure Management. Anesthesiology 2021;134:250–61.

11. Saugel B, Kouz K, Meidert AS, et al. How to measure blood pressure using an arterial catheter: a systematic 5-step approach. Crit Care 2020;24:172.

12. Handlogten KS, Wilson GA, Clifford L, et al. Brachial artery catheterization: an assessment of use patterns and associated complications. Anesth Analg 2014; 118:288–95.

13. Scheer BV, Perel A, Pfeiffer UJ. Clinical review: complications and risk factors of peripheral arterial catheters used for haemodynamic monitoring in anaesthesia and intensive care medicine. Crit Care 2002;6:198–204.

14. Roach JK, Thiele RH. Perioperative blood pressure monitoring. Best Pract Res Clin Anaesthesiol 2019;33:127–38.

15. Forouzanfar M, Dajani H, Groza V, et al. Oscillometric blood pressure estimation: past, present, and future. IEEE Rev Biomed Eng 2015;8:44–63.

16. Yelderman M, Ream A. Indirect measurement of mean blood pressure in the anesthetized patient. Anesthesiology 1979;50:253–6.

17. Kouz K, Scheeren TWL, de Backer D, et al. Pulse Wave Analysis to Estimate Cardiac Output. Anesthesiology 2020;134:119–26.

18. Saugel B, Hoppe P, Nicklas JY, et al. Continuous noninvasive pulse wave analysis using finger cuff technologies for arterial blood pressure and cardiac output monitoring in perioperative and intensive care medicine: a systematic review and meta-analysis. Br J Anaesth 2020;125:25–37.

19. Saugel B, Kouz K, Scheeren TWL, et al. Cardiac output estimation using pulse wave analysis-physiology, algorithms, and technologies: a narrative review. Br J Anaesth 2021;126:67–76.

20. Rogge DE, Nicklas JY, Schön G, et al. Continuous noninvasive arterial pressure monitoring in obese patients during bariatric surgery: an evaluation of the vascular unloading technique. Anesth Analg 2019;128:477–83.

21. Berkelmans GFN, Kuipers S, Westerhof BE, et al. Comparing volume-clamp method and intra-arterial blood pressure measurements in patients with atrial fibrillation admitted to the intensive or medium care unit. J Clin Monit Comput 2018;32:439–46.

22. Shah P, Louis M. Physiology, central venous pressure.. In: StatPearls [Internet]. 2020. Available at: https://www.ncbi.nlm.nih.gov/books/NBK519493/. Accessed November 19, 2020.

23. Magder S. How to use central venous pressure measurements. Curr Opin Crit Care 2005;11:264–70.

24. Guyton A. Determination of cardiac output by equating venous return curves with cardiac response curves. Physiol Rev 1955;35:123–9.

25. Kumar A, Anel R, Bunnell E, et al. Pulmonary artery occlusion pressure and central venous pressure fail to predict ventricular filling volume, cardiac performance, or the response to volume infusion in normal subjects. Crit Care Med 2004;32:691–9.

26. Boldt J, Lenz M, Kumle B, et al. Volume replacement strategies on intensive care units: results from a postal survey. Intensive Care Med 1998;24:147–51.

27. Michard F, Alaya S, Zarka V, et al. Global end-diastolic volume as an indicator of cardiac preload in patients with septic shock. Chest 2003;124:1900–8.

28. Hofer CK, Furrer L, Matter-Ensner S, et al. Volumetric preload measurement by thermodilution: a comparison with transoesophageal echocardiography. Br J Anaesth 2005;94:748–55.

29. Marik PE, Baram M, Vahid B. Does central venous pressure predict fluid responsiveness? A Systematic Review of the Literature and the Tale of Seven Mares. Chest 2008;134:172–8.

30. Marik PE, Cavallazzi R. Does the central venous pressure predict fluid responsiveness? An updated meta-analysis and a plea for some common sense. Crit Care Med 2013;41:1774–81.

31. Pinsky M, Kellum J, Bellomo R. Central venous pressure is a stopping rule, not a target of fluid resuscitation. Crit Care Resusc 2015;17:56.

32. Van Beest P, Wietasch G, Scheeren T, et al. Clinical review: use of venous oxygen saturations as a goal - a yet unfinished puzzle. Crit Care 2011;15:232.

33. Vincent JL. The pulmonary artery catheter. J Clin Monit Comput 2012;26:341–5.

34. Bootsma I, Boerma E, de Lange F, et al. The contemporary pulmonary artery catheter. Part 1: placement and waveform analysis. J Clin Monit Comput 2021. https://doi.org/10.1007/s10877-021-00662-8.

35. O'Quin R, Marini J. Pulmonary artery occlusion pressure: clinical physiology, measurement, and interpretation. Br J Psychother 1983;128:319–26.

36. Shah M, Hasselblad V, Stevenson L, et al. Impact of the pulmonary artery catheter in critically ill patients: meta-analysis of randomized clinical trials. JAMA 2005; 294:1664–70.

37. Rajaram S, Desai N, Kalra A, et al. Pulmonary artery catheters for adult patients in intensive care (Review). Cochrane Database Syst Rev 2013;2:CD003408.

38. Harvey S, Harrison DA, Singer M, et al. Assessment of the clinical effectiveness of pulmonary artery catheters in management of patients in intensive care (PAC-Man): a randomised controlled trial. Lancet 2005;366:472–7.

39. Cohen MG, Kelly RV, Kong DF, et al. Pulmonary artery catheterization in acute coronary syndromes: insights from the GUSTO IIb and GUSTO III trials. Am J Med 2005;118:482–8.

40. Rapoport J, Teres D, Steingrub J, et al. Patient characteristics and ICU organizational factors that influence frequency of pulmonary artery catheterization. J Am Med Assoc 2000;283:2559–67.

41. Koo KKY, Sun JCJ, Zhou Q, et al. Pulmonary artery catheters: evolving rates and reasons for use. Crit Care Med 2011;39:1613–8.

42. Ospina-Tascón GA, Cordioli RL, Vincent JL. What type of monitoring has been shown to improve outcomes in acutely ill patients? Intensive Care Med 2008; 34:800–20.

43. Rothe CF. Mean circulatory filling pressure: its meaning and measurement. J Appl Physiol 1993;74:499–509.

44. Maas JJ, Pinsky MR, Geerts BF, et al. Estimation of mean systemic filling pressure in postoperative cardiac surgery patients with three methods. Intensive Care Med 2012;38:1452–60.

45. Wijnberge M, Sindhunata DP, Pinsky MR, et al. Estimating mean circulatory filling pressure in clinical practice: a systematic review comparing three bedside methods in the critically ill. Ann Intensive Care 2018;8:73.

46. Maas JJ, Geerts BF, Van Den Berg PCM, et al. Assessment of venous return curve and mean systemic filling pressure in postoperative cardiac surgery patients. Crit Care Med 2009;37:912–8.

47. Fessler HE, Brower RG, Wise RA, et al. Effects of positive end-expiratory pressure on the canine venous return curve. Am Rev Respir Dis 1991;143:19–24.

48. Parkin WG, Leaning MS. Therapeutic control of the circulation. J Clin Monit Comput 2008;22:391–400.

49. Guyton A, Lindsey A, Abernathy B, et al. Venous return at various right atrial pressures and the normal venous return curve. Am J Physiol 1957;189:609–15.

50. Saugel B, Vincent JL. Cardiac output monitoring: how to choose the optimal method for the individual patient. Curr Opin Crit Care 2018;24:165–72.

51. Monnet X, Teboul JL. Transpulmonary thermodilution: advantages and limits. Crit Care 2017;21:147.

52. Reuter DA, Huang C, Edrich T, et al. Cardiac output monitoring using indicator-dilution techniques: basics, limits, and perspectives. Anesth Analg 2010;110:799–811.

53. Jozwiak M, Monnet X, Teboul J-L. Pressure waveform analysis. Anesth Analg 2018;126:1930–3.

54. Esper SA, Pinsky MR. Arterial waveform analysis. Best Pract Res Clin Anaesthesiol 2014;28:363–80.

55. Slagt C, Malagon I, Groeneveld ABJ. Systematic review of uncalibrated arterial pressure waveform analysis to determine cardiac output and stroke volume variation. Br J Anaesth 2014;112:626–37.

56. Saugel B, Cecconi M, Wagner JY, et al. Noninvasive continuous cardiac output monitoring in perioperative and intensive care medicine. Br J Anaesth 2015;114:562–75.

57. Appel P, Kram H, Mackabee J, et al. Comparison of measurements of cardiac output by bioimpedance and thermodilution in severely ill surgical patients. Crit Care Med 1986;14:933–5.

58. Marik P, Pendelton J, Smith R. A comparison of hemodynamic parameters derived from transthoracic electrical bioimpedance with those parameters obtained by thermodilution and ventricular angiography. Crit Care Med 1997;25:1545–50.

59. Sageman W, Amundson D. Thoracic electrical bioimpedance measurement of cardiac output in postaortocoronary bypass patients. Crit Care Med 1993;21:1139–42.

60. Chamos C, Vele L, Hamilton M, et al. Less invasive methods of advanced hemodynamic monitoring: principles, devices, and their role in the perioperative hemodynamic optimization. Perioper Med 2013;2:19.

61. Critchley LAH, Calcroft RM, Tan PYH, et al. The effect of lung injury and excessive lung fluid, on impedance cardiac output measurements, in the critically ill. Intensive Care Med 2000;26:679–85.

62. Wallace AW, Salahieh A, Lawrence A, et al. Endotracheal cardiac output monitor. Anesthesiology 2000;92:178–89.

63. Marik PE. Noninvasive cardiac output monitors: a state-of the-art review. J Cardiothorac Vasc Anesth 2013;27:121–34.

64. Marik PE, Cavallazzi R, Vasu T, et al. Dynamic changes in arterial waveform derived variables and fluid responsiveness in mechanically ventilated patients: a systematic review of the literature. Crit Care Med 2009;37:2642–7.

65. Jozwiak M, Teboul JL, Monnet X. Extravascular lung water in critical care: recent advances and clinical applications. Ann Intensive Care 2015;5:38.

66. Sakka SG, Rühl CC, Pfeiffer UJ, et al. Assessment of cardiac preload and extravascular lung water by single transpulmonary thermodilution. Intensive Care Med 2000;26:180–7.

67. Marik PE. Fluid Responsiveness and the Six Guiding Principles of Fluid Resuscitation. Crit Care Med 2016;44:1920–2.

68. Renner J, Scholz J, Bein B. Monitoring fluid therapy. Best Pract Res Clin Anaesthesiol 2009;23:159–71.
69. Michard F, Teboul JL. Predicting fluid responsiveness in ICU patients: a critical analysis of the evidence. Chest 2002;121:2000–8.
70. Bendjelid K, Romand JA. Fluid responsiveness in mechanically ventilated patients: a review of indices used in intensive care. Intensive Care Med 2003; 29(3):352–60.
71. Calvin J, Driedger A, Sibbald W. The hemodynamic effect of rapid fluid infusion in critically ill patients. Surgery 1981;90:61–76.
72. Michard F, Boussat S, Chemla D, et al. Relation between respiratory changes in arterial pulse pressure and fluid responsiveness in sepsis. Am J Respir Crit Care Med 2000;162:134–8.
73. Carsetti A, Cecconi M, Rhodes A. Fluid bolus therapy: monitoring and predicting fluid responsiveness. Curr Opin Crit Care 2015;21:388–94.
74. Guerin L, Monnet X, Teboul JL. Monitoring volume and fluid responsiveness: from static to dynamic indicators. Best Pract Res Clin Anaesthesiol 2013;27:177–85.
75. Jozwiak M, Monnet X, Teboul J-L. Prediction of fluid responsiveness in ventilated patients. Ann Transl Med 2018;6:352.
76. Monnet X, Marik PE, Teboul JL. Prediction of fluid responsiveness: an update. Ann Intensive Care 2016;6:111.
77. Vos JJ, Poterman M, Salm PP, et al. Noninvasive pulse pressure variation to predict fluid responsiveness at multiple thresholds: a prospective observational study. Can J Anaesth 2015;62:1153-60.
78. Michard F, Chemla D, Teboul JL. Applicability of pulse pressure variation: how many shades of grey? Crit Care 2015;19:144.
79. Kramer A, Zygun D, Hawes H, et al. Pulse pressure variation predicts fluid responsiveness following coronary artery bypass surgery. Chest 2004;126: 1563–8.
80. Tavernier B, Makhotine O, Lebuffe G, et al. Systolic pressure variation as a guide to fluid therapy in patients with sepsis-induced hypotension. Anesthesiology 1998;89:1313–21.
81. Cannesson M, Attof Y, Rosamel P, et al. Respiratory variations in pulse oximetry plethysmographic waveform amplitude to predict fluid responsiveness in the operating room. Anesthesiology 2007;106:1105–11.
82. Cannesson M, Besnard C, Durand PG, et al. Relation between respiratory variations in pulse oximetry plethysmographic waveform amplitude and arterial pulse pressure in ventilated patients. Crit Care 2005;9:R562–8.
83. Natalini G, Rosano A, Franceschetti M, et al. Variations in arterial blood pressure and photoplethysmography during mechanical ventilation. Anesth Analg 2006; 103:1182–8.
84. Solus-Biguenet H, Fleyfel M, Tavernier B, et al. Non-invasive prediction of fluid responsiveness during major hepatic surgery. Br J Anaesth 2006;97:808–16.
85. Cannesson M, Delannoy B, Morand A, et al. Does the pleth variability index indicate the respiratory- induced variation in the plethysmogram and arterial pressure waveforms? Anesth Analg 2008;106:1189–94.
86. Cannesson M, Desebbe O, Rosamel P, et al. Pleth variability index to monitor the respiratory variations in the pulse oximeter plethysmographic waveform amplitude and predict fluid responsiveness in the operating theatre. Br J Anaesth 2008;101:200–6.
87. Zimmermann M, Feibicke T, Keyl C, et al. Accuracy of stroke volume variation compared with pleth variability index to predict fluid responsiveness in

mechanically ventilated patients undergoing major surgery. Eur J Anaesthesiol 2010;27:555–61.

88. Perel A. Automated assessment of fluid responsiveness in mechanically ventilated patients. Anesth Analg 2008;106:1031–3.

89. Broch O, Bein B, Gruenewald M, et al. Accuracy of the pleth variability index to predict fluid responsiveness depends on the perfusion index. Acta Anaesthesiol Scand 2011;55:686–93.

90. Aditianingsih D, George YWH. Guiding principles of fluid and volume therapy. Best Pract Res Clin Anaesthesiol 2014;28:249–60.

Neuromuscular Blockade Monitoring

Stephan R. Thilen, MD, MS[a],*, Wade A. Weigel, MD[b]

KEYWORDS

- Neuromuscular monitoring
- Neuromuscular block or neuromuscular blocking or neuromuscular blockade
- Nerve stimulation • Anesthesia recovery period or anesthesia recovery
- Postoperative or residual neuromuscular weakness

KEY POINTS

- Neuromuscular blocking drugs (NMBDs) continue to be associated with an unacceptable incidence of adverse outcomes, most importantly postoperative residual neuromuscular blockade and also accidental awareness under general anesthesia.
- Routine quantitative neuromuscular monitoring is the only method of assuring satisfactory recovery from NMBDs and patient safety.
- A prereversal assessment should always be obtained from the adductor pollicis, which is the gold standard site for monitoring. A valid prereversal assessment is necessary for proper planning of the reversal.
- Patients with full spontaneous recovery can be identified by quantitative monitoring, and they should not be exposed to pharmacologic reversal drugs.
- Electromyography has advantages over other kinds of quantitative technologies; it does not require free movement of the thumb and provides valid measurements without the need for normalization.

BACKGROUND

The introduction of neuromuscular blocking drugs (NMBDs) to anesthesiology practice in the early 1940s was an enormously important milestone.[1] NMBDs are a central part of anesthesiology practice; however, these drugs are also associated with serious complications. An early seminal report by Beecher and Todd[2] found a mortality rate of 1:2100 with anesthetics that did not include the use of curare and a mortality rate of 1:370 when curare was used. The most important mechanism linking NMBDs to increased mortality and morbidity is widely recognized as postoperative residual

---

[a] Department of Anesthesiology & Pain Medicine, University of Washington, 325 Ninth Avenue, Box 359724, Seattle, WA 98104, USA; [b] Department of Anesthesiology, Virginia Mason Medical Center, 1100 9th Avenue, Mailstop B2-AN, Seattle, WA 98101, USA
* Corresponding author.
E-mail address: sthilen@uw.edu

Anesthesiology Clin 39 (2021) 457–476
https://doi.org/10.1016/j.anclin.2021.05.001
1932-2275/21/© 2021 Elsevier Inc. All rights reserved.

neuromuscular blockade (rNMB). rNMB has been well documented for decades, and it remains a common complication of NMBDs today, occurring in 30% or more of cases.[3,4] There is now consensus among experts that the key to improved care and safety with NMBDs is implementation of appropriate neuromuscular monitoring.[5] Fortunately, ongoing educational efforts, expert statements and guidelines, as well as more user-friendly monitoring equipment have created momentum toward improving routine perioperative neuromuscular monitoring.[6]

TYPES OF ASSESSMENT

Broadly, there are 3 types of assessments of recovery from NMBDs: (1) observation using clinical tests, (2) use of a peripheral nerve stimulator (PNS) for qualitative monitoring, and (3) use of a neuromuscular monitor for quantitative monitoring. Arguably, only quantitative monitoring should be considered "monitoring."

Clinical Observation and Clinical Tests

Clinical observation involves observing patient movement, spontaneous respiratory effort, tidal volumes, and the patient's ability to perform a task. The diaphragm is the most resistant muscle to NMBDs, and when it shows contractions this only indicates that the patient is not deeply paralyzed (now referred to as having *complete block*, see later discussion for definitions of different levels of block). A patient requires only minimum recovery of paralysis to maintain normal tidal volumes while still intubated. Therefore, assessment of respirations and tidal volumes lacks clinical value when determining if a patient is ready for extubation. Furthermore, evaluation of respiration should not be used to plan for an optimal reversal strategy including selection of drug, neostigmine or sugammadex, and dose.

The most commonly used clinical test has probably been the head lift test, which involves asking the patient to lift the head for 5 seconds. This test is often difficult to use before extubation because it requires that the patient be awake enough to follow commands while also tolerating the presence of the endotracheal tube. The head lift test has been formally evaluated and was found to have low sensitivity for residual paralysis. Kopman and colleagues[7] reported that 10 volunteers could all pass the head lift test with individual train-of-four (TOF) ratios in the range 0.45 to 0.75. Debaene and colleagues[8] estimated the sensitivity for diagnosing residual paralysis in 331 patients and found that it was 11%. Therefore, the head lift test, as well as all other clinical tests, are no longer considered an acceptable standard for determining readiness for extubation.

Peripheral Nerve Stimulators and Qualitative Assessment of Neuromuscular Function

PNSs are used to evoke muscle responses (twitches) that are subjectively evaluated, and this form of assessment has therefore been referred to as *subjective monitoring*. In this article we use the term *qualitative assessment* as opposed to *quantitative monitoring,* which is discussed in later section. Although the first PNS for perioperative assessment of neuromuscular function became commercially available in 1958, the adoption of these devices for routine neuromuscular assessments has been slow.[9] There are several reasons for this; first, for many years there was a lack of equipment and anesthesiologists were forced to use clinical observation and tests because no other approach was available. Second, although PNS units were widely available in US hospitals by the 1970s, the frequency and severity of rNMB was underappreciated and therefore the use of a PNS was often not considered important. An international survey of anesthesia providers conducted in 2008 reported that 19% of Europeans and 9% of Americans were still never using instrumental devices (PNS or quantitative monitor).[10]

PNS is useful for the assessment of depth of block, but it is not ideal for guiding reversal, and it is unequivocally inadequate for confirmation of recovery.

Technical aspects of peripheral stimulation

Peripheral nerve stimulation is the application of an electrical current across the skin over a nerve to initiate an action potential down that nerve resulting in activation of the innervated muscle. The nerve-muscle response most studied and most acceptable for clinical evaluation is the ulnar nerve and adductor pollicis. Electrodes are placed over the ulnar nerve, which lies next to the ulnar artery in the ulnar groove at the wrist (**Fig. 1**). Cleansing and degreasing of the skin with alcohol and abrasion with a gauze optimizes the adhesive connection to the skin as well as the transfer of current from the silver-silver chloride interface of the applied pads. The pads can be simple electrocardiography pads or specialized pads for this application. The negative (black) electrode should be placed distally, approximately 1 cm proximal to the wrist skin crease, whereas the positive (red) electrode should be 3 to 6 cm more proximal ("red to the heart," see **Fig. 1**).[11,12] The range of current on most nerve stimulators and monitors is 0 to 80 mA. Electrical bursts are delivered as a square wave pulse (ie, constant current) with a duration of 200 to 300 μs. As current is increased more muscle fibers are recruited strengthening the muscle response incrementally up to a point at which the muscle response peaks. Once this peak muscular response is reached, higher currents do not elicit any greater muscle contraction; this is known as the maximal current. Supramaximal current, generally 20% more than the maximal current, ensures consistent activation of all muscle fibers; this is important to ensure that any subsequent decrement in muscle contraction is not caused by increases in skin resistance or other causes of inadequate electrical stimulation.

Modes of stimulation

Current delivered as isolated single pulses is known as single twitch (ST) and is usually applied to the nerve at frequencies of 0.1 or 0.15 Hz, that is, 1 twitch every 10 or 6.7 s, respectively. With neuromuscular block, the degree of *twitch depression* is measured.

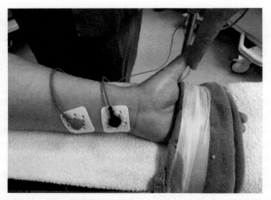

Fig. 1. Tactile assessment with use of a PNS for ulnar nerve stimulation. The electrodes are properly placed, and the hand and fingers are immobilized so that the isolated thumb movement can be assessed.

ST has been used to monitor the onset of block and the intraoperative depth of block when using a depolarizing NMBD, that is, succinylcholine. To use ST optimally, control amplitude should be measured initially, before administration of NMBD, which should be preceded by stabilization and calibration. These requirements have made ST monitoring less popular for routine practice, especially after TOF monitoring (see later discussion) became available. ST is now primarily used for determining drug potency (evaluation of the dose response). Conventionally, ED_{95} represents the effective dose of a drug for 95% of patients, whereas ED_{50} is the effective dose for 50% of patients. NMB drug potency follows a different convention, which incorporates 95% depression of the ST amplitude in half the patients. A more accurate way to convey this using traditional nomenclature would be $ED_{50}95\%$, relaying that for 50% of patients there is a 95% twitch depression. NMB literature, however, simply uses ED_{95} and relies on the reader to know the actual meaning.

The most clinically relevant mode of stimulation is the TOF and consists of 4 sequential ST stimuli delivered at a rate of 2 stimuli per second (2 Hz). TOF can be repeated every 12 to 20 seconds without significant potentiation. TOF is used to evaluate the fade of a nondepolarizing block caused by NMB binding to prejunctional acetylcholine receptors, which limits Ach vesicle migration thereby reducing Ach release into the neuromuscular junction. This fade, quantified by the magnitude of the fourth twitch compared with the first twitch (T4/T1 ratio [TOFR]), serves as the fundamental means used clinically to determine return of strength after a nondepolarizing blockade. Satisfactory return of strength has been set at a TOFR 0.90, meaning the fourth twitch is 90% the magnitude of the first twitch. Although there is no need to obtain a control value, it is good practice to start monitoring before administration of NMBs.

Benefits are as follows:
- Confirms proper placement of the electrodes that the PNS or monitor works and gives the provider a clear indication of baseline twitches (which should appear the same before extubation)
- Helps to prevent the situation wherein the anesthesia provider finds no twitch response at the end of the surgical procedure and may be in doubt whether the monitor works properly.
- Some monitors self-calibrate and determine the supramaximal current at start-up; these processes can be run only before paralysis, and they allow for optimized performance
- May be helpful for assessment of onset and determination of time for intubation
- Early recovery, for example, return of T1, indicates the individual patient's rate of spontaneous recovery
- May be helpful for early identification of infiltrating intravenous cannula because the delayed onset of neuromuscular block will be obvious

Close observation of the 4 responses will allow the clinician to appreciate significant fade; however, it is known that both visual and tactile assessments of fade lack precision; this means that we are not able to subjectively identify more subtle but still clinically significant fade. With increasing depth of block there is a progressive loss of twitches with the fourth twitch first to disappear (B and C in **Fig. 2**). During recovery there is return of twitches in the reverse order (see F and G in **Fig. 2**). The number of evoked responses (twitches) is referred to as the *train-of-four count* (TOFC). When subjectively assessed, the TOFC has 6 possible classifications, namely, 0, 1, 2, 3, 4 with fade, and 4 without fade. The term *four out of four* encompasses 2 distinct classifications and should be avoided. Studies have compared the TOF count based

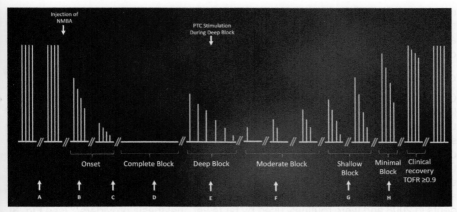

Fig. 2. Monitoring of neuromuscular block by TOF and posttetanic count (PTC). Before administration of NMBD there are 4 equal twitches (A in figure). With onset after a typical intubating dose ($2\times$ ED_{95}) of NMBD there will first be diminishing twitch amplitude (B) and then loss of twitches (C). Most often there is a brief period of complete block during which no twitches can be evoked, not even after a tetanic stimulation (D). Complete block often lasts for 20 to 30 min following a usual intubating dose, although prediction in an individual patient is unreliable, and this is an important reason to always monitor. Deep block is defined as block with train-of-four count (TOFC) = 0. At this depth PTC can be determined; PTC = 6 here (E). TOFC 1 to 3 is considered moderate block, and many types of surgeries are successfully facilitated with this depth of block (F). TOFC of 4 with a TOFR less than 0.4 is considered a shallow block (G), whereas a block with TOFC of 4 and TOFR greater than 0.4 is a minimal block (H). Note that minimal block cannot be distinguished from full recovery by visual or tactile assessment; this determination requires quantitative monitoring.

on qualitative assessment versus quantitative assessment.[13,14] Mechanomyography (MMG) was found to be more sensitive than palpation for counting TOF twitches, electromyography (EMG) was comparable to palpation, and acceleromyography (AMG) was less sensitive than palpation or EMG. It is not clear if these differences in TOFC are of clinical significance. The authors believe that any carefully used method of obtaining the TOFC at adductor pollicis is useful for assessing the intraoperative depth of block and for guiding a successful reversal. The exception is the distinction between TOFC with fade and TOFC without fade, which was not tested in these studies. Although it is possible to subjectively determine whether there is fade, this does not correlate with an accurate TOFR measurement. When the TOFR is higher than 0.4 experienced clinicians cannot reliably identify fade. Consequently, residual paralysis with a TOFR in the range 0.4 to 0.9, the range between visually or manually detectable fade and full return of strength, is a blind zone of subjective assessment. This important limitation with PNS and qualitative assessment cannot be overcome with anything other than quantitative monitoring. At the other end of the spectrum, when no twitches are present (TOFC = 0) there is a way to further define the depth of block by using a phenomenon known as posttetanic potentiation. This phenomenon invokes sustained intense electrical stimulation with a tetanic stimulation at 50 Hz, or 50 electrical impulses per second, delivered for 5 seconds, which causes the release of large amounts of acetylcholine (Ach) into the synaptic cleft. Posttetanic potentiation also leads to increased migration of Ach to the nerve ending, which allows for greater release of Ach with subsequent depolarizations over the next 2 to 5 minutes. When single twitches, one per second, are delivered 3 seconds after the tetanus then muscle responses may occur that were not present with TOF stimulation. Counting these twitches produces the posttetanic count (PTC). Complete block is the absence of any tetanus potentiated twitches (PTC = 0). See **Table 1** for consensus defined levels of block.

Quantitative Monitoring

Quantitative monitoring, which is sometimes referred to as objective monitoring, allows for a precise measurement of the evoked muscle response and the display of these measurements in real time. Note that the ulnar nerve is stimulated in the exact same manner as when qualitative assessment is used. The great advantage with quantitative monitoring is that it overcomes the main limitation of qualitative monitoring, which is the inability to identify subtle but clinically significant fade. Thus, the so-called zone of blind paralysis, when TOFRs are in the range 0.4 to 0.9, does not apply (**Fig. 3**).[3] Quantitative monitors were available to only 23% of American respondents in 2008 and were routinely used by far fewer anesthesia providers[10] (see **Fig. 3**).

WHY IS NEUROMUSCULAR MONITORING IMPORTANT

The evidence supporting quantitative monitoring for improved care has been mounting over the past 2 decades, and this pertains in particular to the prevention of rNMB.

Postoperative Residual Neuromuscular Blockade

Residual paralysis is a significant patient safety issue. There is now sufficient literature to provide irrefutable evidence that rNMB is associated with adverse outcomes. These outcomes include impaired pharyngeal function with increased risk of aspiration, airway obstruction, respiratory failure and reintubation, hypoxemic events, and postoperative pulmonary complications including pneumonia. It is beyond the scope of this article on neuromuscular monitoring to discuss in detail the literature on outcomes associated with rNMB. Shortly after TOF monitoring was first introduced by Ali and colleagues[15] in 1970, it was suggested that the threshold for adequate recovery should be a TOF ratio of 0.7 at the adductor pollicis muscle. This suggestion was based on studies showing that the forced vital capacity approached normal values at this degree of neuromuscular recovery.[16] However, later volunteer studies clearly showed that a TOF ratio of 0.7 is not adequate.[7] The muscles of the pharynx and upper airway are sensitive to NMBDs, and it was shown that swallowing and protection of the

Table 1		
Levels of Neuromuscular Block		
Depth of Block	**PNS and Qualitative Assessment**	**Quantitative Monitor**
Complete	PTC = 0	PTC = 0
Deep block	PTC ≥1, TOFC = 0	PTC ≥1, TOFC = 0
Moderate block	TOFC = 1–3	TOFC = 1–3
Shallow block	TOFC = 4; TOF fade present	TOFR < 0.4
Minimal block	TOFC = 4; TOF fade absent	TOFR 0.4–0.9
Acceptable recovery	Cannot be determined	TOFR ≥ 0.9

Note that the 2 most superficial levels of block cannot be distinguished by subjective (visual or tactile/manual) assessments but require quantitative monitoring.

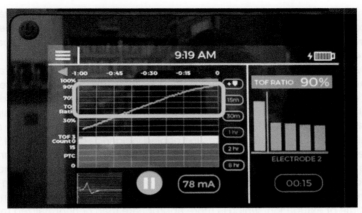

Fig. 3. Screenshot from a TwitchView (Blink Device Company, Seattle, USA) EMG quantitative monitor. The orange line shows a patient's progressive recovery of the TOF ratio over 1 hour. The yellow box highlights the range of TOF ratios from 0.4 to 0.9. With qualitative (subjective) assessments, the anesthesia provider will find a TOF count of 4 without fade throughout this range and will not know when the patient has fully recovered to a TOF ratio of at least 0.9. Quantitative monitoring allows for precise measurements and display of the TOF ratio in real time.

upper airway was significantly impaired unless the TOF ratio was at least 0.9.[17] The genioglossus muscle is an important upper airway dilator and is also sensitive to NMBDs. Eikermann and colleagues[18] conducted a study on healthy volunteers; the subjects were only slightly paralyzed and their airways were examined by MRI. **Fig. 4** is from this study and illustrates the profoundly narrowed airway at TOF ratios of 0.5 and 0.8, which are levels of block often seen with residual paralysis. It is obvious how this could impact the clinical picture, especially for patients with a difficult airway, those with OSA, or those who have undergone surgery potentially associated with edema of the airway. Upper airway edema may occur after nasopharyngeal surgery, after a lengthy spine procedure in the prone position or after a procedure in the steep

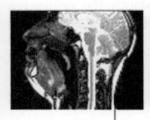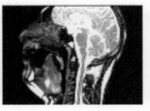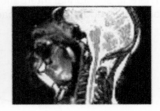

Fig. 4. (*Left*) The airway, including retropalatal and retroglossal dimensions, before paralysis. (*Middle*) A volunteer with TOF ratio = 0.5, and (*right*) a volunteer with TOF ratio = 0.8. Note that these degrees of paralysis cannot be identified without quantitative monitoring. (Eikermann M, Vogt FM, Herbstreit F, et al. The predisposition to inspiratory upper airway collapse during partial neuromuscular blockade. Am J Respir Crit Care Med. 2007;175(1):9-15. doi:10.1164/rccm.200512-1862OC. Reprinted with permission of the American Thoracic Society. Copyright © 2021 American Thoracic Society. All rights reserved. The American Journal of Respiratory and Critical Care Medicine is an official journal of the American Thoracic Society.)

Trendelenburg position. However, all patients should have an optimized airway at the time of extubation, and an international consensus now exists regarding the importance of recovery to a TOF ratio of at least 0.9 for all patients before extubation[5,12] (see **Fig. 4**).

rNMB was reported in a 1979 seminal study that found a 42% incidence on arrival to the postanesthesia care unit (PACU).[19] Although some things have changed since then (we do not use long-acting NMBDs in routine care and the threshold for full recovery has been raised to TOF ratio 0.9), the incidence of rNMB has remained unacceptably high. rNMB is an iatrogenic problem that is entirely preventable. In a recent meta-analysis including 12,664 patients the pooled incidence of rNMB was 31% when subjective monitoring with PNS was used and 12% when quantitative monitoring was used. The incidence depends on several factors, and among these is the type of surgery. A recent multicenter US study focusing on elective abdominal surgery in 2012 to 2013 found the incidence to be 64.7%.[4] This study reported normalized measurements at time of extubation, which is more appropriate than nonnormalized measurements, which have often been reported in other studies and which yield a lower incidence of rNMB. Severe residual paralysis with TOFR less than 0.6 was present in 31% of patients.

Prevention of Postoperative Residual Blockade

Todd and colleagues[20,21] published 2 reports from a Quality Improvement project at University of Iowa in which they implemented routine quantitative monitoring. The project was prompted by a notably high incidence of reintubations. The interventions included comprehensive education about monitoring as well as performance feedback. **Fig. 5** shows that the percent of patients with TOFR 90% or less upon arrival to the PACU was halved, although the final percentage was still almost 15% after a 34-month period. The more severe levels or residual paralysis, TOFR 0.8 or less and TOFR 0.5 or less were also reduced. Importantly, these gains were associated with a reduction in the incidence of reintubations.

A recent systematic review concluded that quantitative monitoring outperforms subjective monitoring in reducing rNMB as defined by a TOF ratio of less than 0.9.[22]

The Effect of Neuromuscular Blocking Drugs Is Unpredictable for the Individual Patient

There is substantial interpatient variation in response to NMBDs. This variation has been well recognized for decades; in a classical article, Katz[23] reported the paralyzing

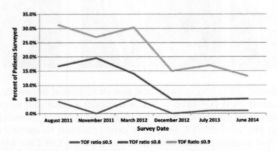

Fig. 5. Trends in the incidence of inadequate reversal from neuromuscular blockade. The graph shows the incidences of TOF ratios in studied patients on arrival to the PACU. Data are shown for the fraction of patients with TOF ratios 0.5 or less, 0.8 or less, and 0.9 or less. (Todd et al, Anesth Analg 2015 Sep;121(3):836-8.)

effects of administering 0.1 mg D-tubocurarine to 100 patients. Six patients had no measurable paralysis, and 7 patients had complete depression of the evoked response. The remaining 87 patients responded to this dose with variable degrees of twitch depression. The investigator determined that the individual patient response could not be predicted based on age, gender, body build, or physical status (American Society of Anesthesiologists classification). In another study using a single dose of rocuronium ($<2\times$ ED_{95}) to facilitate intubation 120 patients were enrolled to receive neostigmine after spontaneous recovery from the NMB. The surgery durations ranged from 119 to 212 minutes, yet 24 patients (21%) could not be included in the study because the TOFR remained less than 90% at the conclusion of surgery.[24]

Fig. 6 illustrates the great variation in response to NMBDs. In this study more than 400 patients received a single dose of 0.6 mg/kg rocuronium. Note that even as far out as 350 minutes there are still patients with TOFR less than 0.9. Conversely, there are outliers on the other end of the spectrum with TOFR greater than 0.9 after 30 minutes. It is useful to consider that each patient has a unique, individual, rate of spontaneous recovery, which cannot be reliably assumed or predicted. Therefore, management of paralysis needs to be individualized by monitoring the depth of the neuromuscular block.

An early indication of an individual patient's rate of spontaneous recovery is the time to return of the first twitch in TOF response (referred to as T1) after a standard intubating dose of $2\times$ ED_{95}. Dubois and colleagues reported that the time interval between administration of the intubating dose and return of T1 is highly correlated with other

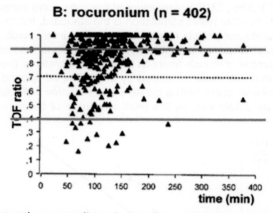

Fig. 6. Plot illustrates the extraordinary interpatient variation in response to rocuronium. The plot shows 402 patients who each received a standard intubating dose of rocuronium 0.6 mg/kg at time 0. No additional doses were given, and none of these patients were reversed. Quantitative measurements are made at time of admission to the postanesthesia care unit. We see how patients have recovered to different TOF ratios, and in general the recovery is obviously better with more time. We see some patients with complete spontaneous recovery to 1.0, whereas others have a low TOF ratio even after several hours. Variation would have been reduced to some degree if ideal body weight had been used for dosage calculations and if the intubating dose had been adjusted for gender (ED_{95} for rocuronium is 15%–25% lower for females). However, a substantial interindividual variation in effect of NMBDs is always present and the effect and duration for an individual patient is unpredictable. Patients with TOF ratios in the range between the 2 red lines (0.4–0.9) have residual paralysis, which cannot be diagnosed with use of a peripheral nerve stimulator and qualitative assessment. (*From* Debaene et al, Anesthesiology 2003; 98:1042-8.)

parameters of recovery, including TOF ratio 0.75 and full clinical recovery to TOF ratio 0.90. **Fig. 7** is adapted from this study. Although this early indication of the recovery rate is useful and can be determined by PNS and qualitative assessment, it does not allow prediction of time to full recovery with adequate precision for patient safety.

QUANTITATIVE NEUROMUSCULAR MONITORING TECHNOLOGIES

The term neuromuscular monitoring should strictly pertain to quantitative monitoring as the only modality that offers valid, reproducible measurements to assess return of muscle function after muscle paralysis.[12] There are multiple different types of monitors using different measuring techniques. Not all types of monitors are commercially available, and the breadth of commercial offerings differs between technologies. The technologies that will be discussed include MMG, EMG, AMG, and kinemyography. Phonomyography is not addressed.

The only noncommercially available technology that will be discussed is MMG. MMG has traditionally been reserved as a research tool because the equipment tended to be bulky and careful setup was required. This technology measures the isometric force of the thumb under a preload (150–300 g) via a transducer. The apparatus is cumbersome in the clinical setting, and the technology is not widely available. In a recent study measuring MMG the researchers built their own MMG.[25] The accuracy of MMG is touted to represent the "gold standard" for measuring muscle strength, although this may be changing in favor of newer technologies. Most technologies are compared with MMG for accuracy and precision.

EMG is the only technology which will be discussed that does not rely on or require thumb movement. Rather, EMG is a measure of the compound action potential of the muscle of interest. As ulnar nerve stimulation is the standard, the muscles of interest for EMG are the adductor pollicis muscle and the first interosseus muscle; these 2 muscles have similar response to NMBDs. Transfer of signal occurs from the nerve to an increasing number of muscle fibers as the current increases, producing the muscle compound action potentials measured by EMG. The compound action potential manifests as a biphasic curve with a positive and negative deflection. The strength of the signal can be determined by the peak amplitude of the curve or by the area

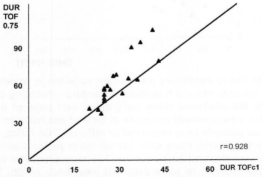

Fig. 7. Correlation between early (DUR TOFc1 = duration to return of first twitch) and late (DUR TOF 0.75 = duration to spontaneous recovery to TOF ratio 0.75); 20 patients who received rocuronium 0.6 mg/kg at time 0. Time scales are expressed in minutes, r is the Pearson correlation coefficient. (*From* Dubois et al. Early and late parameters describing the offset of neuromuscular blockade are highly intercorrelated. Acta Anaesthesiol Scand. 2012 Jan;56(1):76-82. doi: 10.1111/j.1399-6576.2011.02596.x.)

under the curve. This technology is the one that most closely resembles MMG in terms of accuracy and precision, although the correlation may differ by a TOFR 0.05.[25,26] Owing to the accuracy, EMG may replace MMG as the gold standard. Although this technology does not require thumb movement, it is prone to electrical interference from sources such as electrocautery. Examples of currently available EMG-based monitors are shown in **Fig. 8**.

EMG monitors are not dependent on the free movement of the thumb. Ideally, monitoring data should be automatically entered in the anesthesia record, and it is expected that in the future we will be able to routinely review anesthesia records and determine whether there was rNMB or not at the time of extubation.

AMG was developed in the 1980s and has been the dominant form of quantitative monitoring both for routine care and for clinical research. This technology is based on Newton's second law, force = mass × acceleration, where the mass (the thumb) is constant and the force is proportional to measured acceleration. Acceleration is measured by use of a piezoelectric transducer, which generates an electrical signal. The TOF-Watch (Organon, Ireland) (see **Fig. 5**) was a common type of monitor that measured the acceleration in a single vector. This uniaxial measurement meant the transducer needed to be positioned in line with the vector of the thumb range of movement. The device thus required meticulous setup and attention. The TOF-Watch is no longer available. The Stimpod (Xavant, Pretoria, South Africa) (**Fig. 9**) is a newer-generation AMG device that uses triaxial transducer technology. This device captures acceleration in 3 dimensions, rendering it less dependent on precise setup and hence more reliable. A critical feature of all AMG devices is that they require unencumbered motion of the thumb. Acceleration cannot be measured without free movement. In addition, limiting wrist and hand movement during testing improves accuracy by isolating the acceleration caused by the adductor pollicis after ulnar nerve stimulation.

The main drawback of AMG is the overestimation of TOFR when compared with MMG and EMG, although it still correlates well.[27,28] Baseline (no paralysis given) TOFR measured by AMG is frequently in the range between 1.10 and 1.15 but can be as high as 1.47.[29] Normalization and preload are 2 ways that have been advocated to improve AMG accuracy.[30] Normalization is a process in which a baseline TOFR is measured before administration of an NMBD, and all subsequent measurements are calculated as a fraction of that baseline to compensate for the overestimation. As an example, if the baseline TOFR is 1.15 and the postoperative TOFR is 0.95, then the normalized TOFR is 0.95/1.15 = 0.83. In this example, the nonnormalized value (TOFR = 0.95) would not classify the patient as having rNMB but the normalized value

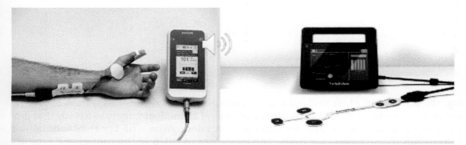

Fig. 8. Two EMG-based monitors. (*Left*) TetraGraph by Senzime AB, Sweden and (*right*) TwitchView. Note that all forms of neuromuscular monitoring stimulate the ulnar nerve in the same manner; it is only the evaluation of the response that sets them apart.

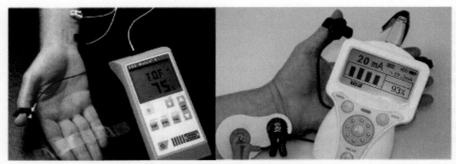

Fig. 9. Acceleromyography monitors. (*Left*) TOF-Watch SX; (*right*) the Stimpod 450 triaxial acceleromyograph.

(TOFR = 0.83) is <0.9 and therefore the patient will be classified as having rNMB after normalization. Thus, normalization usually yields lower TOF ratios, and when the incidence of rNMB in a cohort of patients is estimated based on normalized values it will be higher than it would be if nonnormalized (raw) values were used (**Fig. 10**). When normalization is not feasible because the baseline value was not measured or recorded the threshold for full recovery should be a nonnormalized TOFR of 1.0.[31]

Kinemyography is another commercially available technology, although it has not gained the same degree of popularity as AMG or EMG. This technology uses a strip of isoelectric polymer material spanning the space between the thumb and index finger. When the thumb moves this strip of material deforms, which produces an electrical signal. This technology seems to be measuring a component of thumb range of motion rather than acceleration or force.[32] The data comparing KMG to EMG or MMG has yielded inconsistent results, some studies showing good correlation, whereas others indicating that KMG overestimates by as much as TOFR 0.10.[33–36]

CHALLENGES WITH USE OF QUANTITATIVE MONITORING

There are challenges with acquisition of any new monitoring modality that may impede widespread adoption into routine anesthetic practice. This challenge partially hinges

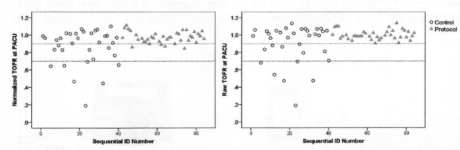

Fig. 10. Scatterplots of normalized and nonnormalized (also called "raw") train-of-four ratios at arrival to the PACU for 72 patients undergoing abdominal surgery in a study that prospectively evaluated a protocol for reversal with neostigmine. The upper horizontal line corresponds to the criteria for rNMB. The incidences of rNMB in the control and protocol groups are 41% and 13%, respectively, when normalized values are used (*Left*). The incidences are 38% and 0%, respectively, when nonnormalized values are used (*Right*). (*From* Thilen et al, British Journal of Anaesthesia 2018; 121:367-77.)

on clinicians' unwillingness to change practice because they believe that current practice is safe and effective. Overcoming this requires education as well as unlearning previously taught concepts.[37]

Another barrier is the cost of acquiring and using new equipment, and this can only be overcome when the recognized benefits to patient well-being and hospital costs are sufficient to justify use of the monitors. Experts around the world recognize the need to use quantitative monitoring, and some anesthesia societies are now issuing statements for its use (**Table 2**).[38–40] The cost of a quantitative monitor varies between approximately $1000 and $2000 per unit. For EMG monitors using disposable arrays each array costs approximately $10 to $20 (personal experience). The cost can be substantially offset by savings in drug costs. Only quantitative monitoring makes it possible to reliably identify the patients who have a full spontaneous recovery and therefore should not be exposed to the cost and potential side effects of a reversal drug that they do not need.

On the practical side of getting providers to use the equipment the problems range from setting up the equipment to believing the information to acting on the information.[24] Setting up the equipment has been shown to be easy to learn and requires about 1 minute.[42] The calibration required for some monitors, namely, AMG if normalization is desired, can take another 30 seconds. To accomplish quantitative monitoring within the daily workflow of an anesthesiologist it is ideal to place the monitor before induction. Calibration and baseline measurements can be done while the patient is awake or after induction before NMB administration. Pain from neural stimulation is modest (VNRS≤4) at 30 mA and less but increases to verbal numerical rating

Table 2 Recommendations from International Guidelines and Consensus Statement	
2018 International Consensus Statement[5]	Objective monitoring (documentation of train-of-four ratio ≥0.90) is the only method of assuring that satisfactory recovery of neuromuscular function has taken place
Association of Anaesthetists of Great Britain and Ireland guideline[38]	Quantitative neuromuscular monitoring should be used whenever neuromuscular blocking (NMB) drugs are administered, throughout all phases of anaesthesia from before initiation of neuromuscular blockade until recovery of the train-of-four ratio to > 0.9 has been confirmed.
Canadian Anesthesiologists' Society guideline[39]	Cautious dosing, vigilant monitoring, and the appropriate reversal of neuromuscular blocking drugs are all essential for patient safety. Neuromuscular monitoring must be used when neuromuscular blocking agents are administered
French Society of Anesthesia and Intensive Care Medicine guideline[40]	The use of quantitative adductor pollicis monitoring of the neuromuscular blockade is probably recommended for diagnosing a residual neuromuscular blockade and obtaining a ratio of ≥ 0.9 for the fourth to first TOF response (T4/T1 ratio) at the adductor pollicis to eliminate the possibility of diagnosing a residual neuromuscular blockade
Australian and New Zealand College of Anaesthetists[41]	Quantitative neuromuscular function monitoring must be available for every patient in whom neuromuscular blockade has been induced and should be used whenever the anesthetist is considering extubation following the use of nondepolarizing neuromuscular blockade

scale (VNRS) 5 to 6 with 40 to 50 mA current. It is noteworthy that nerve stimulation, even at low levels of current, may elicit significant pain in select patients.[43] Another option is to induce anesthesia, wait for the patient to be verbally nonresponsive and for the lid reflex to abate, and then initiate the calibration sequence before muscle relaxant injection. If a baseline is not attained, quantitative TOFR monitoring can still be used, and the precision offered by all quantitative monitors far exceeds that of clinical assessment with or without a PNS.

Getting the equipment to function during cases in which the arms are tucked is possible even with AMG, although EMG technology is ideally suited for this situation because thumb movement is not required. Getting AMG to work properly requires special attention to the tucking procedure and possibly equipment to maintain thumb movement within the tuck. A tubular device has been made for this purpose.[44] Alternatively, a nonsterile glove can be inflated and placed in the palm of the hand (**Fig. 11**).

Clinicians wary of new technology tend to compare it with the status quo, which in this case is clinical signs with or without PNS. Fluctuating values and error messages were cited as the top 2 frustrations for clinicians using first-generation AMG.[45] As technology has advanced these issues are improving. The main advantage of quantitative monitors is the precise measurement of the TOFR; however, they also provide a count of twitches (TOFC). When an acceleromyograph is used to measure the TOFC, this is often lower than the subjectively observed TOFC.[13] The clinical significance of

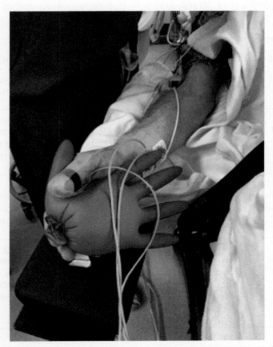

Fig. 11. A standard nonsterile glove is inflated and taped in the patient's hand, allowing for thumb movement also when the arm and hand are tucked. The acceleration transducer is secured at the distal phalanx of the thumb. This method has not been formally validated but was used at the authors' institutions before transitioning to EMG monitoring for cases with tucked arms.

this difference is not clear, and counting twitches by observation or by monitoring are both useful for following deeper levels of block.

Changing practice can be difficult particularly when a monitor reveals residual paralysis after care has been delivered, consistent with years of practice. In this instance there is a tendency to assert monitor inaccuracy. This is particularly difficult when neostigmine is used for reversal because many clinicians do not realize the strict limitations of its effectiveness. Perhaps this explains why less than 5 years of clinical experience correlates with higher use of quantitative monitors.[45]

Last, having expertise and enthusiasm for quantitative monitoring present in a department increases use.[20,45] Someone to advocate for the technology and to be available to troubleshoot problems is helpful.

SITE OF MONITORING

When AMG or a PNS is used and the adductor pollicis is unavailable bilaterally, it has been common practice to conduct assessments on the face. However, facial nerve monitoring and evaluation of eye muscle twitches is difficult and unreliable. In a prospective cohort study, 150 patients who received NMBDs during anesthesia were assessed for residual paralysis using AMG on arrival to the PACU.[46] In this study, 52% of patients who had intraoperative facial nerve stimulation by PNS and subjective assessments of eye muscle twitches had rNMB (nonnormalized TOFRs <0.9) compared with 22% of patients who had subjective assessments of the adductor pollicis. One potential explanation for this result is that muscles surrounding the eye, especially the corrugator supercilii, are relatively resistant to NMBDs compared to the adductor pollicis and studies have consistently documented an earlier recovery of twitches at this site.[47–55] It is possible that direct muscle stimulation, which circumvents the neuromuscular block, plays a role in some cases. Importantly, if facial nerve monitoring is used intraoperatively, it is essential to move monitoring to the ulnar nerve/adductor pollicis at the end of the procedure and before administration of pharmacologic reversal.[56,57] An evidence-based approach to reversal requires a valid prereversal assessment, which can be obtained only at the gold standard site of the ulnar nerve and adductor pollicis. Notably, it has been shown that the usual dosing guidelines for sugammadex do not apply when eye muscle twitches are assessed.[58]

When monitoring of adductor pollicis is not possible, the next best site is stimulation of the posterior tibial nerve and evaluation of the great toe twitch, if it can be easily and safely accessed. Several studies have compared posterior tibial and ulnar nerve stimulation and have found a more rapid recovery of the TOF response at the great toe.[59–62] Monitoring of the great toe may, therefore, result in a relative underestimation of the neuromuscular blockade (similar to monitoring at the face). Therefore, with great toe monitoring it is also recommended to move monitoring to the adductor pollicis for the prereversal assessment when the arms become accessible again at the end of the surgical procedure.

PARETIC EXTREMITIES

Twitch responses, and TOFRs, are exaggerated in paretic limbs, and assessing neuromuscular function by PNS or quantitative monitoring in a paretic extremity is likely to underestimate the degree of neuromuscular blockade and may contribute to administration of a relative overdose of NMBD.[63,64] One study reported that the exaggerated response is further increased when a limb has been paretic for more than 3 weeks.[65]

SUMMARY

NMBDs have important adverse effects that continue to be too common, including rNMB and accidental awareness with general anesthesia; these are iatrogenic complications and are completely preventable. A PNS can be used to determine when to administer additional NMBDs and the appropriate dose of reversal agent at the end of the procedure. However, quantitative monitoring is the only available method of ensuring full recovery of neuromuscular function before final emergence and extubation at the end of surgical procedures. Quantitative monitoring also makes it possible to identify patients who have a complete spontaneous recovery and who do not need to be pharmacologically reversed. There is currently an international momentum to adopt routine quantitative monitoring, and several international societies endorse the use of quantitative monitoring.

CLINICS CARE POINTS

- Routine use of neuromuscular monitoring is essential for optimizing the perioperative management of NMBDs.

- Quantitative monitoring provides real-time measurements of the TOF ratio and has important advantages compared with PNS with subjective assessment. Most importantly, tactile or visual assessments do not allow for identification of subtle but clinically significant fade in the TOF response. Only quantitative monitoring can confirm that satisfactory recovery of neuromuscular function has taken place.

- A recent systematic review concluded that quantitative monitoring outperforms subjective monitoring in reducing rNMB as defined by a TOF ratio of less than 0.9.

- The adductor pollicis is the gold standard and the preferred site for neuromuscular monitoring.

- A valid prereversal assessment is essential for planning a timely and successful reversal, and it should always be based on an assessment of the adductor pollicis response to ulnar nerve stimulation.

- Patients with spontaneous recovery to a TOF ratio of at least 0.9 can be identified by quantitative monitoring and should not receive pharmacologic reversal.

- EMG has advantages over AMG. EMG provides valid measurements even when movement of the thumb is constrained.

- It is best practice to routinely confirm a TOF ratio of at least 0.9 at the adductor pollicis before extubation.

DISCLOSURE

The authors have nothing to disclose.

REFERENCES

1. Griffith HR, Johnson GE. The use of curare in general anesthesia. Anesthesiology 1942;3:418–20.
2. Beecher HK, Todd DP. A study of the deaths associated with anesthesia and surgery: based on a study of 599, 548 anesthesias in ten institutions 1948-1952, inclusive. Ann Surg 1954;140(1):2–35.
3. Plaud B, Debaene B, Donati F, et al. Residual paralysis after emergence from anesthesia. Anesthesiology 2010;112(4):1013–22.

4. Saager L, Maiese EM, Bash LD, et al. Incidence, risk factors, and consequences of residual neuromuscular block in the United States: The prospective, observational, multicenter RECITE-US study. J Clin Anesth 2019;55:33–41.

5. Naguib M, Brull SJ, Kopman AF, et al. Consensus statement on perioperative use of neuromuscular monitoring. Anesth Analg 2018;127(1):71–80.

6. Nemes R, Renew J. Clinical practice guideline for the management of neuromuscular blockade: what are the recommendations in the USA and other countries? Curr Anesthesiol Rep 2020;10:90–8.

7. Kopman AF, Yee PS, Neuman GG. Relationship of the train-of-four fade ratio to clinical signs and symptoms of residual paralysis in awake volunteers. Anesthesiology 1997;86(4):765–71.

8. Debaene B, Plaud B, Dilly MP, et al. Residual paralysis in the PACU after a single intubating dose of nondepolarizing muscle relaxant with an intermediate duration of action. Anesthesiology 2003;98(5):1042–8.

9. Christie TH, Churchill-Davidson HC. The St. Thomas's Hospital nerve stimulator in the diagnosis of prolonged apnoea. Lancet 1958;1(7024):776.

10. Naguib M, Kopman AF, Lien CA, et al. A survey of current management of neuromuscular block in the United States and Europe. Anesth Analg 2010;111(1):110–9.

11. Brull SJ, Silverman DG. Pulse width, stimulus intensity, electrode placement, and polarity during assessment of neuromuscular block. Anesthesiology 1995;83(4):702–9.

12. Fuchs-Buder T, Claudius C, Skovgaard LT, et al. Good clinical research practice in pharmacodynamic studies of neuromuscular blocking agents II: the Stockholm revision. Acta Anaesthesiol Scand 2007;51(7):789–808.

13. Bhananker SM, Treggiari MM, Sellers BA, et al. Comparison of train-of-four count by anesthesia providers versus TOF-Watch® SX: a prospective cohort study. Can J Anaesth 2015;62(10):1089–96.

14. Bowdle A, Bussey L, Michaelsen K, et al. Counting train-of-four twitch response: comparison of palpation to mechanomyography, acceleromyography, and electromyography. Br J Anaesth 2020;124(6):712–7.

15. Ali HH, Utting JE, Gray C. Stimulus frequency in the detection of neuromuscular block in humans. Br J Anaesth 1970;42(11):967–78.

16. Ali HH, Wilson RS, Savarese JJ, et al. The effect of tubocurarine on indirectly elicited train-of-four muscle response and respiratory measurements in humans. Br J Anaesth 1975;47(5):570–4.

17. Eriksson LI, Sundman E, Olsson R, et al. Functional assessment of the pharynx at rest and during swallowing in partially paralyzed humans: simultaneous videomanometry and mechanomyography of awake human volunteers. Anesthesiology 1997;87(5):1035–43.

18. Eikermann M, Vogt FM, Herbstreit F, et al. The predisposition to inspiratory upper airway collapse during partial neuromuscular blockade. Am J Respir Crit Care Med 2007;175(1):9–15.

19. Viby-Mogensen J, Jørgensen BC, Ording H. Residual curarization in the recovery room. Anesthesiology 1979;50(6):539–41.

20. Todd MM, Hindman BJ, King BJ. The implementation of quantitative electromyographic neuromuscular monitoring in an academic anesthesia department. Anesth Analg 2014;119(2):323–31.

21. Todd MM, Hindman BJ. The implementation of quantitative electromyographic neuromuscular monitoring in an academic anesthesia department: follow-up observations. Anesth Analg 2015;121(3):836–8.

22. Carvalho H, Verdonck M, Cools W, et al. Forty years of neuromuscular monitoring and postoperative residual curarisation: a meta-analysis and evaluation of confidence in network meta-analysis. Br J Anaesth 2020;125(4):466–82.

23. Katz RL. Neuromuscular effects of d-tubocurarine, edrophonium and neostigmine in man. Anesthesiology 1967;28(2):327–36.

24. Murphy GS, Szokol JW, Avram MJ, et al. Neostigmine administration after spontaneous recovery to a train-of-four ratio of 0.9 to 1.0: a randomized controlled trial of the effect on neuromuscular and clinical recovery. Anesthesiology 2018;128(1): 27–37.

25. Bowdle A, Bussey L, Michaelsen K, et al. A comparison of a prototype electromyograph vs. a mechanomyograph and an acceleromyograph for assessment of neuromuscular blockade. Anaesthesia 2020;75(2):187–95.

26. Engbaek J. Monitoring of neuromuscular transmission by electromyography during anaesthesia. A comparison with mechanomyography in cat and man. Dan Med Bull 1996;43(4):301–16.

27. Itagaki T, Tai K, Katsumata N, et al. Comparison between a new acceleration transducer and a conventional force transducer in the evaluation of twitch responses. Acta Anaesthesiol Scand 1988;32(4):347–9.

28. Werner MU, Kirkegaard Nielsen H, May O, et al. Assessment of neuromuscular transmission by the evoked acceleration response. An evaluation of the accuracy of the acceleration transducer in comparison with a force displacement transducer. Acta Anaesthesiol Scand 1988;32(5):395–400.

29. Suzuki T, Fukano N, Kitajima O, et al. Normalization of acceleromyographic train-of-four ratio by baseline value for detecting residual neuromuscular block. Br J Anaesth 2006;96(1):44–7.

30. Kopman AF. Normalization of the acceleromyographic train-of-four fade ratio. Acta Anaesthesiol Scand 2005;49(10):1575–6.

31. Claudius C, Skovgaard LT, Viby-Mogensen J. Is the performance of acceleromyography improved with preload and normalization? A comparison with mechanomyography. Anesthesiology 2009;110(6):1261–70.

32. Hemmerling TM, Donati F. The M-NMT mechanosensor cannot be considered as a reliable clinical neuromuscular monitor in daily anesthesia practice. Anesth Analg 2002;95(6):1826–7, author reply 1827.

33. Motamed C, Kirov K, Combes X, et al. Comparison between the Datex-Ohmeda M-NMT module and a force-displacement transducer for monitoring neuromuscular blockade. Eur J Anaesthesiol 2003;20(6):467–9.

34. Trager G, Michaud G, Deschamps S, et al. Comparison of phonomyography, kinemyography and mechanomyography for neuromuscular monitoring. Can J Anaesth 2006;53(2):130–5.

35. Stewart PA, Freelander N, Liang S, et al. Comparison of electromyography and kinemyography during recovery from non-depolarising neuromuscular blockade. Anaesth Intensive Care May 2014;42(3):378–84.

36. Khandkar C, Liang S, Phillips S, et al. Comparison of kinemyography and electromyography during spontaneous recovery from non-depolarising neuromuscular blockade. Anaesth Intensive Care 2016;44(6):745–51.

37. Naguib M, Brull SJ, Johnson KB. Conceptual and technical insights into the basis of neuromuscular monitoring. Anaesthesia 2017;72(Suppl 1):16–37.

38. Klein AA, Meek T, Allcock E, et al. Recommendations for standards of monitoring during anaesthesia and recovery 2021: Guideline from the Association of Anaesthetists. Anaesthesia 2021. https://doi.org/10.1111/anae.15501.

39. Dobson G, Chow L, Filteau L, et al. Guidelines to the practice of anesthesia - revised edition 2021. Can J Anaesth 2021;68(1):92–129.
40. Plaud B, Baillard C, Bourgain JL, et al. Guidelines on muscle relaxants and reversal in anaesthesia. Anaesth Crit Care Pain Med 2020;39(1):125–42.
41. Australian and New Zealand College of Anaesthetists. PS18 Guideline on monitoring during anaesthesia 2017. Available at: https://www.anzca.edu.au/getattachment/0c2d9717-fa82-4507-a3d6-3533d8fa844d/PS18-Guideline-on-monitoring-during-anaesthesia. Accessed July 13, 2021.
42. Renew JR, Hex K, Johnson P, et al. Ease of application of various neuromuscular devices for routine monitoring. Anesth Analg 2020. https://doi.org/10.1213/ANE.0000000000005213.
43. Nemes R, Nagy G, Murphy GS, et al. Awake volunteer pain scores during neuromuscular monitoring. Anesth Analg 2020;130(4):941–8.
44. Dubois PE, De Bel M, Jamart J, et al. Performance of acceleromyography with a short and light TOF-tube compared with mechanomyography: a clinical comparison. Eur J Anaesthesiol 2014;31(8):404–10.
45. Söderström CM, Eskildsen KZ, Gätke MR, et al. Objective neuromuscular monitoring of neuromuscular blockade in Denmark: an online-based survey of current practice. Acta Anaesthesiol Scand 2017;61(6):619–26.
46. Thilen SR, Hansen BE, Ramaiah R, et al. Intraoperative neuromuscular monitoring site and residual paralysis. Anesthesiology 2012;117(5):964–72.
47. Stiffel P, Hameroff SR, Blitt CD, et al. Variability in assessment of neuromuscular blockade. Anesthesiology 1980;52(5):436–7.
48. Caffrey RR, Warren ML, Becker KE. Neuromuscular blockade monitoring comparing the orbicularis oculi and adductor pollicis muscles. Anesthesiology 1986;65(1):95–7.
49. Donati F, Meistelman C, Plaud B. Vecuronium neuromuscular blockade at the diaphragm, orbicularis oculi and adductor pollicis muscles. Can J Anaesth 1990;37(4 Pt 2):S13.
50. Sayson SC, Mongan PD. Onset of action of mivacurium chloride. a comparison of neuromuscular blockade monitoring at the adductor pollicis and the orbicularis oculi. Anesthesiology 1994;81(1):35–42.
51. Debaene B, Meistelman C, Beaussier M, et al. Visual estimation of train-of-four responses at the orbicularis oculi and posttetanic count at the adductor pollicis during intense neuromuscular block. Anesth Analg 1994;78(4):697–700.
52. Rimaniol JM, Dhonneur G, Sperry L, et al. A comparison of the neuromuscular blocking effects of atracurium, mivacurium, and vecuronium on the adductor pollicis and the orbicularis oculi muscle in humans. Anesth Analg 1996;83(4):808–13.
53. Abdulatif M, el-Sanabary M. Blood flow and mivacurium-induced neuromuscular block at the orbicularis oculi and adductor pollicis muscles. Br J Anaesth 1997;79(1):24–8.
54. Larsen PB, Gätke MR, Fredensborg BB, et al. Acceleromyography of the orbicularis oculi muscle II: comparing the orbicularis oculi and adductor pollicis muscles. Acta Anaesthesiol Scand 2002;46(9):1131–6.
55. Hattori H, Saitoh Y, Nakajima H, et al. Visual evaluation of fade in response to facial nerve stimulation at the eyelid. J Clin Anesth 2005;17(4):276–80.
56. Donati F. Neuromuscular monitoring: useless, optional or mandatory? Can J Anaesth 1998;45(5 Pt 2):R106–16.
57. Donati F. Neuromuscular monitoring: more than meets the eye. Anesthesiology 2012;117(5):934–6.

58. Yamamoto S, Yamamoto Y, Kitajima O, et al. Reversal of neuromuscular block with sugammadex: a comparison of the corrugator supercilii and adductor pollicis muscles in a randomized dose-response study. Acta Anaesthesiol Scand 2015; 59(7):892–901.

59. Kitajima T, Ishii K, Kobayashi T, et al. Differential effects of vecuronium on the thumb and the big toe muscles evaluated by acceleration measurement. J Anesth 1994;8(2):143–5.

60. Kern SE, Johnson JO, Orr JA, et al. Clinical analysis of the flexor hallucis brevis as an alternative site for monitoring neuromuscular block from mivacurium. J Clin Anesth 1997;9(5):383–7.

61. Saitoh Y, Koitabashi Y, Makita K, et al. Train-of-four and double burst stimulation fade at the great toe and thumb. Can J Anaesth 1997;44(4):390–5.

62. Heier T, Hetland S. A comparison of train-of-four monitoring: mechanomyography at the thumb vs acceleromyography at the big toe. Acta Anaesthesiol Scand 1999;43(5):550–5.

63. Graham DH. Monitoring neuromuscular block may be unreliable in patients with upper-motor-neuron lesions. Anesthesiology 1980;52(1):74–5.

64. Moorthy SS, Hilgenberg JC. Resistance to non-depolarizing muscle relaxants in paretic upper extremities of patients with residual hemiplegia. Anesth Analg 1980;59(8):624–7.

65. Iwasaki H, Namiki A, Omote K, et al. Response differences of paretic and healthy extremities to pancuronium and neostigmine in hemiplegic patients. Anesth Analg 1985;64(9):864–6.

Depth of Anesthesia Monitoring

David Roche, BSc, BM, BS, FCAI, FJFICMI*, Padraig Mahon, MSc, MD, FCARCSI, FJFICMI

KEYWORDS

- Awareness • Bispectral index • Entropy monitoring • Neurosense
- Depth of anesthesia • Electroencephalogram (EEG) • Processed EEG

KEY POINTS

- pEEG monitors provide useful data to the anesthesiologist when interpreted within the clinical context.
- When using a pEEG monitor clinicians should have a basic understanding of that monitor's limitations and be aware that not all drugs administered will produce the effect one might assume.
- With minimal training anesthesiologists are good at interpreting raw EEG data.
- pEEG-guided anesthesia reduces anesthetic consumption but has not been shown to be superior to ETAC-guided anesthesia care at reducing awareness or postoperative complications.

INTRODUCTION

The aim of general anesthesia is the suppression of a patient's experience and explicit memory of the events taking place from induction through to planned emergence.[1] On a day-to-day basis we judge the effectiveness of our interventions using secondary or downstream physiologic parameters including respiratory rate, heart rate, and blood pressure. These parameters exhibit change with time, change that occurs (usually undesirable) as a direct result of a clinician administering a drug (or combination of drugs) with the intention of inducing unconsciousness.[2] The brain is the target organ of our intervention—changes in the electroencephalogram (EEG) are the clinical gold-standard descriptor or measure of our intervention.[3] The EEG can be analyzed in its raw form for characteristic drug-induced patterns of change or summarized using mathematical parameters (processed EEG [pEEG]).[4] After even a short PowerPoint presentation anesthesiologists are surprisingly good at interpreting raw EEG, with the investigators of one study concluding that a combination of pEEG parameters and raw waveform analysis might be the optimal approach.[5]

The authors have nothing to disclose.
Department of Anaesthesiology and Critical Care, Cork University Hospital, Wilton Road, Wilton, Cork T12 DC4A, Ireland
* Corresponding author.
E-mail address: david.g.roche@gmail.com

Anesthesiology Clin 39 (2021) 477–492
https://doi.org/10.1016/j.anclin.2021.04.004   anesthesiology.theclinics.com
1932-2275/21/© 2021 Elsevier Inc. All rights reserved.

The last 2 decades have seen increased interest and uptake in the use of pEEG devices by clinicians. Over this time the bar of expectation has been set high. High-profile studies have generated conflicting and sometimes apparently disappointing results causing confusion.[6,7] However, despite this apparent rocky start, pEEG monitoring seems to be finding its own clinical "feet" and is with us for the future.[8] This article looks at the three commonly available pEEG monitors, we aim to summarise the contemporary clinical literature pertaining to pEEG monitors and their potential pitfalls. We will discuss the effect of commonly used anesthetic drugs on the EEG and pEEG parameters, together with the clinical implications for anesthesia, paediatrics and intensive care.

BACKGROUND
Awareness

The nomenclature surrounding accidental awareness under general anesthesia can be confusing; terms such as wakefulness, connected consciousness, and awareness with and without explicit recall are used to describe the different manifestations of inadequate anesthetic depth. The isolated forearm test is the gold-standard test of connected consciousness (awareness of one's environment and having the ability to respond to cues).[9,10] In a recent multicenter study investigating the incidence of connected consciousness 4.6% of patients responded to verbal cues while anesthetized,[11] The significance of this to us as clinicians is difficult to quantify and at times understand. Inability to recall does not mean the experience did not happen, rather it means the patient cannot recall, as anesthetic agents are amnesic at subhypnotic doses.[12,13] The incidence of awareness with recall (AWR) under general anesthesia is consistently reported between 0.1% and 0.2% when screened for using tools such as the Brice questionnaire. When relying on patients to self-report the incidence decreases dramatically to 1:19,600.[3,14] The consequences of AWR are significant with up to 70% of patients who experience AWR developing posttraumatic stress disorder.[15] The effects of implicit traumatic memories on postoperative long-term behavior and well-being in humans remain unknown.[16]

The Electroencephalogram

Full montage (32 or more channels) EEG is the most widely accepted diagnostic modality for cerebral function monitoring. During anesthesia the EEG exhibits decreased overall neuronal firing, increases in amplitude, increasing synchronicity frontal anteriorization, a reduction in the frequency of the dominant waveforms, and eventual burst suppression.[17,18]

Full multichannel EEG is simply too time consuming to set up for everyday use in the operating room. The last 2 decades have seen a multitude of pEEG devices being brought to market. All these devices acquire one or more frontal EEG channels. The central underlying tenant is that induction and maintenance of anesthesia results in a predominantly slow wave (alpha-delta) pattern, possibly originating in corticothalamic networks that shifts to anterior structures known as frontal anteriorization (**Table 1** for EEG annotation).[18–20] John and colleagues[21] proposed this phenomenon to be an agent agnostic marker of anesthesia-induced loss of consciousness, an assertion that has been recently challenged by Gaskell and colleagues.[22] Using data from the above-mentioned connected consciousness study Gaskell and colleagues[22] identified a subset of patients who responded to commands (demonstrated connected consciousness) in the presence of an alpha-delta pattern on frontal EEG, serving to highlight the danger of general assumption.

Table 1
Classic electroencephalographic frequency ranges

Band or Wave Designation	Frequency Range (Hz)	Clinical Correlation
δ (Delta)	0.5–3.5	Stage III non-REM sleep/deep sleep
θ (Theta)	3.5–7.0	Classic slow wave activity associated with daydreaming Stage 1 non-REM sleep
α (Alpha)	7.0–13.0	Awake quietly resting/relaxed
β (Beta)	13.0–30.0	Awake eyes closed
β2 (overlaps with γ)	30.0–50.0	Awake eyes open

Abbreviation: REM, rapid eye movement.

Periods of burst suppression, that is, isoelectric EEG, alternating with bursts of electrical activity is a well-known EEG activity associated with deepening anesthesia and induced reduction in cortical metabolic rate.[23,24] All the currently available pEEG monitors display a burst suppression ratio (BSR). Periods longer than 0.5 seconds during which the EEG voltage does not exceed ±5 mV are deemed to be suppressed. The BSR is the fraction of the epoch length in which the EEG is suppressed in this way.

PROCESSED ELECTROENCEPHALOGRAPH

Visual changes in the EEG can be identified by trained anesthesiologists[5,25]; alternatively the EEG can be quantified or summarized using time, power, or frequency domain analysis. Time domain analysis is used for amplitude quantification, detection of suppression, and calculation of the BSR. EEG power, the product of voltage and current, first used by Falconer and Brickford to control a halothane vaporizer, has been surpassed by power spectral analysis.

A Fourier analysis converts a time domain waveform into its sine wave components and generates a frequency spectrum—a histogram of amplitudes as a function of frequency (known as the power spectral density [PSD]), and a phase spectrum (discussed later). From this analysis, median frequency, spectral edge frequency 90%/95% (frequency below which 90% or 95% of the spectral power resides), and frequency ratios can be calculated and correlated clinically. Higher order variables such as spectral entropy are also calculated from the PSD. The phase spectrum generated from the Fourier transform measures the phase of component waves (frequencies) relative to the start of the epoch. Bispectral analysis a third-order statistical function measures the correlation of phase between different underlying frequency components of the complex EEG waveform and is a proposed surrogate measure of synchronization.[4] The bispectral or BIS monitor includes this form of analysis, from which it derives its name.

Shannon or spectral entropy is a quantitative EEG variable that mathematically describes the shape or degree of uniformity of the PSD (often described as a measure of disorder). A PSD with a distribution similar to a Bell curve, for instance, will have a low entropy value, and one that is dispersed or uneven will have high entropy, that is, be more visually random. As anesthesia deepens and the EEG becomes limited by frequency, entropy decreases.

Finally, wavelet analysis (WAV) a more recent signal processing development has been applied to the EEG. WAV using very short time intervals can simultaneously track changes in frequency and time. The changes in these variables can then be represented using a probability density function (PDF), which we are familiar with from probability theory. The PDF will assume a stereotypical single spike shape when the EEG is isoelectric and a broad flattened curve shape when awake.[26] The evolution between these 2 extreme shapes is assumed to be consistent with increasing anesthetic drug effect. Other variables influencing the PDF and its shape characteristics might include age, environmental stimulation, and preexisting dementia. The effects of such variables have yet to be described. A brief description of the 3 commonly used pEEG monitors is included in the following sections.

COMMERCIALLY AVAILABLE PROCESSED ELECTROENCEPHALOGRAPHIC MONITORS
BIS

The BIS (Medtronic, Dublin, Ireland) monitor was approved for use in 1996 by the US Food and Drug Administration. At that time, it was brought to market by Aspect Medical, which was subsequently acquired by Covidien, which has since merged with Medtronic. BIS is the most studied and high-profile monitor with currently 3240 citations on PubMed. EEG is acquired (one or more frontal channels) using a disposable electrode array. The EEG is amplified and sampled and undergoes analog to digital conversion and artifact recognition. As discussed earlier, a variety of variables, frequency (β ratio—the log ratio of high-frequency components [30–47 Hz] and classic EEG frequency components [11–20 Hz]), power spectrum, suppression detection, and synchronization, are incorporated into a single proprietary algorithm. The relative contribution of each remains elusive.[27] During development these parameters were calculated for more than 1500 EEG recordings and were correlated with behavioral measures of sedation and anesthesia. These 4 subparameters are combined into a single BIS number, which decreases continuously with decreasing level of consciousness. The original A-1050 monitor produced an average value derived from the previous 60 seconds of useable data.[4] The monitor also provides the suppression ratio and graphical depiction of signal quality and electrical frequencies associated with muscle activity (electromyography [EMG]). A recent "big data" analysis of more than 1000 intraoperative EEGs using 4 known BIS parameters (as previously published by Rampil[4]) for the BIS ranges $0 \leq BIS \leq 21$, $21 < BIS \leq 41$, $41 < BIS \leq 61$, $61 < BIS \leq 78$, and $78 < BIS \leq 98$ concluded that positive predictive values were 100%, 80%, 80%, 85%, and 89% in the order of increasing BIS in the 5 BIS ranges, suggesting a very high probability of burst suppression when $BIS < 21$.[28] The investigators point out that for the fourth BIS parameter QUASI (designed to detect burst suppression in wandering baseline voltage) they made some assumptions in the absence of an explicit definition from the manufacturer. The investigators also suggest that above 60 the BIS value is heavily influenced by high frequencies (via the weighting of the β ratio in the algorithm) associated with muscle activity, potentially explaining the drop in BIS values recorded following administration of muscle relaxants.[29,30] The BIS monitor is now available with dual hemisphere functionality via a bilateral frontal electrode. The clinical utility of this additional feature (outside of carotid surgery as claimed by the manufacturer) remains to be determined. A study comparing patients undergoing electro or magnetic seizure therapy with a bilateral BIS monitor under anesthesia failed to demonstrate a difference in BIS values between the hemispheres.[31]

Entropy

The Entropy monitor was originally brought to market by a Finnish company Datex Ohmeda (since acquired by GE). This monitor uses a concept for summarizing the PSD (discussed previously) developed by Claud Shannon in 1948 as part of his theory of information, thus it is nonproprietary. A description of the methods used in the monitor was published by the company in conjunction with investigators from Helsinki University Hospital in 2004.[32] To overcome the difficulty presented by EMG interference the monitor provides the clinician with spectral entropy values for 2 frequency ranges— one (response entropy [RE] 0.8–47 Hz) that includes typical EMG frequencies and a second without EMG frequencies (state entropy [SE] 0.8–32 Hz). Raw entropy values are transformed using a mathematical spline function to a value range between 0 and 91 for SE and 0 and 100 for RE. The clinician may attribute the value difference between both variables to EMG activity. SE and RE correlate closely as the depth of anesthesia increases (ie, from 91 downward); when both are equal EMG activity can be assumed to be absent.[33] Thus as anesthesia deepens both values should be similar and move in tandem.[34] SE, RE, and BIS have been shown to strongly correlate in the range 30 to 71, with all 3 indices having a similar ability to predict sevoflurane effect site concentration.[35] Similar to the BIS monitor the Entropy monitor also displays a BSR. There are currently more than 100 clinical reports/trials in which the Entropy monitor has been investigated or compared with other modalities. Broadly speaking both BIS and Entropy correlate well over the range of values associated with anesthesia and both monitors have demonstrated the ability to reduce anesthetic drug usage and time in post anaesthetic care unit (PACU). Both monitors together with the Narcotrend-Compact M (MonitorTech-nik, Bad Bramstedt, Germany) have been considered as broadly equivalent by the UK National Institute for Health and Care Excellence.[8]

NeuroSENSE

The NeuroSENSE (NeuroWave Systems Cleveland, OH, USA), differs significantly from both the BIS and Entropy monitors in that it uses analysis of the higher-frequency gamma range (32–64 Hz). A group from the University of British Columbia (2001) first proposed using WAV (a new signal processing approach that can simultaneously track changes in both time and frequency) to track changes occurring in the gamma band during induction—a wavelength-based anesthetic value (WAVcns).[36] The WAV has the advantage that it can be determined in near real time based on 1-second or shorter EEG segments. Both the Entropy and BIS monitors require the PSD to be determined for each epoch, which is computationally intense and requires time, both creating a lag. As discussed previously the WAV integer seen on screen is derived from a probability distribution (PDF), thus the WAVcns can only be said to represent the probability of consciousness or not. The manufacturer claims that WAVcns declines monotonously with increasing burst suppression offering advantages over other monitors. In clinical studies WAVcns correlates with desflurane levels and plateaus at higher concentrations. WAVcns can reliably distinguish loss of and recovery of consciousness during desflurane anesthesia.[37] During propofol anesthesia significant discrepancy (when compared with BIS) occurred during deeper (BIS <40) anesthesia. Propofol has a characteristic EEG signature that may explain this effect.[38] Ketamine, which is known to increase high-frequency EEG activity even at the doses used for postoperative analgesia has recently been shown to significantly increase intraoperative WAVcns values.[39]

CLINICAL PITFALLS

One of the many factors hampering the development of pEEG monitoring is the fact that the mechanism by which hypnotics induce unconsciousness remains unresolved. Gaskell and colleagues[21] describe 3 patients with volitional response using the isolated forearm technique shortly after the induction of anesthesia despite having frontal EEG consistent with anesthesia. It is postulated in the accompanying editorial that disconnection from the outside world caused by anesthesia may not happen in all cortical areas simultaneously.[40] Different anesthetic agents have differing effects on neurobiology and electrical signaling, such that a monitoring system that is validated to detect the unconscious state induced by one anesthetic agent may not reliably detect another.[41] BIS, for example, is unchanged by the hypnotic effects of nitrous oxide and increases with the administration of ketamine.[42,43] The dramatic effect of reduction in EMG frequencies with muscle relaxants and their apparently paradoxic effect on BIS has also been well documented.[30] It has also been suggested that sympathomimetic medications such as ephedrine can increase BIS values.[44] The use of dexmedetomidine has been shown to dramatically slow EEG oscillations and reduce pEEG index values to levels that suggest the patient is deeply unconscious, but they are in fact easily rousable.[45] When using a pEEG monitor clinicians should have a basic understanding of that monitor's limitations, be aware that not all drugs administered will produce the effect one might assume, and use clinical judgment to contextualize the "number" (**Table 2**).

CLINICAL CARE POINTS

- pEEG monitors acquire frontal EEG; recent research suggests that frontal anteriorization of EEG during early stages of anesthesia cannot always be assumed to occur
- Available pEEG monitors provide BSR data that implies very deep anesthesia
- BIS values less than 20 are highly likely to correlate with burst suppression on EEG
- Many pEEG variables are not affected by nitrous oxide
- Ketamine increases high-frequency EEG activity resulting in pEEG variable increases
- Muscle relaxants decrease response entropy and BIS values

Table 2
The effect of different pharmacologic interventions on processed electroencephalographic outputs

Drug	BIS	Entropy	NeuroSENSE
Sevoflurane	Decrease[46]	Decrease[47]	Decrease[38]
Desflurane	Decrease[48]	Decrease[49]	Decrease[37]
Propofol	Decrease[50]	Decrease[51]	Decrease[38]
Opiates	Decrease[52]	Decrease[53]	
Ketamine	Increase[54]	Increase[55]	Increase[39]
Thiopentone	Decrease[56]	Decrease[56]	
Benzodiazepines	Decrease[57]	Decrease[58]	
Dexmedetomidine	Decrease[57]	Decrease[59]	
Neuromuscular blockers	Decrease[60]	Decrease[61]	Decrease[62]
N$_2$O as sole agent	No effect[42]	No effect[63,64]	
N$_2$O + propofol	No effect[65]	No effect[65]	
N$_2$O + sevoflurane	Additive effect (decrease)[65,66]	Additive effect (decrease)[65,66]	

PROCESSED ELECTROENCEPHALOGRAPHIC MONITORS AND AWARENESS

pEEG monitors appear slow to capture the imagination of anesthesiologists in Europe. In the recent National Audit Program 5 audit, pEEG monitors were used in approximately 3% of general anesthetics administered in 2015.[14] Clinicians using a pEEG monitor when administering total intravenous anaesthesia (TIVA) (close to 30%) appear to account for the majority of use. Australian survey data found that 24% of respondents thought pEEG monitoring should be mandatory in all general anesthesia cases with neuromuscular blockade and 74% believed it should be mandatory with TIVA.[67] In North America the American Society of Anaesthesiology (ASA) does not stipulate that pEEG monitors be used as part of routine monitoring; usage estimates or surveys are difficult to find in the literature.[68,69] Given that the estimated global market size for pEEG devices and disposables is currently estimated at $1.64 billion this suggests far greater use of these devices in North America. It is unlikely that economic factors alone account for this difference. In 1994 the BIS monitor became the first widely available commercial depth of anesthesia monitor. An early article published in 1998 by Rampil[4] of UCLA (and a consultant to ASpect Medical Systems) described some of the higher-order spectral and time frequency domain parameters incorporated into the pEEG monitor's proprietary algorithm. Early clinical case reports appeared to show pitfalls with the monitor's use: neuromuscular blockers, montage bias, and poor prediction probability with clinical end points fueling confusion.[60] The high-profile, B-Aware industry-sponsored randomized trial published in the Lancet (2004) demonstrated the capability to reduce the AWR in 2463 at-risk patients; 2 of 1225 (0.17%) patients experienced definite awareness compared with 11 of 1238 (0.91%) in the routine care group ($P = .03$).[7] The statistical analysis became controversial when not all potential confounding factors including type of anesthesia were controlled for, and the stated 82% risk reduction in awareness (in the BIS-guided group) had wide confidence intervals (CI) (95% CI 17%–98%).[70] Interpretation was made more difficult when the effect could not be replicated. The single-center 2008 B-Unaware study randomly assigned 1941 patients to BIS or end-tidal anesthetic gas concentration (ETAC)-guided anesthesia. Two events (definite awareness) occurred in each group.[71] Avidan and colleagues[71] later randomly assigned 6041 patients to structured BIS-guided anesthesia (target range, 40–60) or structured ETAC-guided anesthesia (target range, 0.7–1.3 age-adjusted minimium alveolar concentration [MAC]) in the multicenter BAG-RECALL study. Postoperatively, patients were assessed for explicit recall at 2 time points: 0 to 72 hours and 30 days after extubation using a modified Brice questionnaire. The primary outcome of the trial was awareness with explicit recall. Secondary outcomes included postoperative mortality, psychological symptoms, intensive care and hospital length of stay, average anesthetic gas administration, postoperative pain, nausea and vomiting, and duration of recovery room stay. BAG-RECALL could not establish the superiority of the BIS protocol, with 19 cases of definite or possible intraoperative awareness (0.66%) in the BIS group, versus 8 (0.28%) in the ETAC group, a nonsignificant difference (95% CI, 0.03–0.74; $P = .99$). No difference between groups in the rate of major postoperative adverse outcomes or quantum of anesthetic agent administered was reported.[72]

The MACS (Michigan Awareness Control Study) trial (2012) is the largest unselected prospective randomized effectiveness trial published to date comparing alerts-guided pEEG with alerts-guided ETAC in 21,106 surgical patients. Like the B-Aware trial the MACS trial also included patients receiving TIVA. Conducted over a 2-year period at the University of Michigan the study was unable to determine if a physician alerting protocol based on BIS values or ETAC was superior in preventing definite intraoperative awareness. The study was terminated early due to futility. Definite awareness was 0.12% (11/9376, 95% CI, 0.07%–0.21%) in the ETAC group and 0.08% (8/9460, 95% CI, 0.04%–0.16%) in the BIS group ($P = .48$). The most recent Cochrane review (2019) judged an increased risk of attrition bias as approximately 3000 patients randomized to the BIS intervention did not have BIS values recorded due to technical issues; furthermore, the reviewers were unable to judge the risk of bias for allocation concealment.[73] Post hoc secondary analysis of the MACS trial data suggests that a protocol based on the BIS monitor probably reduces awareness events compared with routine care without any protocol requiring approximately 60,000 (29,900 in each group) patients to show the benefit. Secondary outcomes in the MACS trial including anesthetic dosing neither showed a reduction when alert-driven BIS-guided care was used nor was it associated with reduced recovery room time or reduced incidence of nausea and vomiting compared with routine care.[74]

pEEG MONITORS AND SECONDARY OUTCOMES
Anesthesia Recovery

An early meta-analysis (2004) included 11 small clinical trials in 1380 ambulatory surgical patients randomized to BIS versus routine care. The use of BIS monitoring significantly reduced anesthetic consumption by 19%, reduced the incidence of nausea/vomiting (32% versus 38%; OR, 0.77), and reduced PACU time by a modest 4 minutes. These effects are consistent with the most recent (2019) Cochrane review, with a reduction in time to eye opening and orientation (low certainty with limited patient numbers) and time to PACU discharge reduced by 6.86 minutes in 930 participants (95% CI −11.72 to −2.00; I2 = 79%; 13 studies; low-certainty evidence), across BIS-guided study participants receiving inhalational and intravenous anesthesia.[75]

Morbidity and Mortality

The proposed association between increased depth of anesthesia and poor postoperative outcomes makes intuitive sense. Independent studies published by Radtke and colleagues[76] and the CODA trial group in 2013 helped bolster this. Radtke and colleagues[76] randomly assigned 1277 (>60 years, mini mental state examination >24) patients undergoing a wide range of surgeries to routine (with blinded BIS monitoring) or BIS-guided routine care. Duration of surgery was 60 minutes or more. Patients were assessed at baseline, 1, and 7 days after using CANTAB (Cantab Cognition, Cambridge, UK) for evidence of postoperative cognitive dysfunction (POCD); 95 patients in the BIS-guided compared with 124 patients (16.7% vs 21.4%) in the control group developed delirium ($P = .036$). The percentage of episodes of deep anesthesia (BIS values <20) was independently predictive for postoperative delirium ($P = .006$; odds ratio 1.027). By day 7 BIS guidance was not protective.[76] The CODA Study Group assessed 921 elderly patients on postoperative day 1, 7 days, and 3 months postoperatively using confusion asssesment methods (CAMs) criteria. Median BIS values were significantly lower at 36 (interquartile [IQR] 31–49) in the control group (BIS recorded but not available) versus 53 (IQR 48–59) ($P<.001$) when BIS was available to the anesthesiologist. BIS-guided anesthesia reduced propofol use by 21% and volatile anesthetics by 30%. Significantly less patients in the BIS group compared with routine care (15.6% vs 24.1%, $P = .01$) had evidence of delirium, although cognitive performance was similar between groups at 1 week after surgery. Patients in the BIS group had a significantly lower rate of POCD at 3 months compared with routine care.[77]

Whitlock and colleagues[78] published the results of a single-center (substudy) analysis of 310 cardiothoracic patients enrolled in the previously discussed 2011 BAG-RECALL (n = 6041) trial. Patients were assessed twice daily in the intensive care unit (ICU) using CAMs criteria. The investigators did not demonstrate a statistically significant difference ($P = .58$) in the incidence of delirium in the BIS- versus ETAC protocol-guided groups: 28 of 149 (18.8%) versus 45 of 161 (28.0%), respectively (odds ratio, 0.60; 95% CI, 0.35–1.02).[78] The investigators identified low average volatile anesthetic dose, intraoperative transfusion, ASA physical status, and European System for Cardiac Operative Risk Evaluation as independent predictors of delirium. Whitlock and colleagues called for larger studies using brain monitoring with BIS or an alternative method to determine if such an intervention could change outcomes in cardiac patients. A 2018 meta-analysis including 6 randomized controlled trials and 2929 participants judged the evidence to be of moderate quality that POCD at 3 months could be reduced by optimized anesthesia guided by pEEG indices in patients aged 60 years or older undergoing noncardiac surgical and nonneurosurgical procedures.[79]

Two recent high-profile trials, the international Balanced Anesthesia Study and the single-center ENGAGES (Effect of Electroencephalography-Guided Anesthetic Administration on Postoperative Delirium Among Older Adults Undergoing Major Surgery) study published in the Lancet and JAMA, respectively, seem to further support this view. ENGAGES enrolled 1213 patients, randomized to routine or nonprompted BIS-guided care. There was no significant difference between groups in the median cumulative time with mean arterial pressure less than 60 mm Hg. Median ETAC was significantly lower in the BIS-guided group than the usual care group (0.69 versus 0.80 MAC) and median cumulative time with EEG suppression (ie, the BSR was more than 1%) was significantly less (7 vs 13 minutes). This significant difference did not translate into a significant clinical effect.[80] Four hundred and thirty patients enrolled in ENGAGES study had evidence of preenrollment abnormal cognition. Of these 430 patients, 35% had evidence of postoperative delirium versus 18% in patients without preoperative evidence of abnormal cognition. Patients with preoperative abnormal cognition spent more time in EEG suppression intraoperatively compared with patients without abnormal cognition (13 vs 7 minutes, $P<.001$). A prespecified mediation analysis of data from affected patients, designed to quantify the possible attributable effect of burst suppression to the absolute 17.2% incidence difference, concluded that an absolute 2.4% (99.5% CI, 0.6%–4.8%) was an indirect effect mediated by EEG suppression, whereas an absolute 14.8% was a direct effect of preoperative abnormal cognition. Randomization to pEEG-guided anesthesia did not change the mediated effect size ($P = .078$ for moderation).[81] This finding is consistent with that of recent findings in volunteers (ReCCognition study group).[82]

The 73-center Balanced Anesthesia Trial randomized 6644 patients with significant comorbidities to "deep" aiming for a BIS value of 35 or "light" anesthesia (BIS value 50), the primary outcome being 1-year all-cause mortality. Mean arterial pressure was 3.5 mm Hg higher and volatile anesthetic use 0.26 MAC lower in the BIS 50-guided group (median, 47.2; IQR, 43.7–50.5). One-year mortality and grades 3 and 4 adverse events did not differ significantly between groups.[83]

CLINICAL CARE POINTS

- pEEG-guided anesthesia has not been shown to be superior to ETAC-guided anesthesia care in large randomized studies
- An ETAC protocol is a cost-effective alternative for patients receiving inhaled anesthetics

- BIS-guided care may reduce the incidence of awareness compared with routine care
- pEEG may reduce the incidence of AWR in TIVA cases[73,84]
- These same protocolized RCTs have failed to demonstrate a reduction in mortality, PACU time, or postoperative nausea and vomiting on primary analysis

pEEG in the Intensive Care Unit

Correlation between BIS and clinical assessment of sedation using the sedation agitation scale is poor in critically ill patients, particularly at lighter levels of sedation at which high BIS levels are attributed to EMG activity.[29,85,86] There are some reports from small observational studies that both BIS and Entropy monitoring correlate well with the Richmond Agitation and Sedation Scale,[87,88] with greater correlation at deeper levels of sedation. Despite evidence of some correlation with clinical sedation scales and pEEG outputs in the critically ill, it is difficult to elicit any effect on clinical outcome when used for sedation monitoring alone. A recent Cochrane review (2018) of 4 randomized controlled trials (256 patients) found high-quality evidence lacking on the effect of BIS monitoring on ICU length of stay or ventilator-free days and concluded there is insufficient evidence to support the routine use of pEEG monitoring for patients in the ICU.[89] However, pEEG monitoring may have some limited use in patients receiving critical care following cardiac arrest, in neurologic injury, or in the treatment of seizure disorders. pEEG values have been shown to correlate with Glasgow Coma Scale (GCS) scores in patients with head injury,[90] suggested as a viable evaluation tool for brain injury, particularly when the GCS is <9.[91] Lower pEEG values in the postresuscitation phase of cardiac arrest correlate with increasing mortality. Sedar and colleagues[92] found a BIS less than 10 after cardiac arrest was associated with a 91% mortality, suggesting it has some feasibility as a prognostic marker when combined with other clinical and radiological indicators. pEEG has been used in refractory status epilepticus in which full montage EEG was unavailable to allow sedation to be titrated to burst suppression.[93]

pEEG in Pediatric Care

pEEG monitors are designed to assess the frontal EEG of adults and are not validated for use in pediatric patients.[94] Several studies have shown no benefit of using BIS in the general pediatric population in terms of reducing propofol consumption or reducing emergence agitation. Bhardwaj and Yaddanapudi[95] conducted a randomized trial of standard practice versus BIS-guided anesthesia in 50 patients aged 2 to 12 years; they found no difference in the intraoperative hemodynamic or BIS values between the 2 groups; mean times from termination of anesthesia to eye opening and extubation were similar.[95] Sargin and colleagues[96] did show that in the subgroup of 50 pediatric patients with developmental delay, BIS monitoring reduced time to extubation and time in the PACU when used to titrate anesthesia versus routine care. In an observational study of 400 pediatric patients Faulk and colleagues[97] found no correlation between time spent with a BIS less than 45 versus time spent with a BIS greater than 45 on the incidence of postoperative delirium; this is supported by a small randomized controlled trial by Fredrick and colleagues[98] who randomized pediatric patients to light or deep BIS-guided anesthesia. No difference in emergence delirium between groups was found. A recent study by Beekoo and colleagues[94] studied 135 patients aged 0 to 80 years, with 6 age cutoff points. Anesthesia was maintained at 1.0 MAC of sevoflurane in these patients. BIS values were found to be higher in pediatric patients. Raw EEG analysis was similar across all age groups with dominant theta (slow) activity, suggesting the usefulness of interpreting raw EEG data from pEEG out-puts, particularly in pediatric patients.[94]

TRANSLATION TO CLINICAL PRACTICE

pEEG monitors provide useful data to the anesthesiologist when interpreted within the clinical context. Interpreting the pEEG number in isolation is fraught with pitfalls and is best avoided. The interpretation of raw EEG by the anesthesiologist, preferably ob-tained from 2 or more EEG channels monitoring different cortical regions, combined with summary EEG variables is to our minds the ideal clinical standard. Although ETAC-guided monitoring with alarm prompts is as effective as pEEG monitoring at preventing AWR when using volatile anesthesia, current evidence suggests that pEEG use has the added advantage of reducing overall anesthetic consumption. Many clinicians now support the routine use of pEEG with TIVA. pEEG monitors have been shown to safely decrease the incidence of excessively deep anesthesia; perhaps however, the benefit of this are best judged by anesthesiologists for individual patients.

REFERENCES

1. Goddard N, Smith D. Unintended awareness and monitoring of depth of anaes-thesia. Cont Educ Anaesth Crit Care Pain 2013;13(6):213–7.
2. Bowdle TA. Depth of anesthesia monitoring. Anesthesiol Clin North Am 2006; 24(4):793–822.
3. Avidan MS, Mashour GA. Prevention of intraoperative awareness with explicit recall: making sense of the evidence. Anesthesiology 2013;118(2):449–56.
4. Rampil IJ. A primer for EEG signal processing in anesthesia. Anesthesiology 1998;89(4):980–1002.
5. Barnard JP, Bennett C, Voss LJ, et al. Can anaesthetists be taught to interpret the effects of general anaesthesia on the electroencephalogram? Comparison of per-formance with the BIS and spectral entropy. Br J Anaesth 2007;99(4):532–7.
6. Mashour GA, Avidan MS. Intraoperative awareness: controversies and non-con-troversies. Br J Anaesth 2015;115(Suppl 1):i20–6.
7. Myles PS, Leslie K, McNeil J, et al. Bispectral index monitoring to prevent aware-ness during anaesthesia: the B-Aware randomised controlled trial. Lancet 2004; 363(9423):1757–63.
8. National Institute for Health and Care Excellence. Depth of anaesthesia monitors – Bispectral Index (BIS), E-Entropy and Narcotrend-Compact M. Available at: https://www.nice.org.uk/guidance/dg6. Accessed January 18, 2021.
9. Tunstall ME. Detecting wakefulness during general anaesthesia for caesarean section. Br Med J 1977;1(6072):1321.
10. Russell IF, Sanders RD. Monitoring consciousness under anaesthesia: the 21st century isolated forearm technique. Br J Anaesth 2016;6:738–40.
11. Sanders RD, Gaskell A, Raz A, et al. Incidence of connected consciousness after tracheal intubation: a prospective, international, multicenter cohort study of the isolated forearm technique. Anesthesiology 2017;126(2):214–22.
12. Sanders RD, Tononi G, Laureys S, et al. Unresponsiveness ≠ unconsciousness. Anesthesiology 2012;116(4):946–59.
13. Nordström O, Sandin R. Recall during intermittent propofol anaesthesia. Br J Anaesth 1996;76(5):699–701.

14. Pandit JJ, Andrade J, Bogod DG, et al. 5th National Audit Project (NAP5) on accidental awareness during general anaesthesia: summary of main findings and risk factors. Br J Anaesth 2014;113(4):549–59.

15. Leslie K, Chan MT, Myles PS, et al. Posttraumatic stress disorder in aware patients from the B-aware trial. Anesth Analg 2010;110(3):823–8.

16. Samuel N, Taub AH, Paz R, et al. Implicit aversive memory under anaesthesia in animal models: a narrative review. Br J Anaesth 2018;121(1):219–32.

17. Fahy BG, Chau DF. The technology of processed electroencephalogram monitoring devices for assessment of depth of anesthesia. Anesth Analg 2018; 126(1):111–7.

18. Brown EN, Lydic R, Schiff ND. General anesthesia, sleep, and coma. N Engl J Med 2010;363(27):2638–50.

19. Steriade M, Contreras D, Curró Dossi R, et al. The slow (< 1 Hz) oscillation in reticular thalamic and thalamocortical neurons: scenario of sleep rhythm generation in interacting thalamic and neocortical networks. J Neurosci 1993;13(8): 3284–99.

20. Steriade M, McCormick DA, Sejnowski TJ. Thalamocortical oscillations in the sleeping and aroused brain. Science 1993;262(5134):679–85.

21. John ER, Prichep LS, Kox W, et al. Invariant reversible QEEG effects of anesthetics. Conscious Cogn 2001;10(2):165–83.

22. Gaskell AL, Hight DF, Winders J, et al. Frontal alpha-delta EEG does not preclude volitional response during anaesthesia: prospective cohort study of the isolated forearm technique. Br J Anaesth 2017;119(4):664–73.

23. Akrawi WP, Drummond JC, Kalkman CJ, et al. A comparison of the electrophysiologic characteristics of EEG burst-suppression as produced by isoflurane, thiopental, etomidate, and propofol. J Neurosurg Anesthesiol 1996;8(1):40–6.

24. Woodcock TE, Murkin JM, Farrar JK, et al. Pharmacologic EEG suppression during cardiopulmonary bypass: cerebral hemodynamic and metabolic effects of thiopental or isoflurane during hypothermia and normothermia. Anesthesiology 1987;67(2):218–24.

25. Bottros MM, Palanca BJ, Mashour GA, et al. Estimation of the bispectral index by anesthesiologists: an inverse turing test. Anesthesiology 2011;114(5):1093–101.

26. Zikov T, Bibian S, Dumont GA, et al. Quantifying cortical activity during general anesthesia using wavelet analysis. IEEE Trans Biomed Eng 2006;53(4):617–32.

27. Miller A, Sleigh JW, Barnard J, et al. Does bispectral analysis of the electroencephalogram add anything but complexity? Br J Anaesth 2004;92(1):8–13.

28. Lee H-C, Ryu H-G, Park Y, et al. Data driven investigation of bispectral index algorithm. Sci Rep 2019;9(1):13769.

29. Sackey PV, Radell PJ, Granath F, et al. Bispectral index as a predictor of sedation depth during isoflurane or midazolam sedation in ICU patients. Anaesth Intensive Care 2007;35(3):348–56.

30. Schuller PJ, Newell S, Strickland PA, et al. Response of bispectral index to neuromuscular block in awake volunteers. Br J Anaesth 2015;115(Suppl 1):i95–103.

31. Soehle M, Kayser S, Ellerkmann RK, et al. Bilateral bispectral index monitoring during and after electroconvulsive therapy compared with magnetic seizure therapy for treatment-resistant depression. Br J Anaesth 2014;112(4):695–702.

32. Viertiö-Oja H, Maja V, Särkelä M, et al. Description of the Entropy™ algorithm as applied in the Datex-Ohmeda S/5™ Entropy Module. Acta Anaesthesiol Scand 2004;48(2):154–61.

33. Valjus M, Ahonen J, Jokela R, et al. Response Entropy is not more sensitive than State Entropy in distinguishing the use of esmolol instead of remifentanil in

patients undergoing gynaecological laparoscopy. Acta Anaesthesiol Scand 2006;50(1):32–9.

34. Takamatsu I, Ozaki M, Kazama T. Entropy indices vs the bispectral index for estimating nociception during sevoflurane anaesthesia. Br J Anaesth 2006;96(5): 620–6.

35. Ellerkmann RK, Liermann VM, Alves TM, et al. Spectral entropy and bispectral index as measures of the electroencephalographic effects of sevoflurane. Anesthesiology 2004;101(6):1275–82.

36. Bibian S, Zikov T, Dumont G, et al. Estimation of the anesthetic depth using wavelet analysis of electroencephalogram. 2001 conference proceedings of the 23rd annual international conference of the IEEE engineering in medicine and biology society. Istanbul, Turkey, October 25-28, 2001.

37. Görges M, West NC, Cooke EM, et al. Evaluating NeuroSENSE for assessing depth of hypnosis during desflurane anesthesia: an adaptive, randomized-controlled trial. Can J Anaesth Mar 2020;67(3):324–35. Une évaluation du moniteur Neuro-SENSE pour mesurer la profondeur de l'hypnose pendant une anesthésie au desflurane : une étude randomisée contrôlée adaptable.

38. Bresson J, Gayat E, Agrawal G, et al. A randomized controlled trial comparison of NeuroSENSE and bispectral brain monitors during propofol-based versus sevoflurane-based general anesthesia. Anesth Analg 2015;121(5):1194–201.

39. van Heusden K, Cooke E, Brodie S, et al. Effect of ketamine on the NeuroSENSE WAV(CNS) during propofol anesthesia; a randomized feasibility trial. J Clin Monit Comput 2020. https://doi.org/10.1007/s10877-020-00511-0.

40. Mashour GA, Avidan MS. Black swans: challenging the relationship of anaesthetic-induced unconsciousness and electroencephalographic oscillations in the frontal cortex. Br J Anaesth 2017;4:563–5.

41. Purdon PL, Sampson A, Pavone KJ, et al. Clinical electroencephalography for anesthesiologists: part I: background and basic signatures. Anesthesiology 2015; 123(4):937–60.

42. Barr G, Jakobsson JG, Owall A, et al. Nitrous oxide does not alter bispectral index: study with nitrous oxide as sole agent and as an adjunct to i.v. anaesthesia. Br J Anaesth 1999;82(6):827–30.

43. Hirota K, Kubota T, Ishihara H, et al. The effects of nitrous oxide and ketamine on the bispectral index and 95% spectral edge frequency during propofol-fentanyl anaesthesia. Eur J Anaesthesiol 1999;16(11):779–83.

44. Ishiyama T, Oguchi T, Iijima T, et al. Ephedrine, but not phenylephrine, increases bispectral index values during combined general and epidural anesthesia. Anesth Analg 2003;97(3):780–4.

45. Akeju O, Pavone KJ, Westover MB, et al. A comparison of propofol- and dexmedetomidine-induced electroencephalogram dynamics using spectral and coherence analysis. Anesthesiology 2014;121(5):978–89.

46. Revuelta M, Paniagua P, Campos JM, et al. Validation of the index of consciousness during sevoflurane and remifentanil anaesthesia: a comparison with the bispectral index and the cerebral state index. Br J Anaesth 2008;101(5):653–8.

47. Kim YS, Won YJ, Jeong H, et al. A comparison of bispectral index and entropy during sevoflurane anesthesia induction in children with and without diplegic cerebral palsy. Entropy (Basel) 2019;21(5):498.

48. Sudhakaran R, Makkar JK, Jain D, et al. Comparison of bispectral index and end-tidal anaesthetic concentration monitoring on recovery profile of desflurane in patients undergoing lumbar spine surgery. Indian J Anaesth 2018;62(7):516–23.

49. Han SS, Han S, Kim BG, et al. The concentration of desflurane preventing spectral entropy change during surgical stimulation: a prospective randomized trial. J Clin Anesth 2017;37:86–91.

50. Kreuer S, Bruhn J, Larsen R, et al. Comparability of Narcotrend index and bispectral index during propofol anaesthesia. Br J Anaesth Aug 2004;93(2):235–40.

51. Mahon P, Kowalski RG, Fitzgerald AP, et al. Spectral entropy as a monitor of depth of propofol induced sedation. J Clin Monit Comput 2008;22(2):87–93.

52. Egan TD, Minto CF, Hermann DJ, et al. Remifentanil versus alfentanil: comparative pharmacokinetics and pharmacodynamics in healthy adult male volunteers. Anesthesiology 1996;84(4):821–33.

53. Kim HT, Heo HE, Kwon YE, et al. Effect of remifentanil on consumption of sevoflurane in entropy monitored general anesthesia. Korean J Anesthesiol 2010; 59(4):238–43.

54. Sakai T, Singh H, Mi WD, et al. The effect of ketamine on clinical endpoints of hypnosis and EEG variables during propofol infusion. Acta Anaesthesiol Scand 1999; 43(2):212–6.

55. Hans P, Dewandre PY, Brichant JF, et al. Comparative effects of ketamine on Bispectral Index and spectral entropy of the electroencephalogram under sevoflurane anaesthesia. Br J Anaesthr 2005;94(3):336–40.

56. Park HS, Kim YS, Kim SH, et al. Comparison of electroencephalogram between propofol- and thiopental-induced anesthesia for awareness risk in pregnant women. Sci Rep 2020;10(1):6192.

57. Gencer M, Sezen O. A study comparing the effect of premedication with intravenous midazolam or dexmedetomidine on ketamine-fentanyl sedoanalgesia in burn patients: a randomized clinical trial. Burns 2021;47(1):101–9.

58. Jeon S, Lee HJ, Do W, et al. Randomized controlled trial assessing the effectiveness of midazolam premedication as an anxiolytic, analgesic, sedative, and hemodynamic stabilizer. Medicine (Baltimore) 2018;97(35):e12187.

59. Kumar NRR, Jonnavithula N, Padhy S, et al. Evaluation of nebulised dexmedetomidine in blunting haemodynamic response to intubation: a prospective randomised study. Indian J Anaesth 2020;64(10):874–9.

60. Messner M, Beese U, Romstöck J, et al. The bispectral index declines during neuromuscular block in fully awake persons. Anesth Analg 2003;97(2):488–91, table of contents.

61. Xing Y, Xu D, Xu Y, et al. Effects of neuromuscular blockages on entropy monitoring during sevoflurane anesthesia. Med Sci Monit 2019;25:8610–7.

62. Christ B, Guerci P, Baumann C, et al. Influence of neuromuscular block and reversal on bispectral index and NeuroSense values. Eur J Anaesthesiol 2014; 31(8):437–9.

63. Anderson RE, Jakobsson JG. Entropy of EEG during anaesthetic induction: a comparative study with propofol or nitrous oxide as sole agent. Br J Anaesth 2004;92(2):167–70.

64. Spijkerman S, Smith FJ, Becker PJ. Effect of nitrous oxide on spectral entropy during sevoflurane anaesthesia at an altitude of 1 400 metres. South Afr J Anaesth Analgesia 2007;13(2):46.

65. Ozcan MS, Ozcan MD, Khan QS, et al. Does nitrous oxide affect bispectral index and state entropy when added to a propofol versus sevoflurane anesthetic? J Neurosurg Anesthesiol 2010;22(4):309–15.

66. Hans P, Dewandre PY, Brichant JF, et al. Effects of nitrous oxide on spectral entropy of the EEG during surgery under balanced anaesthesia with sufentanil and sevoflurane. Acta Anaesthesiol Belg 2005;56(1):37–43.

67. Ben-Menachem E, Zalcberg D. Depth of anesthesia monitoring: a survey of attitudes and usage patterns among Australian anesthesiologists. Anesth Analg 2014;119(5):1180–5.
68. of AS, Anesthesiologists Task Force on Intraoperative Awareness. Practice advisory for intraoperative awareness and brain function monitoring: a report by the american society of anesthesiologists task force on intraoperative awareness. Anesthesiology 2006;104(4):847–64.
69. American Society of Anesthesiologists- Committee on Standards and Practice Parameters. Standards for basic anesthetic monitoring. Available at: https://www.asahq.org/standards-and-guidelines/standards-for-basic-anesthetic-monitoring. Accessed January 18, 2021.
70. Deem S, Souter MJ. B-Aware: recall of intraoperative events. Lancet 2004;9437: 840–1 [author reply: 841–2].
71. Avidan MS, Zhang L, Burnside BA, et al. Anesthesia awareness and the bispectral index. N Engl J Med 2008;358(11):1097–108.
72. Avidan MS, Jacobsohn E, Glick D, et al. Prevention of intraoperative awareness in a high-risk surgical population. N Engl J Med 2011;365(7):591–600.
73. Lewis SR, Pritchard MW, Fawcett LJ, et al. Bispectral index for improving intraoperative awareness and early postoperative recovery in adults. Cochrane Database Syst Rev 2019;9(9):Cd003843.
74. Mashour GA, Shanks A, Tremper KK, et al. Prevention of intraoperative awareness with explicit recall in an unselected surgical population: a randomized comparative effectiveness trial. Anesthesiology 2012;117(4):717–25.
75. Liu S. Effects of bispectral index monitoring on ambulatory anesthesia: a meta-analysis of randomized controlled trials and a cost analysis. Anesthesiology 2004;101:311–5.
76. Radtke FM, Franck M, Lendner J, et al. Monitoring depth of anaesthesia in a randomized trial decreases the rate of postoperative delirium but not postoperative cognitive dysfunction. Br J Anaesth 2013;110(Suppl 1):i98–105.
77. Chan MT, Cheng BC, Lee TM, et al. BIS-guided anesthesia decreases postoperative delirium and cognitive decline. J Neurosurg Anesthesiol 2013;25(1):33–42.
78. Whitlock EL, Torres BA, Lin N, et al. Postoperative delirium in a substudy of cardiothoracic surgical patients in the BAG-RECALL clinical trial. Anesth Analg 2014;118(4):809–17.
79. Punjasawadwong Y, Chau-In W, Laopaiboon M, et al. Processed electroencephalogram and evoked potential techniques for amelioration of postoperative delirium and cognitive dysfunction following non-cardiac and non-neurosurgical procedures in adults. Cochrane Database Syst Rev 2018;5(5):Cd011283.
80. Wildes TS, Mickle AM, Ben Abdallah A, et al. Effect of electroencephalography-guided anesthetic administration on postoperative delirium among older adults undergoing major surgery: the ENGAGES randomized clinical trial. JAMA 2019;321(5):473–83.
81. Fritz BA, King CR, Ben Abdallah A, et al. Preoperative cognitive abnormality, intraoperative electroencephalogram suppression, and postoperative delirium: a mediation analysis. Anesthesiology 2020;132(6):1458–68.
82. Shortal BP, Hickman LB, Mak-McCully RA, et al. Duration of EEG suppression does not predict recovery time or degree of cognitive impairment after general anaesthesia in human volunteers. Br J Anaesth 2019;123(2):206–18.
83. Short TG, Campbell D, Frampton C, et al. Anaesthetic depth and complications after major surgery: an international, randomised controlled trial. Lancet 2019; 394(10212):1907–14.

84. Zhang C, Xu L, Ma YQ, et al. Bispectral index monitoring prevent awareness during total intravenous anesthesia: a prospective, randomized, double-blinded, multi-center controlled trial. Chin Med J (Engl) 2011;124(22):3664–9.
85. Nasraway SS Jr, Wu EC, Kelleher RM, et al. How reliable is the Bispectral Index in critically ill patients? A prospective, comparative, single-blinded observer study. Crit Care Med 2002;30(7):1483–7.
86. Fraser GL, Riker RR. Bispectral index monitoring in the intensive care unit provides more signal than noise. Pharmacother 2005;25(5 Pt 2):19s–27s.
87. Karamchandani K, Rewari V, Trikha A, et al. Bispectral index correlates well with Richmond agitation sedation scale in mechanically ventilated critically ill patients. J Anesth 2010;24(3):394–8.
88. Sharma A, Singh PM, Trikha A, et al. Entropy correlates with Richmond Agitation Sedation Scale in mechanically ventilated critically ill patients. J Clin Monit Comput 2014;28(2):193–201.
89. Shetty RM, Bellini A, Wijayatilake DS, et al. BIS monitoring versus clinical assessment for sedation in mechanically ventilated adults in the intensive care unit and its impact on clinical outcomes and resource utilization. Cochrane Database Syst Rev 2018;2(2):Cd011240.
90. Ebtehaj M, Yaqubi S, Seddighi AS, et al. Correlation between BIS and GCS in patients suffering from head injury. Irish J Med Sci 2012;181(1):77–80.
91. Li S, Fei Z, Zhang J, et al. Bispectral index values are accurate diagnostic indices correlated with glasgow coma scale scores. J Neurosci Nurs 2019;51(2):74–8.
92. Seder DB, Dziodzio J, Smith KA, et al. Feasibility of bispectral index monitoring to guide early post-resuscitation cardiac arrest triage. Resuscitation 2014;85(8):1030–6.
93. Musialowicz T, Mervaala E, Kälviäinen R, et al. Can BIS monitoring be used to assess the depth of propofol anesthesia in the treatment of refractory status epilepticus? Epilepsia 2010;51(8):1580–6.
94. Beekoo D, Yuan K, Dai S, et al. Analyzing Electroencephalography (EEG) waves provides a reliable tool to assess the depth of sevoflurane anesthesia in pediatric patients. Med Sci Monit 2019;25:4035–40.
95. Bhardwaj N, Yaddanapudi S. A randomized trial of propofol consumption and recovery profile with BIS-guided anesthesia compared to standard practice in children. Paediatr Anaesth 2010;20(2):160–7.
96. Sargin M, Uluer MS, Ozmen S. The effects of bispectral index monitoring on hemodynamics and recovery profile in developmentally delayed pediatric patients undergoing dental surgery. Paediatr Anaesth 2015;25(9):950–5.
97. Faulk DJ, Twite MD, Zuk J, et al. Hypnotic depth and the incidence of emergence agitation and negative postoperative behavioral changes. Paediatr Anaesth 2010;20(1):72–81.
98. Frederick HJ, Wofford K, de Lisle Dear G, et al. A randomized controlled trial to determine the effect of depth of anesthesia on emergence agitation in children. Anesth Analg 2016;122(4):1141–6.

Intraoperative Nociception Monitoring

Harsha Shanthanna, MD, FRCPC, PhD[a],*, Vishal Uppal, MBBS, FRCA, MSc[b],
Girish P. Joshi, MBBS, MD, FFARCSI[c]

KEYWORDS

- Nociception • Monitoring • Opioid use • Surgical pain

KEY POINTS

- Nociception refers to the process of encoding and processing noxious stimuli. Under the state of general anesthesia, a patient cannot feel pain. However, nociceptive signals are generated in the periphery and reach the central nervous system.
- Nociception can lead to autonomic effects in the form of variability in the heart rate, blood pressure, skin permeability; reflex movements; and increased stress response.
- Nociception monitoring can have several potential benefits during surgery.
- Available nociception monitoring systems depend on the identification and measurement of indirect effects of nociception. Depending on the type of input and technology, available monitors are based on algorithms, and the output is usually a signal between a range of dimensionless values, interpreted to indicate nociception-antinociception balance.
- Among the available technologies, Surgical Pleth Index (SPI) has been more widely studied. Although some studies indicate decreased opioid use, it is not consistent, and the decrease in opioids may not be clinically relevant.
- Despite advances in nociception monitoring technology and availability, their limitations presently override their benefits in routine anesthesia care.

NOCICEPTION AND PAIN AND THEIR RELEVANCE TO THE STATE OF ANESTHESIA

Nociception refers to the neural process of encoding and processing noxious stimuli,[1] whereas pain is a perceptual experience in a conscious individual as a result of information resembling actual or potential tissue damage.[2] The concept of anesthesia does not have a set definition. The term anesthesia was coined by Sir Oliver Wendell Holmes (1846) to describe the state that renders a patient insensible to the trauma of surgery. Presently, most agree that the concept of balanced anesthesia includes three

[a] Department of Anesthesia, and Department of Health Research Methods, Evidence and Impact, McMaster University, 1280 Main Street West, Hamilton, Ontario L8S 4K1, Canada; [b] Department of Anesthesia, Dalhousie University, Nova Scotia Health Authority and IWK Health Centre, 5th Floor, Halifax Infirmary Site, Room 5452, 1796 Summer Street, Halifax B3H 3A7, Canada; [c] The University of Texas Southwestern Medical Center, 5323 Harry Hines Boulevard, Dallas, TX 75390-9068, USA
* Corresponding author.
E-mail address: shanthh@mcmaster.ca

Anesthesiology Clin 39 (2021) 493–506
https://doi.org/10.1016/j.anclin.2021.03.008   **anesthesiology.theclinics.com**
1932-2275/21/© 2021 Elsevier Inc. All rights reserved.

components: (1) unconsciousness, (2) immobility, and (3) antinociception.[3] Effectively, it aims to produce amnesia (lack of recall) and hypnosis (being unaware), and lack of response to nociceptive stimuli and its consequent effects.[4] Because an individual is unconscious, the perception of pain is absent, but nociceptive signals can continue to be registered with consequent physiologic reactions. Besides the dimension of consciousness, pain can exist without nociception (perceived damage) and all nociception need not result in pain (many wounded soldiers experience no pain despite nociceptive signals).[5] This differentiation becomes necessary to appreciate when one considers surgery under general anesthesia (GA) versus only regional anesthesia (presence of conscious state) or sedation.

PHYSIOLOGY OF NOCICEPTION AND ITS EFFECTS

Like any other sensory modality, nociception is initiated by specific receptors called nociceptors. There is clear evidence of distinct classes of nociceptors activated by noxious stimuli in humans, which include extremes of temperature, intense pressure, and chemicals signaling potential or actual tissue damage, such as during inflammation or injury. The nociceptive information is encoded as all or none action potentials in the periphery that gets transmitted to higher centers in specific neural pathways, depending on the frequency of action potentials and temporal summation of synaptic signals. Signals are carried by Aδ fibers, myelinated with velocities of 5 to 30 m/s, for fast-onset pain and small-diameter C fibers, unmyelinated with velocities of 0.4 to 1.4 m/s, for dull or visceral pain. The primary neuron with its cell body in the dorsal root ganglia ends in levels I, II, and V of the spinal dorsal horn.[3] The second-order neuron projects up within the anterolateral spinothalamic tract to synapse at the level of the thalamus with the third-order neurons. Signals from this level project to somatosensory and anterior cingulate cortices to provide sensory-discriminative and affective-cognitive aspects of pain, respectively. Third-order neurons also connect with structures within the medulla, midbrain, amygdala, and hypothalamus.[3] Signal transmission at all synaptic connections within the central nervous system are modulated by descending facilitatory and inhibitory circuits. Although the quantification is challenging, the presence of nociception as nociceptive activity registered within the central nervous system is captured directly using electromyography (EMG) for spinal reflex responses, and cortical responses using functional MRI, along with the recording of somatosensory evoked potentials (SSEP) and electroencephalography (EEG). However, as we explain later, the commonly used monitoring approach involves measuring the effects of nociception (reactions) and not direct nociception. Because many of these effects are potentially influenced by factors other than nociception under GA, their responses may not be directly proportional to the degree of nociception. There is also evidence to suggest that despite the administration of clinically sufficient doses of opioids, nociceptor activation may persist under GA, although their clinical effects may be abolished.[6] This not only has implications for the measurement and interpretation of nociceptive signals in clinical practice but potentially also for the influence of intraoperative nociception on the persistence of pain after surgery.

EFFECTS OF NOCICEPTION THAT FORM THE BASIS OF NOCICEPTIVE MONITORING

The effects of noxious stimulation on the physiologic systems of a patient broadly include somatic, autonomic, neuroendocrine, and stress responses (**Table 1**).[3] These responses are involuntary and are used as surrogate responses to indicate nociception. Although muscle relaxation is not an expected requirement of every anesthetic, muscle relaxants are routinely administered to facilitate surgery, and this, in turn, interferes with the ability to infer antinociception using movements or respiratory changes. Most of these changes are as a result of increase in sympathetic activity or the corresponding decrease in parasympathetic tone. If not controlled, they result in increases in heart rate, blood pressure, cold and sweaty hands, dilated pupils, and an increase in galvanic skin conductance. With appropriate technology and assessment, one can observe changes in these variables, apart from changes to EEG and EMG patterns. However, the same variables can also be used to indicate the depth of anesthesia, such as using PRST (P [systolic blood pressure], R [heart rate], S [sweating], and T [tears]) scores.[7,8] In addition, other factors can also influence the observed clinical responses. Studies have indicated that arousal and emotional state can variably affect or modulate levels of nociception and pain. Under GA, patient, surgical, and drug factors could play a role.[9,10] Patients on β-blockers, older patients, and those with a pacemaker may demonstrate no significant tachycardia; blood loss caused by surgery may result in tachycardia, and deep inhalation anesthesia can cause bradycardia. An ideal nociceptor monitor should have the following characteristics: (1) to be able to objectively and unambiguously distinguish patients having signs of nociception versus those without; (2) reflect changes in the noxious stimulation, presence, and also a graded effect on the measurement of nociception; and (3) react to changes in the level of analgesic effect of a drug or technique in the presence of a standard stimulus.

BENEFITS OF NOCICEPTIVE MONITORING

Nociceptive monitoring could have several benefits for clinical and research purposes, within and outside of the operating room.

1. Measurement of antinociception can allow titrated doses of drug administration and achievement of nociception-antinociception balance. This becomes especially

Table 1
Effects of nociception and their use in monitoring technology

Effects of Nociception	Monitoring Technology
A. Somatic	
Motor: movements[a]	Nociceptive flexion response
Sensory: information relayed to CNS	Cortical recordings
B. Autonomic	
Breathing: tachycardia[a]	Heart rate variability with respiration
Hemodynamic: increased heart rate, blood pressure	NoL, ANI
Sudomotor: sweating, skin conductance changes	Skin conductance
Pupillary changes	Pupillometry
Neuroendocrine: increased stress response	Surgical Stress Index

Abbreviations: ANI, Analgesia Nociception Index; CNS, central nervous system; NoL, Nociception Level Index.
[a] These changes are influenced by administration of muscle relaxants.

relevant with paradigms of opioid-minimizing anesthesia and reducing opioid-related side effects.[11]

2. Nociceptive monitoring could be useful for the development and use of automated closed loop multimodal anesthesia systems in the future.

3. A better understanding of the link between intraoperative nociception levels and postoperative pain could allow for personalized medicine care pathways.

4. Nociceptive monitoring could be of benefit in noncommunicable states, other than GA, such as patients in the intensive care unit.[12]

5. Nociceptive monitoring could be used to study the effects of nontraditional analgesics (analgesic adjuncts), such as α_2 agonists (eg, dexmedetomidine), systemic magnesium, and systemic lidocaine.

6. Nociceptive monitoring could be used to assess effects of regional analgesic techniques particularly when the spread of sensory blockade does not necessarily reflect the analgesic effectiveness, such as novel fascial plane blocks.

7. The complex and differential effects of placebo and affective states on pain and nociception can be assessed and better understood.

8. Nociception monitoring can potentially help to better understand the influence of acute surgical pain and its intensity on persistent postsurgical pain.

UNDERSTANDING THE AVAILABLE NOCICEPTIVE MONITORING TECHNOLOGIES AND THEIR APPLICABILITY DURING SURGERY

There have been numerous devices developed to measure nociception and to be used specifically in patients under GA. The absence of a gold standard makes the assessment of the efficacy of each of these monitors challenging. For this review, we discuss some of the commercially available devices.[12] These devices are classified as monitors based on single parameters, two parameters, or multiple parameters. **Table 2** lists the names of these monitors, their mechanism of action, advantages, and disadvantages. The following section describes these monitors, their technology, and suggested application parameters. Besides the commercially available devices, there are reports of other scores or indexes that have not been extensively studied, such as the Clinical Signs–Stimulus–Antinociception score, which combines the clinical signs, remifentanil effect-site concentrations, and an approximate of the intensity of skin incision (stimulus).[13]

Single-Parameter Monitors

Analgesia Nociception Index
The Analgesia Nociception Index (ANI; MDoloris Medical Systems, Loos, France) system generally includes sensors applied to the chest wall to measure parasympathetic activity. The monitor produces a score ranging from 0 to 100 based on the area under the curve analysis of heart rate variability. A higher score indicates a parasympathetic response and, therefore, less nociception. It is one of the more extensively investigated approaches. However, the clinical studies have shown conflicting results regarding its efficacy in reducing postoperative pain and predicting hemodynamic changes during surgery. This may be caused by various factors affecting parasympathetic activity under GA. It seems to be ineffective in awake patients because of emotional influences and has only weak psychometric properties to detect pain in intensive care unit patients.[14]

Fluctuations in skin conductance
Fluctuations in skin conductance (MedStorm Innovation, Oslo, Norway) involves the application of sensors to the palm or sole. It is based on the principle that sympathetic

Table 2
Summary of common nociceptive monitoring technology published in literature

Technology	Mechanism of Action	Advantages	Disadvantages
Analgesic Nociception Index	Analysis of heart rate variability by sensors applied on chest wall	Easy to use Better studied than other monitors	Affected by factors affecting parasympathetic activity Conflicting results regarding its efficacy
Skin conductance	Changes in skin conductance of palm and sole with sympathetic stimulation	Easy to use	Affected by factors affecting parasympathetic activity May not be able to predict response to analgesics
Pupillometry	Pupillary diameter controlled by sympathetic and parasympathetic inputs	Noninvasive Some initial promising reports	Affected by depth of anesthesia and drugs Requires repeated eye opening and measurements
Polysynaptic reflex (withdrawal reflex), R-III threshold	A polysynaptic spinal withdrawal reflex at biceps femoris in response to nociceptive stimulation of sural nerve	Independent of autonomic influences	Predictive value for withdrawal reaction not better than BIS
Cardiovascular Depth of Analgesia Index	This monitor is based on the principle that the nociceptive stimulus depresses the cardiac baroreflex via subcortical structures	Noninvasive Possibly reduces clinically unpredictable movements	Limited comparative data available on this technique
Surgical Pleth Index, previously called Surgical Stress Index	A finger probe measures pulse wave amplitude (peripheral autonomic tone) and heartbeat interval (cardiac autonomic tone)	Easy to use, no consumables Evidence suggests it lowers opioid consumption and shorter times to tracheal extubation	No widely accepted cutoff threshold values
qNOX	Analysis of EEG and EMG using mathematical models	Single forehead monitor measures depth and nociception Independent of autonomic influences	Limited data on its efficacy
Composite Variability Index	Frontal EEG electrodes are used to measure variability of the BIS and EMG measured	Limited information available	Limited information available

(continued on next page)

Table 2 (continued)			
Technology	Mechanism of Action	Advantages	Disadvantages
Nociception Level Index	A finger probe measures parameters from multiple different information sources including photoplethysmogram, skin conductance, skin conductance fluctuation, heart rate, and heart rate variability	Easy to use Uses multiple parameters to provide guidance Initial studies show promising results	Limited data on its efficacy

Abbreviations: BIS, Bispectral Index.

stimulation leads to rapid changes in the water permeability of the excreting ducts, affecting skin conductance. This technology has been used in lie detection tests. An increase in the number of skin conductance fluctuations per second of more than 0.2 units is associated with severe pain or nociception. Considering that several factors, such as depth of anesthesia, affect the sympathetic response under GA, this method's clinical value has been questioned. Intraoperative opioid use did not reduce skin conductance in a study indicating that this method may respond to nociception but not antinociception interventions.[15]

Pupillometric assessment of nociception
The currently available pupillometer (AlgiScan, IDMed, Marseille, France) is a portable device with a sterilizable eyepiece that requires intermittent measurement with an open eye. It measures pupil diameter using infrared rays as the extent of pupillary reflex dilation (PRD) for an electric nociceptive stimulus. The device is based on the principle that sympathetic and parasympathetic inputs control the pupillary diameter. Studies that have used this technique have considered the change from baseline in the PRD and typically an increase of greater than 30% as a sign of nociception stimulation needing analgesic.[16] These findings require further confirmation. This technique's downside is that the index is affected by medications used intraoperatively and the need for repeated measurement.

Nociceptive flexion reflex threshold
In the nociceptive flexion reflex (NFR) threshold method (also known as RIII reflex; NFTS Paintracker, Dolosys, Berlin, Germany), transcutaneous electrical stimulation is applied at the lateral malleolus to stimulate nociceptive afferents of the sural nerve. The EMG electrodes at the ipsilateral biceps femoris measure the polysynaptic spinal withdrawal reflex. The mechanism of action of this technique is independent of sympathetic and parasympathetic stimulation. A higher intensity of electrical stimulation required at the sural nerve to elicit spinal withdrawal reflex indicates increased analgesia or antinociception. In theory, this technique may predict sudden movement as a result of a noxious stimulus. However, a study found that the NFR threshold had a lower predictive value for withdrawal reaction under GA when compared with the bispectral index (BIS), thus limiting its clinical utility.[17] Recently, the NRF model has been revised to improve predictability.[18]

Cardiovascular depth of analgesia

The cardiovascular depth of analgesia monitor (CARDEAN) index (Alpha-2, Lyon, France) is based on the principle that the nociceptive stimulus depresses the cardiac baroreflex via subcortical structures.[19] A nociceptive stimulus generally causes transient tachycardia and hypertension. If analgesia is adequate, baroreflex-mediated bradycardia (longer R-R interval) follows hypertension. Whereas, if antinociception is not adequate, the hypertension is followed by tachycardia (short R-R interval). This index (0%–100%) measures the degree of inhibition of the baroreflex caused by an inadequate antinociception using systolic blood pressure and R-R interval. CARDEAN value of less than 60 indicates little or no nociception, and CARDEAN value of more than or equal to 60 indicates nociception. The calculation of the index number is based on the area under the curve for the R-R interval. Although there are limited comparative data available on this technique, a study found that when used along with a BIS monitor, CARDEAN-guided opioid administration was associated with a reduction of clinically unpredictable movements in unparalyzed patients undergoing colonoscopy.[20]

Two-Parameter Monitors

Surgical Pleth Index

Initially developed as Surgical Stress Index, Surgical Pleth Index (SPI; General Electric Healthcare, Helsinki, Finland) is measured using a proprietary oxygen saturation (SpO$_2$) finger probe and does not require any consumables. A 0 to 100 score is produced using the pulse wave amplitude (peripheral autonomic tone) and heartbeat interval (cardiac autonomic tone). The method, as described by the manufacturer, initially produces normalized heart rate and the plethysmographic amplitude to decrease interpatient variability and then computes a score based on normalized numbers. The manufacturer recommends aiming for a score of less than 50 intraoperatively as an indicator of adequate antinociception. However, there is considerable heterogeneity in the studies regarding the cutoff thresholds for the index and type of general anesthetic technique used. The output values are not considered useful for awake patients.

qNOX

This EEG/EMG-based monitor (qCON 2000 monitor, Fresenius Kabi, Mataro, Spain) is marketed as a "two monitoring solutions in one device, using one single sensor." The sensor is applied to the forehead like a BIS monitor. The display shows qCON and qNOX scores. The former is almost identical to a BIS index measuring the depth of anesthesia. In contrast, the latter is thought to measure nociception. The mathematical models used in qCON and qNOX are derived from the Adaptive Neuro-Fuzzy Inference System.[21] The output for qNOX display ranges from 0 to 99 values with less than 40 implying a low likelihood of movement in response to a noxious stimulus. A small study showed that the qCON and qNOX were different in the detection of loss of consciousness and loss of response to stimuli during induction and emergence from GA.[22] Similar to the NFR threshold, this system is independent of autonomic responses making it an attractive option. However, data on its efficacy are lacking. Studies have shown no association or correlation of qNOX with acute postsurgical pain soon after emergence.[23]

Composite Variability Index

The Composite Variability Index (CVI) is a weighted combination of BIS, sBIS (sBIS is the standard deviation of the BIS signal over the previous 3 minutes), and sEMG (standard deviation of the EMG over the previous 3 minutes). The resulting value ranges between 0 and 10; it is a dimensionless number with lower values indicating an ideal balance between nociception and antinociception. When BIS and CVI were used with differing remifentanil target site concentrations and BIS values, it was noticed that unstimulated CVI values were more representative of hypnotic depth, although CVI seemed to correlate with somatic responses.[24]

Multiparameter System

Nociception Level Index

The Nociception Level Index (NoL; Medasense, Ramat Gan, Israel) sensor is similar to the peripheral finger SpO_2 probe. The sensor uses multiple different information sources that include finger photoplethysmogram, skin conductance, skin conductance fluctuation, heart rate, and heart rate variability. These parameters are nonlinearly combined with the statistical technique random forest regression to produce a score that ranges from 0 to 100. The score value between 10 and 25 is recommended for titration when using this monitor.[25] The monitor's initial experience suggested that the NoL was a reliable measure of noxious stimulation and performed better than simple clinical measures.[26] A recent small study showed that compared with standard care, intraoperative remifentanil administration was lower in the NoL-guided group (mean difference, 0.039 μg/kg/min; 95% confidence interval [CI], 0.025 to 0.052 μg/kg/min; $P < .001$). Furthermore, the NoL group experienced less intraoperative hypotension (2 of 40 episodes vs 11 of 40 patients in the control group).[25] Although the initial reports on this technology are promising, the studies evaluating this technology have several limitations including investigators' conflicts of interests. Future independent assessments will determine if these differences translate into an improvement in any clinically meaningful outcomes.

REVIEW OF EXISTING LITERATURE
Intraoperative Nociceptive Monitoring Compared with Standard Care

So far, four different systematic reviews of randomized controlled trials have evaluated the existing evidence in using nociception monitoring technology compared with standard control for improving nociception-antinociception balance and in reducing opioid use. Gruenewald and Dempfle[27] reported seven trials that used three different modalities (CARDEAN, SPI, and ANI) of nociception monitoring. Despite the heterogeneity in the technique and outcomes reported, meta-analyses of included studies were performed. They observed a statistically significant decrease in movement events with no other differences for pain or opioid use, either during or after surgery. Won and colleagues[28] considered only trials evaluating the use of SPI versus standard care and included five trials. They noted significantly reduced intraoperative opioid use with SPI (standardized mean difference, −0.41; 95% CI, −0.70 to −0.11), and shortened emergence time by nearly 2 minutes. Jiao and colleagues[29] evaluated 10 studies. Although they pooled all studies together and observed statistically lower use of intraoperative opioid administration, statistical and clinical heterogeneity make these findings difficult to interpret. As a subgroup analysis, they also reported SPI guidance to reduce intraoperative opioid use as compared with standard care (standardized mean difference, −0.37; 95% CI, −0.57 to −0.18), but this was not observed with ANI.[29] In the most recent review, Meijer and colleagues[30] included 12 trials using five different techniques including SPI, ANI, NoL, CARDEAN, and pupillometry. Six of the included studies reported intraoperative opioid consumption as their primary outcome. Only SPI, used in six studies, was associated with an intraoperative opioid-sparing effect with a reduction of morphine by −0.06 mg/kg/h (95% CI, −0.12 to −0.00). Despite the small reduction in intraoperative opioid use studies have found similar or more opioid use in the postoperative period. In effect, there may be little overall benefit when one considers the entire perioperative period with regard to pain control or opioid use.

Nociceptive Monitoring Systems that Have Not Been Compared with Standard Care

We observe that there are other monitoring technologies that have been used in other studies that have never been compared with the standard care to establish their validity in being able to measure nociception and also help titrate the use of intraoperative opioid or analgesics. Ledowski and colleagues[31] tested skin conductance as a measure of sympathetic tone reflective of nociception. Although initial tests on the postoperative pain cohort indicated a correlation between pain intensity and the number of skin conductance fluctuations per second as the measure of skin conductance, subsequent studies have shown limited sensitivity and specificity in identifying patients with moderate or severe pain.[32] Compared with many other monitors, NFR does not depend on variables from the autonomic nervous system and relies on spinal reflex responses. Despite this difference, studies have indicated that predicting reflexes or movements may not be independent of the anesthetic or hypnotic depth.[33] von Dincklage and colleagues[34] compared the NFR, BIS, CVI, Noxious Stimulation Response Index (derived from drug effect-site concentrations), and also the calculated propofol/remifentanil effect compartment concentrations as predictors of movement and heart rate responses in 50 female subjects at laryngeal mask airway insertion and skin incision. For both these responses, NFR was better than any other modality for prediction.[34] Fascial muscle EMG activity has been used to study inadequate anesthetic depth or analgesia. Edmonds and colleagues[35] noted that high amplitude surface EMG could be observed in individuals under ketamine anesthesia or with inadequate analgesia. The amplitude of those surface EMGs decreased with opioid treatment; this was not consistently associated with lowered vigilance or analgesia, but they were predictive of opioid drug effects. Others have used such EMG signals to predict imminent arousal and the potential for decreased anesthetic depth.[36] Additionally, researchers have attempted to combine EEG signals with EMG signals to increase the specificity of nociception-related responses using signal data and combining them in linear and nonlinear measures.[36] Existing technology using such combined measures independent of autonomic signals includes CVI[24] and qNOX,[21] both of which have not been compared with the standard in a randomized controlled trial. NoL is the only multicomponent measure that has been studied for nociception monitoring and has been shown to be better at discriminating between noxious and nonnoxious stimulus and also to show a graded response,[37] including responses to opioids.[38]

Nociceptive Monitoring Using Direct Measure of Cortical Activity

Some studies have attempted to evaluate direct measures of nociceptive cortical activity. Schmidt and colleagues[39] compared remifentanil, propofol, and placebo in three double-blind sessions on healthy volunteers and observed for changes in the SSEPs and intracutaneous pain-evoked potentials. As expected, pain ratings were decreased by remifentanil and sedation ratings by propofol. Although early components of SSEPs were unaffected by medications, the amplitudes of the long latency SSEP components increased significantly with remifentanil, decreased with propofol, and remained unchanged with placebo. Untergehrer and colleagues[40] studied nociception-related evoked potentials in 60 healthy male volunteers, divided into four groups of 15 receiving subanesthetic but increasing concentrations of propofol, sevoflurane, remifentanil, and (s)-ketamine. They recorded neurophysiologic potentials separately during baseline and drug exposure, including midlatency auditory-evoked potentials (to assess levels of consciousness), visceral pain-evoked potentials generated by a bipolar electrode in distal esophagus, and contact heat-evoked potentials generated by contact heat applied to skin. Without any global suppression of cortical activity indicated by auditory-evoked potentials, the potentials for visceral pain-evoked potentials generated by a bipolar electrode in distal esophagus were decreased with increasing concentrations of propofol, sevoflurane, remifentanil, and (s)-ketamine. Liley and colleagues[41] separately analyzed the cortical state (a measure of cortical responsiveness) and cortical input (a measure of the magnitude of cortical input) with effect site measurement of propofol and remifentanil, using EEG data from a previously published study.[42] They observed that with increasing effect-site remifentanil concentration, cortical input decreased significantly with no such changes to cortical state, whereas the latter decreased with increasing effect-site concentration of propofol. These studies indicate that perhaps directly measuring the cortical evoked potentials and states allow one to establish the differential effects of drugs on the state of hypnosis and nociception.

Using Nociceptive Monitoring Technology in the Regional Blockade

In theory, measures of nociception can allow one to study the extent of afferent blockade from regional analgesia techniques. Huybrechts and colleagues[43] used PRD to assess the blockade of thoracic epidural in thoracotomy patients and observed that they were able to separate blocked segments from unblocked segments and that a PRD of 0.5 mm was predictive of the incomplete block and a PRD greater than 1 mm was highly predictive of an inadequate block. Similarly, PRD was used by Isnardon and colleagues[44] to assess blockade of popliteal sciatic nerve block, and by Duceau and colleagues[45] for evaluating thoracic paravertebral block. However, we did not come across any studies assessing the completeness of afferent sensory blockade with fascial plane blocks, which are known to have inherent inconsistencies in their blockade.

LIMITATIONS AND DISADVANTAGES

1. Because there is no gold standard, validation of a nociceptive monitor is difficult to achieve.
2. Depending on the input variables, a specific monitoring technology may be responsive to nociceptive inputs or antinociceptive inputs alone. Hence, this would be inadequate as a tool to measure the balance.
3. The use of pain response and its intensity to study the effects of nociception is inappropriate. Apart from the obvious differences in pain versus nociception, different kinds of stimulus to evoke pain can have differential responses to surrogate measures of nociception used in available technologies.
4. Despite attempts to use nociceptive monitoring application for its specific stated purpose, hypnotic and antinociceptive components of anesthesia are interconnected at some levels.[3] Either could have an effect on the other domain depending on the dose, quantity, type of stimulation, or the state of consciousness within the spectrum of unconscious to conscious.
5. Considering the inconsistent and small differences in intraoperative opioid reduction, the benefit of nociception monitoring for opioid-free or -sparing approaches is questionable.[11]
6. There is some evidence suggesting analgesic potential for vasoactive drugs, such as β-blockers.[46] Such administration of vasoactive agents for opioid sparing will directly interfere with the working of nociceptive monitoring, making it unreliable.
7. Although this is not well appreciated, there is differing understanding and expectations between abolishing/reducing nociceptive-induced effects versus actually

abolishing/reducing nociception. The premise of what is clinically relevant can be challenged.

SUMMARY

There have been significant advances in the understanding and development of nociception monitoring technology. However, significant limitations remain, including lack of consistency in effectively reducing opioid requirements or predicting acute postoperative pain. Hence, their applicability in present-day anesthesia care is uncertain and questionable. Future technologies might hold promise for truly personalized care with an automated closed-loop multimodal anesthesia system, which includes the component of hypnotic and analgesic balance for a patient.

CLINICS CARE POINTS

- Nociception refers to the process of encoding and processing noxious stimuli.
- Nociception can lead to effects on the autonomic nervous system, reflex movements, and increased stress response.
- Available nociception monitoring systems depend on the identification and measurement of indirect effects of nociception to indicate nociception-antinociception balance.
- Among the available technologies, Surgical Pleth Index (SPI) has been more widely studied.
- Despite advances in nociception technologies, their limitations presently override their benefits for routine use. Hence, their utility and applicability in present-day anesthesia care is uncertain.

DISCLOSURE

Girish Joshi has received honoraria from Baxter Pharmaceuticals and Pacira Pharmaceuticals. Harsha Shanthanna and Vishal Uppal have no financial or commercial conflicts of interest. No funding to disclose.

REFERENCES

1. Sneddon LU. Comparative physiology of nociception and pain. Physiology (Bethesda) 2018;33(1):63–73.
2. Raja SN, Carr DB, Cohen M, et al. The revised International Association for the Study of Pain definition of pain: concepts, challenges, and compromises. Pain 2020;161(9):1976–82.
3. Cividjian A, Petitjeans F, Liu N, et al. Do we feel pain during anesthesia? A critical review on surgery-evoked circulatory changes and pain perception. Best Pract Res Clin Anaesthesiol 2017;31(4):445–67.
4. Prys-Roberts C, Anesthesia. a practical or impractical construct? Br J Anaesth 1987;59(11):1341–5.
5. Beecher HK. Pain in men wounded in battle. Ann Surg 1946;123(1):96–105.
6. Lichtner G, Auksztulewicz R, Velten H, et al. Nociceptive activation in spinal cord and brain persists during deep general anaesthesia. Br J Anaesth 2018;121(1): 291–302.
7. Smajic J, Praso M, Hodzic M, et al. Assessment of depth of anesthesia: PRST score versus bispectral index. Med Arh 2011;65(4):216–20.

8. Evans JM, Bithell JF, Vlachonikolis IG. Relationship between lower oesophageal contractility, clinical signs and halothane concentration during general anaesthesia and surgery in man. Br J Anaesth 1987;59(11):1346–55.

9. Edwards L, Ring C, McIntyre D, et al. Increases in arousal are associated with reductions in the human nociceptive flexion reflex threshold and pain ratings. J Psychophysiology 2006;20(4):259–66.

10. Rhudy JL, Williams AE, McCabe KM, et al. Affective modulation of nociception at spinal and supraspinal levels. Psychophysiology 2005;42(5):579–87.

11. Shanthanna H, Ladha KS, Kehlet H, et al. Perioperative opioid administration: a critical review of opioid-free versus opioid-sparing approaches. Anesthesiology 2021;134(4):645–59.

12. Ledowski T. Objective monitoring of nociception: a review of current commercial solutions. Br J Anaesth 2019;123(2):e312–21.

13. Rantanen M, Yli-Hankala A, van Gils M, et al. Novel multiparameter approach for measurement of nociception at skin incision during general anaesthesia. Br J Anaesth 2006;96(3):367–76.

14. Chanques G, Tarri T, Ride A, et al. Analgesia nociception index for the assessment of pain in critically ill patients: a diagnostic accuracy study. Br J Anaesth 2017;119(4):812–20.

15. Ledowski T, Pascoe E, Ang B, et al. Monitoring of intra-operative nociception: skin conductance and surgical stress index versus stress hormone plasma levels. Anaesthesia 2010;65(10):1001–6.

16. Sabourdin N, Barrois J, Louvet N, et al. Pupillometry-guided intraoperative remifentanil administration versus standard practice influences opioid use: a randomized study. Anesthesiology 2017;127(2):284–92.

17. Jakuscheit A, Posch MJ, Gkaitatzis S, et al. Utility of nociceptive flexion reflex threshold and bispectral index to predict movement responses under propofol anaesthesia. Somatosens Mot Res 2017;34(2):139–44.

18. Jurth C, Dorig TM, Lichtner G, et al. Development, validation and utility of a simulation model of the nociceptive flexion reflex threshold. Clin Neurophysiol 2018; 129(3):572–83.

19. Nosaka S. Modifications of arterial baroreflexes: obligatory roles in cardiovascular regulation in stress and poststress recovery. Jpn J Physiol 1996;46(4):271–88.

20. Martinez JY, Wey PF, Lions C, et al. A beat-by-beat cardiovascular index, CARDEAN: a prospective randomized assessment of its utility for the reduction of movement during colonoscopy. Anesth Analg 2010;110(3):765–72.

21. Jensen EW, Valencia JF, Lopez A, et al. Monitoring hypnotic effect and nociception with two EEG-derived indices, qCON and qNOX, during general anaesthesia. Acta Anaesthesiol Scand 2014;58(8):933–41.

22. Melia U, Gabarron E, Agusti M, et al. Comparison of the qCON and qNOX indices for the assessment of unconsciousness level and noxious stimulation response during surgery. J Clin Monit Comput 2017;31(6):1273–81.

23. Ledowski T, Schmitz-Rode I. Predicting acute postoperative pain by the Qnox score at the end of surgery: a prospective observational study. Br J Anaesth 2020;124(2):222–6.

24. Sahinovic MM, Eleveld DJ, Kalmar AF, et al. Accuracy of the composite variability index as a measure of the balance between nociception and antinociception during anesthesia. Anesth Analg 2014;119(2):288–301.

25. Meijer FS, Martini CH, Broens S, et al. Nociception-guided versus standard care during remifentanil-propofol anesthesia: a randomized controlled trial. Anesthesiology 2019;130(5):745–55.

26. Martini CH, Boon M, Broens SJ, et al. Ability of the nociception level, a multiparameter composite of autonomic signals, to detect noxious stimuli during propofol-remifentanil anesthesia. Anesthesiology 2015;123(3):524–34.
27. Gruenewald M, Dempfle A. Analgesia/nociception monitoring for opioid guidance: meta-analysis of randomized clinical trials. Minerva Anestesiol 2017; 83(2):200–13.
28. Won YJ, Lim BG, Kim YS, et al. Usefulness of Surgical Pleth Index-guided analgesia during general anesthesia: a systematic review and meta-analysis of randomized controlled trials. J Int Med Res 2018;46(11):4386–98.
29. Jiao Y, He B, Tong X, et al. Intraoperative monitoring of nociception for opioid administration: a meta-analysis of randomized controlled trials. Minerva Anestesiol 2019;85(5):522–30.
30. Meijer FS, Niesters M, van Velzen M, et al. Does nociception monitor-guided anesthesia affect opioid consumption? A systematic review of randomized controlled trials. J Clin Monit Comput 2020;34(4):629–41.
31. Ledowski T, Bromilow J, Paech MJ, et al. Monitoring of skin conductance to assess postoperative pain intensity. Br J Anaesth 2006;97(6):862–5.
32. Ledowski T, Ang B, Schmarbeck T, et al. Monitoring of sympathetic tone to assess postoperative pain: skin conductance vs surgical stress index. Anaesthesia 2009;64(7):727–31.
33. Seitsonen ER, Korhonen IK, van Gils MJ, et al. EEG spectral entropy, heart rate, photoplethysmography and motor responses to skin incision during sevoflurane anaesthesia. Acta Anaesthesiol Scand 2005;49(3):284–92.
34. von Dincklage F, Correll C, Schneider MH, et al. Utility of nociceptive flexion reflex threshold, bispectral index, composite variability index and noxious stimulation response index as measures for nociception during general anaesthesia. Anaesthesia 2012;67(8):899–905.
35. Edmonds HL Jr, Couture LJ, Paloheimo MP, et al. Objective assessment of opioid action by facial muscle surface electromyography (SEMG). Prog Neuropsychopharmacol Biol Psychiatry 1988;12(5):727–38.
36. Melia U, Vallverdu M, Borrat X, et al. Prediction of nociceptive responses during sedation by linear and non-linear measures of EEG signals in high frequencies. PLoS One 2015;10(4):e0123464.
37. Edry R, Recea V, Dikust Y, et al. Preliminary intraoperative validation of the nociception level index: a noninvasive nociception monitor. Anesthesiology 2016; 125(1):193–203.
38. Renaud-Roy E, Stockle PA, Maximos S, et al. Correlation between incremental remifentanil doses and the nociception level (NOL) index response after intraoperative noxious stimuli. Can J Anaesth 2019;66(9):1049–61.
39. Schmidt GN, Scharein E, Siegel M, et al. Identification of sensory blockade by somatosensory and pain-induced evoked potentials. Anesthesiology 2007;106(4): 707–14.
40. Untergehrer G, Jordan D, Eyl S, et al. Effects of propofol, sevoflurane, remifentanil, and (S)-ketamine in subanesthetic concentrations on visceral and somatosensory pain-evoked potentials. Anesthesiology 2013;118(2):308–17.
41. Liley DT, Sinclair NC, Lipping T, et al. Propofol and remifentanil differentially modulate frontal electroencephalographic activity. Anesthesiology 2010;113(2): 292–304.
42. Ferenets R, Vanluchene A, Lipping T, et al. Behavior of entropy/complexity measures of the electroencephalogram during propofol-induced sedation: dose-dependent effects of remifentanil. Anesthesiology 2007;106(4):696–706.

43. Huybrechts I, Barvais L, Ducart A, et al. Assessment of thoracic epidural analgesia during general anesthesia using pupillary reflex dilation: a preliminary study. J Cardiothorac Vasc Anesth 2006;20(5):664–7.

44. Isnardon S, Vinclair M, Genty C, et al. Pupillometry to detect pain response during general anaesthesia following unilateral popliteal sciatic nerve block: a prospective, observational study. Eur J Anaesthesiol 2013;30(7):429–34.

45. Duceau B, Baubillier M, Bouroche G, et al. Pupillary reflex for evaluation of thoracic paravertebral block: a prospective observational feasibility study. Anesth Analg 2017;125(4):1342–7.

46. Gelineau AM, King MR, Ladha KS, et al. Intraoperative esmolol as an adjunct for perioperative opioid and postoperative pain reduction: a systematic review, meta-analysis, and meta-regression. Anesth Analg 2018;126(3):1035–49.

Cerebral Perfusion and Brain Oxygen Saturation Monitoring with

Jugular Venous Oxygen Saturation, Cerebral Oximetry, and Transcranial Doppler Ultrasonography

Georgia Tsaousi, MD, MSc, PhD[a], Alessio Tramontana, MD[b],
Farouk Yamani, MD[b], Federico Bilotta, MD, PhD[b],*

KEYWORDS

- Cerebral perfusion • Oxygen saturation monitoring
- Jugular venous oxygen saturation • Cerebral oximetry • Transcranial doppler

KEY POINTS

- Multimodal cerebral monitoring can provide real-time information on cerebral hemodynamics and oxygenation.
- Jugular bulb oxygen saturation provides a gross indicator of global cerebral perfusion, yet focal ischemic processes could not be detected accurately.
- Cerebral near-infrared spectroscopy (NIRS) gained clinical interest because of noninvasiveness, although several pitfalls and inaccuracies need critical appraisal.
- Current evidence concerning the impact of NIRS on outcomes as well as NIRS-based clinical management algorithms remains inconclusive.
- Transcranial Doppler ultrasonography sonography provides relevant perioperative information in patients at high risk for cerebral hyperperfusion, hypoperfusion, or embolization.

INTRODUCTION

Maintaining the integrity of brain function through oxygen delivery optimization is a pivotal objective of perioperative anesthetic management.[1] Shortages in blood supply, oxygen delivery, or metabolic substrate, as well as a combination of these factors, might result in brain performance failure; however, the brain remains one of the least

[a] Department of Anesthesiology and ICU, School of Medicine, Faculty of Health Sciences, Aristotle University of Thessaloniki, University Campus, 54124 Thessaloniki, Greece; [b] Department of Anesthesiology, Critical Care and Pain Medicine, Policlinico Umberto I, "Sapienza" University of Rome, viale del Policlinico 151, 00185 Rome, Italy
* Corresponding author.
E-mail address: bilotta@tiscali.it

Anesthesiology Clin 39 (2021) 507–523
https://doi.org/10.1016/j.anclin.2021.03.009
1932-2275/21/© 2021 Elsevier Inc. All rights reserved.

anesthesiology.theclinics.com

monitored organs during anesthesia.[2–5] Accumulating evidence indicates that in the perioperative period cerebral desaturation occurs relatively frequently.[3,4] Thus, monitoring of cerebral perfusion status may be useful for detecting and possibly correcting perioperative perturbations in oxygen supply or metabolic demand ratio and thus may hinder overt or subtle neurologic sequelae.

This article aims to outline the commonly used technologies for monitoring cerebral perfusion or oxygenation status: jugular bulb oxygen saturation (Sjo$_2$), near-infrared spectroscopy (NIRS), and transcranial Doppler ultrasonography (TCD).

DISCUSSION
Jugular Bulb Oximetry

Basic principles of technology

Sjo$_2$ monitoring constitutes a nonquantitative estimate of the balance between global cerebral oxygen delivery and utilization and, therefore, may serve as a clinical indicator of the adequacy of cerebral perfusion.[1,6] Under normal circumstances, cerebral blood flow (CBF) is coupled with the cerebral metabolic rate for oxygen; therefore, regional CBF is modified to meet tissue metabolic requirements.[1,2] The Sjo$_2$ monitoring relies on the principle that any oxygen delivery and supply mismatch affects cerebral oxygen extraction ratio and jugular venous oxygen saturation originally described by Gibbs and colleagues[7] in healthy volunteers.

Venous blood drainage from each hemisphere is performed predominantly through the ipsilateral internal jugular vein. Monitoring the oxygenation status of jugular bulb ipsilateral to the focal brain lesion might be considered a preferable choice to obtain valid readings. Cerebral venous drainage is characterized by extremely high interindividual variability, so the venous outflow representation of specific brain areas to a particular jugular bulb cannot be estimated accurately.[8,9] Hence, in patients with focal brain injuries, the more appropriate side for jugular bulb catheterization cannot be determined definitely (**Table 1**).[9]

Of importance, in individuals with no intracranial pathology, the Sjo$_2$ from either side serves as an estimate of global cerebral oxygenation status, considering that the values obtained in the normal brain represent the drainage of all regions of the brain and not only the ipsilateral ones.[13] On the contrary, in cases of brain pathology, the coupling of regional blood supply to metabolic demands is disturbed and thus a disagreement of bilateral Sjo$_2$ values typically is encountered.[14] From a technical perspective, Sjo$_2$ monitoring can be achieved by ultrasound-guided insertion of a catheter in the jugular bulb via retrograde cannulation of the internal jugular vein, while Sjo$_2$ determination can be accomplished either by intermittent blood sampling or continuously using a fiberoptic oximetry catheter.[1,6,8] Taking into account anatomic interindividual variability, proper catheter positioning should be ascertained by lateral cervical radiograph or angiographic catheterization of the jugular bulb.[9,15] The correctly positioned catheter tip should be above the second cervical vertebra and lie within a distance less than 2 cm from the upper margin of the jugular bulb. This practice is employed to eliminate the risk of falsely high Sjo$_2$ recordings, attributed to the substantial contamination with oxygen-rich blood from extracranial tissues drained by the facial vein and possibly from the inferior petrosal sinus, which are in close proximity to the jugular bulb.[15] Another source of contamination of a properly positioned catheter could be the rapid withdrawal of blood (faster than 2 mL/min), particularly when CBF is low.[16] Likewise, erroneous readings also could be obtained from the interference of wall artifacts when a fiberoptic catheter is used for continuous Sjo$_2$ monitoring (see **Table 1**).[15,17] Complications of jugular bulb cannulation are rare,

Table 1
Cerebral perfusion pressure monitoring during surgical procedures with an enhanced risk of neurologic injury

Technique	Advantages	Disadvantages	Normal Values	Thresholds for Intervention
Cerebral oxygenation				

Jugular venous oximetry	• Global, flow-weighted measure
	• Straightforward to perform
	• Easy to interpret
	• Real-time, continuous
	• High specificity
	• Low-cost monitoring in intermittent sampling
		• Invasive
		• Insensitive to regional ischemia
		• Low sensitivity
		• Inaccurate readings due to contamination from extracranial tissues
		  ○ Catheter not properly positioned
		  ○ Rapid blood withdrawal
		• Inaccurate readings due to wall artifacts
			Sjo_2 57.1%
			(95% CI, 52.3–61.1)[10]
				• $Sjo_2 \leq 44.7$% (95% CI, 36.5–53) risk of ischemic brain damage[10]
				• $Sjo_2 > 69.5$% (95% CI, 61.2–77.7) risk of hyperemia[10]

NIRS cerebral oximetry	• Noninvasive • Real-time, continuous • Assessment of regional • Cerebral tissue oxygenation • High spatial and temporal resolution • Valid also in nonpulsatile CBF	• Signals affected by extracranial blood and ambient light • Lack of standardization between • Commercial devices • Interindividual baseline variability dynamic error of readings • Ischemic thresholds not clearly defined	$rSco_2$ 70% ±6% (range 47%–83%)[11]	• <50%–60% absolute values or • >20% decrease compared with baseline[12]
Cerebral blood flow				

(continued on next page)

Table 1
(continued)

Technique	Advantages	Disadvantages	Normal Values	Thresholds for Intervention
Transcranial Doppler	• Noninvasive • Real-time, continuous	• Relative rather than absolute CBF • Operator dependent • Failure rate in 8% to 20% of TCD examinations; absent acoustic window • Inaccurate readings due to probe dislocation in 20% of continuous TCD examinations	Mean flow velocity • MCA 55 ±12 cm/s • ACA 50 ±11 cm/s • PCA 40 ±10 cm/s PI 1.1–1.5	• CBFV <60% to baseline—hypoperfusion • CBFV <80%—risk of stroke • PI >1.5—high resistance • PI <0.5—below normal resistance • Resistance index >0.8—high resistance
TCCD	Technically advanced and accurate tool	Inappropriate for prolonged continuous monitoring of CBF		Not determined

and no association with intracranial pressure (ICP) augmentation has been demonstrated.[10,14,16,17]

Data interpretation

Normal Sjo_2 determination remains a matter of controversy. Although relevant studies indicate Sjo_2 values of 57.1% as an average estimate of normal cerebral oxygenation status, the definition of the lower limit of normal Sjo_2 values is more challenging due to the high variability encountered among relevant studies (see **Table 1**).[8,16,18] In general terms, global cerebral hypoperfusion could be speculated at Sjo_2 readings below 55%.[9,10,19] Although this ischemic threshold has been identified repeatedly as a prognostic indicator of poor neurologic outcome, its validity has been questioned by several investigators.[8,15,18] In patients with head injuries, it has been shown that secondary brain damage occurs only when jugular bulb desaturation is below 45%.[20]

On the other hand, the presence of an elevated Sjo_2 is a heterogeneous condition, and Sjo_2 recordings greater than 75% should be regarded as a warning sign of eminent neurologic impairment.[6,16] Typically, high Sjo_2 values have been related to scenarios associated with arteriovenous shunting or disproportional excess of CBF and oxygen delivery relative to cerebral metabolic demands, leading to hyperemia.[6] It is advisable to interpret both the absolute values and trends of Sjo_2 within the clinical context of the individual patient.[1,6]

Clinical applications

In the perioperative clinical setting, Sjo_2 monitoring has been used for the optimization of cerebral oxygen delivery, mainly during surgical procedures incurring an augmented risk of postoperative neurologic morbidities, such as thoracic[19] or cardiovascular surgery.[8,21–24] Clinical evidence indicates that patients undergoing normothermic cardiopulmonary bypass (CPB) are at greater risk of cerebral desaturation and hypothermic CPB,[8] whereas jugular bulb desaturation occurs more frequently during off-pump compared with conventional coronary artery surgery (coronary artery bypass graft [CABG]).[23] This derangement of the cerebral oxygenation status, however, during off-pump CABG, which is induced by surgical displacement of the heart, seems to be transient and is reversed almost completely in the immediate postoperative period.[21,22] Moreover, Sjo_2 has been suggested as a useful physiologic marker for guiding the use of selective cerebral perfusion to enhance cerebral protection during aortic arch repair surgery.[25,26]

Yet, the association between jugular bulb desaturation during cardiac surgery and postoperative neurologic or neurocognitive sequelae, as well as the possible effect of Sjo_2-guided optimization of cerebral oxygen supply to metabolic demand ratio on neurologic outcomes, could not be demonstrated due to lack of robust evidence.[8,23,24]

Furthermore, only sparse data are available on the use of Sjo_2 for the detection of cerebral desaturation episodes in carotid artery endarterectomy (CEA),[27] major abdominal procedures,[28] or surgeries performed in beach chair position (BCP).[29] Due to the diversity of outcomes assessed, the role of Sjo_2 monitoring during noncardiac procedures could not be defined clearly.

Although Sjo_2 has been valued as a global, flow-weighted measure, incidents of critical regional ischemia might go undetected. Furthermore, it is characterized by low sensitivity and an enhanced risk of missing low saturation recordings. It is characterized, however, by high specificity and is considered a low-cost monitoring modality when intermittent sampling is applied (see **Table 1**). Sjo_2 monitoring was highly investigated and implemented into clinical practice for almost 4 decades, but thereafter the scientific interest declined sharply, and noninvasive technologies became a more attractive alternative for the estimation of cerebral oxygenation status.

Cerebral Oximetry

Basic principles of technology

Monitoring cerebral oximetry with NIRS technology provides an absolute and continuous measure of regional cerebral tissue oxygen saturation ($rSco_2$) in a region of interest, in a noninvasive manner.[1,2,5] The underlying concept of measuring oxygen saturation of hemoglobin in brain tissue was introduced by Frans Jöbsis in the late 1970s[30]; however, the first cerebral oximeters were commercially available no earlier than the 1990s.[31]

The NIRSs quantify the relative concentrations of oxyhemoglobin and deoxyhemoglobin within the target tissue through reliance on the transmission and absorption of near-infrared light as it passes through tissue, based on the modified Beer-Lambert law.[2,32] Thus, it may be viewed as an estimate of the balance between cerebral oxygen supply and demand.[2,32]

Extracranial blood constitutes a considerable source of error in $rSco_2$ measurements (see **Table 1**).[33] To offset this, newer NIRS technologies employ the spatially resolved spectroscopy technique by integrating into their sensors 2 closely spaced detectors (optodes) at a certain distance from the emitter (4–5 cm).[6,33] This arrangement enables the subtraction of signals received by the proximal detector from those received by the distal one, corresponding to photons reflected from superficial (skin and skull) and deeper tissue layers (brain), respectively.[34] Because the depth of photon penetration is related directly to the source-detector distance, the signal received by the distal detector penetrates the brain tissue at a depth of approximately 2 cm to 3 cm.[34,35] Thus, multidistance NIRS techniques refine the recorded oxyhemoglobin/deoxyhemoglobin signals, yielding more accurate estimates of cerebral oxygenation disturbances.[34,35]

When the adhesive sensors of the NIRS device are attached bilaterally on the forehead, the $rSco_2$ values represent the cerebral oxygen supply/demand in the so-called watershed area of the frontal cortex, supplied by the anterior and middle cerebral arteries (MCAs), a region of the brain susceptible to hypoxemia (see **Table 1**).[1,2,35]

The measurement of blood hemoglobin oxygen saturation is limited to the intravascular compartment (microvessels of a diameter <100 μm) and combines measures of arterial, venous, and capillary blood within the field of view, depending on the wavelengths of light and tissue, oxyhemoglobin, and deoxyhemoglobin.[1,2,35] It has been suggested that $rSco_2$ values obtained by NIRS devices are concordant with CBF variations when arterial oxygen saturation and cerebral oxygen consumption are constant and when the arterial-to-venous blood volume ratios remain stable.[1,2] In contrast to pulse oximetry, NIRS technology can receive signals from both pulsing and nonpulsing blood under the optodes and, therefore, can be used when there is nonpulsatile CBF, such as during CPB (see **Table 1**).[36]

Recent advances in NIRS technology include frequency (or domain)-resolved spectroscopy and time-resolved spectroscopy, which incorporate emission of intensity-modulated light and information on individual photon time of flight, to allow more accurate measurement of oxyhemoglobin/deoxyhemoglobin ratio as compared with continuous wave methods.[31]

Data interpretation

Cerebral oximetry readings principally reflect venous blood oxygenation, given the predominance of the venous system in circulating blood.[2] Consequently, most devices calibrated by the manufacturer assuming a fixed ratio of the contribution of 70% to 75% venous blood and 25% to 30% arterial blood to the signal, while the blood volume from the capillary network is neglected.[2,31] Nevertheless, this fixed ratio may be affected by individual variability, arterial blood contribution, changes in body position (such as Trendelenburg or beach chair), or hypoxia.[1,32,37] Over and above, the measured ratio of venous and arterial blood in brain tissue is approximately 50:50, implying that the assumptions about the constancy of arterial to venous blood volumes easily are violated.[38]

The normal $rSco_2$ values range between 58% and 82% (70% ±6%).[39] Clinical data acquired from healthy individuals subjected to tilting table maneuvers indicate that decrease of $rSco_2$ greater than 20% compared with baseline could induce loss of consciousness due to serious cerebral perfusion failure.[40] Likewise, absolute perioperative levels of $rSco_2$ below 50% to 60% have been linked to adverse neurologic outcomes and increased mortality (see **Table 1**).[11,41]

Nonetheless, the interdevice variability regarding sensor technology and mathematical algorithms used prohibit absolute $rSco_2$ value comparisons between commercially available devices, whereas interindividual baseline variability and dynamic error of readings render cerebral oximeters more suitable as trend monitors.[32] It is strongly recommended to interpret perioperative cerebral oximetry measurements in the context of the preinduction baseline value, patient-specific, and disease-specific characteristics as well as alterations of physiologic variables (see **Table 1**).[1]

Clinical applications
Cardiac surgery. Cardiac surgery incurs an enhanced risk of postoperative neurologic sequelae, eliciting symptoms ranging from minor disorders to major disabilities, or even death.[11,41] Low preoperative $rSco_2$ recordings have been linked to a higher probability of mortality, or postoperative delirium, implying that $rSco_2$ could serve as a preoperative risk stratification marker.[11,12]

Although NIRS technology, and NIRS-based algorithms have been adopted by cardiac surgery centers worldwide, current evidence concerning the impact of these practices on the modulation of cerebral morbidity and remote outcomes remains inconclusive, yet.[11,42–44] In the context of patient care optimization, 3 relevant meta-analyses failed to provide any evidence that personalized optimization of cerebral oxygenation by implementing NIRS-based algorithms or interventions could be beneficial to postoperative cognitive outcomes of adult cardiac surgery patients.[11,42,43] Over and above, damage to organs distant to the brain, such as the heart or kidneys, seems to remain unaffected by the improved overall perfusion using the brain as the index organ.[42] Likewise, a recent Cochrane review reported a lack of high-quality evidence to support any profound effect of active cerebral NIRS monitoring on postoperative nervous system injury, delirium, cognitive function deterioration, and death.[44]

Based on available evidence, only a weak recommendation regarding the implementation of intraoperative cerebral oximetry–guided interventional algorithm to reverse acute intraoperative cerebral perfusion deterioration and reduce the length of stay in the cardiosurgical care unit, could be supported.[45]

It is recommended, however, to use this technology in adult patients undergoing aortic arch surgery[1,45–47] and in the pediatric cardiac surgical population.[48] In aortic arch surgery, it has been shown that intraoperative cerebral desaturation higher than 80% of the baseline value was a major determinant of postoperative neurologic dysfunction, whereas cerebral saturation emerged as a strong predictor of major complications.[46,47]

Carotid artery endarterectomy. Emerging evidence in the vascular literature advocates the possible role of NIRS technology for cerebral ischemia monitoring during CEA, as a valid adjunct tool to the gold standard technologies in this area, namely TCD and electroencephalograph (EEG) monitoring.[32,49] Interpretation of EEG abnormalities might become a difficult task in the context of general anesthesia administration, whereas the routine use of EEG for lowering the incidence of intraoperative stroke could not be routinely recommended.[50] In the largest cohort study to date assessing the validity of NIRS and TCD compared with EEG to assess cerebral hypoperfusion requiring shunt placement during CEA under general anesthesia, a decrease of 16% in $rSco_2$ and of 48% in cerebral blood flow velocity (CBFV) had moderate positive predictive value but high negative predictive value for cerebral ischemia during CEA.[49] Therefore, these findings indicate that NIRS and TCD could be used independently to decrease the rate of unnecessary shunting. Nonetheless, TCD could not provide data on cerebral oxygenation and may not be useful in approximately 15% to 20% of patients with a poor temporal bone window.[50] This further emphasizes the importance of developing NIRS technology, which eventually could be applied as a single monitoring option to detect cerebral desaturation events during vascular surgery. Clinical trials in awake patients undergoing CEA have documented that a decline of regional brain oxygenation of 15% to 20% could detect the occurrence of cerebral ischemia.[51,52] The predictive value of NIRS-assessed cerebral oxygenation disturbances was comparable to that of stump pressure deterioration.[52]

In terms of outcome prognosis, a cohort study involving 466 patients subjected to CEA under general anesthesia, reported an association of $rSco_2$ deterioration of at least 20% during temporary internal carotid artery clipping with a 10-fold and 8-fold enhanced risk of ischemic stroke and postoperative cognitive dysfunction (POCD), respectively.[53] Moreover, baseline $rSco_2$ values lower than 50% promoted a 6-fold higher likelihood of ischemic stroke in the early postoperative period.[53]

Considering that hypoxemic stroke is a major contributor to postoperative morbidity and mortality, NIRS technology is potentially attractive monitoring during CEA, yet its application as a routine practice and its possible benefits are disputed.[32] Studies have not been powered sufficiently to determine the relationship between cerebral NIRS and stroke, while in current practice the use of shunting is left to the discretion of surgeons.

Beach chair surgery. Considering that hemodynamic compromise is a common consequence of the BCP, a profound deterioration of CBF and cerebral oxygenation is to be expected, further enhancing the risk of brain ischemia.[1] The average incidence of cerebral desaturation events during BCP as detected with NIRS ranges from 30% to 40%, and their onset is expected within 8 minutes after transitioning from a postinduction supine position to the BCP.[54] To date, no robust evidence exists to support the application of protocols designed to maintain cerebral perfusion, to minimize the risk of cerebral desaturation development, or to associate these events with a worsened neurologic outcome.[55,56] Thus, no clear recommendations of the routine use of NIRS monitoring in BCP surgery could be made.

High-risk noncardiac surgery. In elderly patients undergoing major abdominal surgery or arthroplasty procedures, changes of cerebral saturation were found significantly correlated with POCD, whereas NIRS-guided interventions modulated neurologic outcome in a favorable manner.[57,58] Although the underlying low-perfusion state and brain oxygen delivery deterioration can be inferred from cerebral oximetry, no robust evidence substantiates the routine use of cerebral NIRS technologies in the aforementioned surgical settings, to predict mortality or cerebral ischemia events implicated in long-term neurologic sequelae.

The main argument in favor of cerebral NIRS technology is its noninvasiveness. Nonetheless, several pitfalls, such as signal contamination by extracranial tissues and ambient light, the dependence of readings by the sample volume, and the lack of reference standard or index test to validate r $rSco_2$ values per se, should be appraised during data interpretation (see **Table 1**).[2]

Transcranial Doppler Ultrasonography

Basic principles of technology

Brain ultrasonography has been extensively implemented into clinical practice for approximately 4 decades for the bedside assessment of brain parenchyma, and cerebral hemodynamics, in a real-time, continuous, and noninvasive fashion.[59] This monitoring modality can be performed by either transcranial M-mode TCD or B-mode transcranial color-coded duplex (TCCD) ultrasound technology, through the 4 main acoustic windows (transtemporal, occipital, submandibular, and transorbital).[59] The temporal acoustic window constitutes the most common approach to the insonation of the basal cerebral arteries, such as the MCA, anterior cerebral artery (ACA), and posterior cerebral artery (PCA).[59–61] MCA is responsible for approximately 75% of CBF to 1 hemisphere, whereas its straight course to the doppler probe renders MCA a suitable candidate for continuous TCD monitoring.[59,60]

TCD employs 2-MHz ultrasound waves to determine CBFV in large cerebral vessels by examining the Doppler shift caused by red blood cells moving through the field of view, based on the spectral display and standard criteria, such as arterial depth, arterial blood flow direction, and waveform analysis.[5,60] The TCD waveform resembles an arterial pulse wave, because it encompasses peak systolic, end-diastolic, and mean components, all of which are used for the quantitative analysis of CBFV.[61] Mean CBFV could be considered an accurate estimate of CBF provided that vessel cross-sectional area and angle of insonation remain constant during the period of measurement, so it essentially measures relative changes rather than actual CBF.[61,62]

Aiming to enhance the validity of the gained information, several TCD-derived indices have been developed (see **Table 1**). In this context, the pulsatility index (PI), which represents the difference between systolic and diastolic flow velocities divided by the mean velocity, serves as a valid descriptor of distal cerebrovascular resistance.[62] Another useful parameter is the resistivity index, which represents flow resistance distal to the site of insonation and is calculated by subtracting diastolic from systolic flow velocity and dividing the value by systolic flow velocity.[59]

Based on the physiologic relationship between CBFV and pressure in cerebral vessels with compliant walls, an increase of ICP affects the CBFV waveform obtained by TCD, with low diastolic flow velocity, peaked waveform, and a higher PI constituting the most prominent markers of disturbed CBF.[63] Thereby, CBFV waveform analysis could aim to estimate noninvasive ICP (nICP). Existing evidence favors PI as a sensitive noninvasive surrogate of raised ICP—although its specificity is low—in cases of criteria for the institution of invasive ICP monitoring not met or the insertion of ICP catheter contraindicated.[64]

Over and above, advanced parameters of the cerebral circulation obtained from TCD signal processing, such as cerebral autoregulation (CA), noninvasive cerebral perfusion pressure (nCPP), critical closing pressure (CrCP), and cerebral compliance, have been studied extensively as markers of cerebral hemodynamics and cerebrovascular reactivity assessment in different intracranial pathologies.[59,62,63]

TCCD technology incorporates color-coded Doppler vessel representation in bidimensional pulsed-wave Doppler ultrasound imaging and enables visualization of the main cerebral structures and vessels and high-precision identification of the individual arteries of the circle of Willis. The duplex imaging systems can provide basic information regarding the 3 components of CBFV in an insonated artery as well as the PI.[59] Compared with conventional TCD, TCCD is a more technically advanced and accurate tool, yet it does not allow prolonged continuous monitoring of CBF (see **Table 1**).[59]

Data interpretation

Several physiologic factors, such as age, hematocrit, gender, fever, metabolic factors, pregnancy, menstruation, exercise, and brain activity, seem to affect CBFV. In detail, female gender, anemia, hypertension, and hypercapnia increase CBFV, whereas advanced age (>60 years) or pregnancy (third trimester) exerts an adverse impact on CBFV.[60]

Under normal circumstances, the highest mean flow velocity values are registered in MCA, followed by ACA and PCA (see **Table 1**).[59,60] A decrease in CBFV of more than 60% compared with baseline has been linked to hypoperfusion, whereas flow deterioration above 80% incurs an increased risk of perioperative stroke.[65] PI is independent of the angle of insonation, and a value of more than 1.5 represents high-resistance blood flow.[59] Any resistivity index value above 0.8, however, indicates increased downstream resistance (see **Table 1**).[60,64]

Limitations of TCD waveform analysis are (1) continuous monitoring is disturbed by artifacts caused by probe dislocation, in greater than 20% of the cases,[66] and (2) inappropriate evaluation of intracranial hemodynamic changes occurs in 8% to 20% of TCD examinations, due to the profound ultrasonic attenuation through the temporal window.[67]

Clinical applications

Cardiac surgery. Brain sonography can play a role in multimodal neurologic monitoring during cardiac surgery.[68] Periprocedural neurologic injury is attributed mainly to CBP-induced cerebral microemboli or cerebral hypoperfusion/hyperperfusion, in conjunction with CA impairment, calling for a more individualized hemodynamic management.[68,69] TCD technology has allowed accurate monitoring of cerebral perfusion during cardiac arrest,[68] low-flow CBP,[69-74] or off-pump CABG[71] as well as detection of improper cannulation or cross-clamping of aortic arch vessels.[68,70] The release of both air and solid emboli (ie, fat, clots, platelet aggregates, and atherosclerotic plaque material) could be identified by the ultrasonic characteristics of the embolus–blood interface in the form of high-intensity transient signals (HITSs).[72] Typically, TCD techniques reveal a large number of HITSs representing microparticles released during CBP, which might be implicated in neurologic morbidity.[70,72] Although the likelihood of stroke seems to be higher when solid embolic material enters the cerebral circulation, the impact of embolic signals on the pathogenesis of POCD remains debatable.[71-74] Considering that current TCD technology cannot discriminate between true emboli from false-positive artifacts or solid and air microemboli, the full effects related to HITSs counts on a patient's neurologic outcome would be milder than expected.[74]

Ensuring adequate cerebral perfusion pressure constitutes a top-priority in aortic arch surgery and procedural success depends on the efficacy of selective cerebral perfusion during hypothermic circulatory arrest.[69] Besides the detection of cerebral embolic microparticles, the use of brain ultrasonography in aortic arch surgery enables confirmation of the adequacy of selective cerebral perfusion strategy and timely intervention when it is jeopardized.[68–74]

Carotid artery endarterectomy. In the same fashion as cardiac surgery, CEA is complicated commonly by perioperative neurologic disturbances, caused by cerebral hypoperfusion after carotid cross-clamping or embolization secondary to atheromatous plaque disruption during the initial dissection phase.[75] Embolization is the predominant predisposing factor to intraoperative ischemic events (80%), whereas hemodynamic factors compromise cerebral perfusion in the minority of the CEA cases (80% and 20%, respectively), both of which can be detected reliably by TCD monitoring.[75]

A recent meta-analysis, including 25 studies in a total of 4705 patients, validated the efficacy of intraoperative TCD monitoring in predicting perioperative strokes after CEA.[75] The investigators reported a 4-times higher likelihood of changes involving MCA-CBFV or the presence of cerebral microembolic signals, in patients presenting an intraoperative stroke (4%) compared with nonstroke cases. Moreover, a Cochrane review[76] assessed the comparable efficacy of monitoring cerebral hemodynamics (TCD and carotid stump back pressure), cerebral oxygen metabolism (Sjo$_2$ and NIRS), or cerebral functional state (EEG and somatosensory evoked potentials) in CEA surgeries, in terms of selective shunting use and neurologic outcome optimization. No clear superiority of 1 form of monitoring over another could be demonstrated.

Beach chair surgery. Current literature lacks robust evidence on the use of TCD for the assessment of cerebral hemodynamics during BCP.[63,77,78] It has been reported that after the establishment of BCP CBFV in MCA declines by 22% ±7% (range 6%–33%), corresponding to mean arterial pressure deterioration varying between 22% and 52%.[77] More recently, a thorough assessment of cerebral hemodynamics using a multiparameter TCD-derived approach in patients undergoing shoulder surgery demonstrated a decreasing trend between positioning changes for MCA-CBFV (6%), nICP (29%), nCPP (12%), and CrCP (9%), with a concomitant increase of PI (11%).[63] Although the reported CBFV reduction in MCA during BCP is considerably lower compared with cerebral ischemia threshold (60%), it might be of utmost importance in patients with clinically overt or covert cerebrovascular disease, in whom the neurologic sequelae may be more catastrophic.[63]

High-risk noncardiac surgery. Surgical procedures performed in steep head-down positions and laparoscopic procedures necessitating the creation of a pneumoperitoneum might promote reduced venous return and consequent intracranial hypertension.[79,80] Existing studies substantiate the use of intraoperative TCD to identify CBF changes in such clinical settings, whereas optic nerve sheath diameter measurement has been suggested as an accurate estimate of ICP elevations during laparoscopy.[79,80] In patients subjected to major orthopedic surgery under general anesthesia, the use of TCD revealed a 600% increase of cerebral embolic load perioperatively, the nature of cerebral microembolism being primarily of gaseous origin.[81] TCD ultrasonography, when used in conjunction with bubble studies on transthoracic echocardiography, presents excellent sensitivity and specificity in quantifying the severity of right-to-left shunting (compared with transesophageal echocardiography)[82] or to screen patients before sitting-position craniotomy.[83] TCD has been used increasingly to assess changes in cerebral hemodynamics and to monitor subsequent ventriculoperitoneal shunt function in patients with hydrocephalus. PI has been shown to correlate well with the ventricular size and serve as a useful indicator of elevated ICP.[84]

TCD is reliable at detecting events of CBF deviations during surgical or anesthetic procedures, which incur an augmented risk for cerebral hyperperfusion or hypoperfusion, embolization, or their combined effects. Currently, TCD sonography has gained renewed interest due to the increasing experience especially with point-of-care ultrasound, and availability of more powerful ultrasound systems. Nonetheless, routine utilization of TCD is limited by the operator's level of experience and necessity of interpretation (see **Table 1**).[59,60,62]

SUMMARY

Considering the complexity of cerebral function and hemodynamics, it is not surprising that composite approaches toward intraoperative monitoring, that integrates combined measures of cerebral perfusion, oxygenation, and metabolic status, has gained impact on perioperative neurologic injury attenuation. Combining various monitoring modalities reflective of different aspects of cerebral perfusion status, such as NIRS, jugular bulb saturation, and TCD, may provide an extended window for the prevention, early detection, and prompt intervention in ongoing hypoxic/ischemic neuronal injury and, thereby, may improve neurologic outcome. Such an approach would minimize the impact of the inherent limitations of each monitoring modality, while individual components complement each other, thus enhancing the accuracy of the acquired information. Nonetheless, current literature has failed to demonstrate any clear-cut clinical benefit of these monitoring modalities on outcome prognosis or to validate goal-directed treatment protocols.

Technical advances are likely to lead to development of composite approaches toward intraoperative monitoring, because monitoring alone cannot define a patient's outcome. Future studies establishing goal-directed protocols urgently are needed.

CLINICS CARE POINTS

- Sjo_2 monitoring has been used for optimization of cerebral oxygen delivery but it is limited by its invasiveness and lamentable benefits.
- NIRS technology is potentially attractive monitoring during CEA, yet its application in routine clinical practice and its possible benefits are disputed.
- TCD sonography has widening clinical use because of the availability of point-of-care ultrasound and more powerful ultrasound systems.

DISCLOSURE

The authors have nothing to disclose.

REFERENCES

1. Scheeren TWL, Kuizenga MH, Maurer H, et al. Electroencephalography and brain oxygenation monitoring in the perioperative period. Anesth Analg 2019;128:265–77.
2. Khozhenko A, Lamperti M, Terracina S, et al. Can cerebral near-infrared spectroscopy predict cerebral ischemic events in neurosurgical patients? A narrative review of the literature. J Neurosurg Anesthesiol 2019;31:378–84.
3. Patel D, Lunn AD, Smith AD, et al. Cognitive decline in the elderly after surgery and anaesthesia: results from the Oxford project to investigate memory and ageing (OPTIMA) cohort. Anaesthesia 2016;71:1144–52.

4. Mashour GA, Woodrum DT, Avidan MS. Neurological complications of surgery and anaesthesia. Br J Anaesth 2015;114:194–203.
5. Moerman A, De Hert S. Cerebral oximetry: the standard monitor of the future? Curr Opin Anaesthesiol 2015;28:703–9.
6. Smith M. Multimodality neuromonitoring in adult traumatic brain injury: a narrative review. Anesthesiology 2018;128:401–15.
7. Gibbs EL, Lennox WG, Nims LF, et al. Arterial and cerebral venous blood. Arterial-venous differences in man. J Biol Chem 1942;144:325–32.
8. Shaaban Ali M, Harmer M, Latto I. Jugular bulb oximetry during cardiac surgery. Anaesthesia 2001;56:24–37.
9. Stocchetti N, Magnoni S, Zanier ER. My paper 20 years later: cerebral venous oxygen saturation studied with bilateral samples in the internal jugular veins. Intensive Care Med 2015;41:412–7.
10. Goetting MG, Preston G. Jugular bulb catheterization: experience with 123 patients. Crit Care Med 1990;18:1220–3.
11. Schoen J, Meyerrose J, Paarmann H, et al. Preoperative regional cerebral oxygen saturation is a predictor of postoperative delirium in on-pump cardiac surgery patients: a prospective observational trial. Crit Care 2011;15:R218.
12. Ghosal S, Trivedi J, Chen J, et al. Regional cerebral oxygen saturation level predicts 30-day mortality rate after left ventricular assist device surgery. J Cardiothorac Vasc Anesth 2018;32:1185–90.
13. Shenkin HA, Harmel MH, Kety SS. Dynamic anatomy of the cerebral circulation. Arch Neurol Psychiatry 1948;60:240–52.
14. Latronico N, Beindorf AE, Rasulo FA, et al. Limits of intermittent jugular bulb oxygen saturation monitoring in the management of severe head trauma patients. Neurosurgery 2000;46:1131–8.
15. Steiner LA, Andrews PJ. Monitoring the injured brain: ICP and CBF. Br J Anaesth 2006;97:26–38.
16. Chieregato A, Calzolari F, Trasforini G, et al. Normal jugular bulb oxygen saturation. J Neurol Neurosurg Psychiatr 2003;74:784–6.
17. Souter MJ, Andrews PJ. Validation of the Edslab dual lumen oximetry catheter for continuous monitoring of jugular bulb oxygen saturation after severe head injury. Br J Anaesth 1996;76:744–6.
18. Roh D, Park S. Brain multimodality monitoring: updated perspectives. Curr Neurol Neurosci Rep 2016;16:56.
19. Iwata M, Inoue S, Kawaguchi M, et al. Jugular bulb venous oxygen saturation during one-lung ventilation under sevoflurane- or propofol-based anesthesia for lung surgery. J Cardiothorac Vasc Anesth 2008;22:71–6.
20. Chan MT, Ng SC, Lam JM, et al. Re-defining the ischemic threshold for jugular venous oxygen saturation–a microdialysis study in patients with severe head injury. Acta Neurochir Suppl 2005;95:63–6.
21. Tsaousi GG, Pitsis AA, Deliaslani DV, et al. Cerebral oxygenation impairment and S-100β protein release during off-pump coronary artery revascularization. J Cardiothorac Vasc Anesth 2013;27:245–52.
22. Kim JY, Kwak YL, Oh YJ, et al. Changes in jugular bulb oxygen saturation during off-pump coronary artery bypass graft surgery. Acta Anaesthesiol Scand 2005;49:956–61.
23. Diephuis JC, Moons KG, Nierich AN, et al. Jugular bulb desaturation during coronary artery surgery: a comparison of off-pump and on-pump procedures. Br J Anaesth 2005;94:715–20.

24. Kadoi Y, Saito S, Goto F, et al. Decrease in jugular venous oxygen saturation during normothermic cardiopulmonary bypass predicts short-term postoperative neurologic dysfunction in elderly patients. J Am Coll Cardiol 2001;38:1450–5.

25. Kuwabara M, Nakajima N, Yamamoto F, et al. Continuous monitoring of blood oxygen saturation of internal jugular vein as a useful indicator for selective cerebral perfusion during aortic arch replacement. J Thorac Cardiovasc Surg 1992;103: 355–62.

26. Apostolakis E, Akinosoglou K. The methodologies of hypothermic circulatory arrest and of antegrade and retrograde cerebral perfusion for aortic arch surgery. Ann Thorac Cardiovasc Surg 2008;14:138–48.

27. Niinai H, Nakagawa I, Shima T, et al. Continuous monitoring of jugular bulb venous oxygen saturation for evaluation of cerebral perfusion during carotid endarterectomy. Hiroshima J Med Sci 1998;47(4):133–7.

28. Choi SH, Kim SH, Lee SJ, et al. Cerebral oxygenation during laparoscopic surgery: jugular bulb versus regional cerebral oxygen saturation. Yonsei Med J 2013;54:225–30.

29. Jeong H, Jeong S, Lim HJ, et al. Cerebral oxygen saturation measured by near-infrared spectroscopy and jugular venous bulb oxygen saturation during arthroscopic shoulder surgery in beach chair position under sevoflurane-nitrous oxide or propofol-remifentanil anesthesia. Anesthesiology 2012;116(5):1047–56.

30. Jöbsis FF. Noninvasive, infrared monitoring of cerebral and myocardial oxygen sufficiency and circulatory parameters. Science 1977;198:1264–7.

31. Ferrari M, Quaresima V. Near infrared brain and muscle oximetry: from the discovery to current applications. J Near Infrared Spectrosc 2012;20:1–14.

32. Bickler P, Feiner J, Rollins M, et al. Tissue oximetry and clinical outcomes. Anesth Analg 2017;124:72–82.

33. Davie SN, Grocott HP. Impact of extracranial contamination on regional cerebral oxygen saturation: a comparison of three cerebral oximetry technologies. Anesthesiology 2012;116:834–40.

34. Green DW, Kunst G. Cerebral oximetry and its role in adult cardiac, non-cardiac surgery and resuscitation from cardiac arrest. Anaesthesia 2017;72:48–57.

35. Steppan J, Hogue CW Jr. Cerebral and tissue oximetry. Best Pract Res Clin Anaesthesiol 2014;28:429–39.

36. Dullenkopf A, Baulig W, Weiss M, et al. Cerebral near-infrared spectroscopy in adult patients after cardiac surgery is not useful for monitoring absolute values but may reflect trends in venous oxygenation under clinical conditions. J Cardiothorac Vasc Anesth 2007;21:535–9.

37. Sørensen H, Secher NH, Rasmussen P. A note on arterial to venous oxygen saturation as reference for NIRS-determined frontal lobe oxygen saturation in healthy humans. Front Physiol 2014;4:403.

38. Ito H, Ibaraki M, Kanno I, et al. Changes in the arterial fraction of human cerebral blood volume during hypercapnia and hypocapnia measured by positron emission tomography. J Cereb Blood Flow Metab 2005;25:852–7.

39. Kim MB, Ward DS, Cartwright CR, et al. Estimation of jugular venous O2 saturation from cerebral oximetry or arterial O2 saturation during isocapnic hypoxia. J Clin Monit Comput 2000;16:191–9.

40. Chan MJ, Chung T, Glassford NJ, et al. Near-infrared spectroscopy in adult cardiac surgery patients: a systematic review and meta-analysis. J Cardiothorac Vasc Anesth 2017;31:1155–65.

41. Sun X, Ellis J, Corso PJ, et al. Mortality predicted by preinduction cerebral oxygen saturation after cardiac operation. Ann Thorac Surg 2014;98:91–6.

42. Serraino GF, Murphy GJ. Effects of cerebral near-infrared spectroscopy on the outcome of patients undergoing cardiac surgery: a systematic review of randomised trials. BMJ Open 2017;7:e016613.
43. Zheng F, Sheinberg R, Yee MS, et al. Cerebral near-infrared spectroscopy monitoring and neurologic outcomes in adult cardiac surgery patients: a systematic review. Anesth Analg 2013;116:663–6.
44. Yu Y, Zhang K, Zhang L, et al. Cerebral near-infrared spectroscopy (NIRS) for perioperative monitoring of brain oxygenation in children and adults. Cochrane Database Syst Rev 2018;1:CD010947.
45. Thiele RH, Shaw AD, Bartels K, et al. American society for enhanced recovery and perioperative quality initiative joint consensus statement on the role of neuromonitoring in perioperative outcomes: cerebral near-infrared spectroscopy. Anesth Analg 2020;131:1444–55.
46. Yu Y, Lyu Y, Jin L, et al. Prognostic factors for permanent neurological dysfunction after total aortic arch replacement with regional cerebral oxygen saturation monitoring. Brain Behav 2019;9:e01309.
47. Fischer GW, Lin HM, Krol M, et al. Noninvasive cerebral oxygenation may predict outcome in patients undergoing aortic arch surgery. J Thorac Cardiovasc Surg 2011;141:815–21.
48. Spaeder MC, Surma VJ. Cerebral regional oxygen saturation variability in neonates following cardiac surgery. Pediatr Res 2020;23:1–4.
49. Pennekamp CWA, Immink RV, den Ruijter HM, et al. Near-infrared spectroscopy to indicate selective shunt use during carotid endarterectomy. Eur J Vasc Endovasc Surg 2013;46:397–403.
50. Sun Y, Wei C, Cui V, et al. Electroencephalography: clinical applications during the perioperative period. Front Med 2020;7:251.
51. Ritter JC, Green D, Slim H, et al. The role of cerebral oximetry in combination with awake testing in patients undergoing carotid endarterectomy under local anaesthesia. Eur J Vasc Endovasc Surg 2011;41:599–605.
52. Jonsson M, Lindström D, Wanhainen A, et al. Near infrared spectroscopy as a predictor for shunt requirement during carotid endarterectomy. Eur J Vasc Endovasc Surg 2017;53(6):783–91.
53. Kamenskaya OV, Loginova IY, Lomivorotov VV. Brain oxygen supply parameters in the risk assessment of cerebral complications during carotid endarterectomy. J Cardiothorac Vasc Anesth 2017;31:944–9.
54. Salazar D, Hazel A, Tauchen AJ, et al. Neurocognitive deficits and cerebral desaturation during shoulder arthroscopy with patient in beach-chair position: a review of the current literature. Am J Orthop (Belle Mead NJ) 2016;45:E63–8.
55. Meex I, Vundelinckx J, Buyse K, et al. Cerebral tissue oxygen saturation values in volunteers and patients in the lateral decubitus and beach chair positions: a prospective observational study. Can J Anaesth 2016;63:537–43.
56. Mori Y, Yamada M, Akahori T, et al. Cerebral oxygenation in the beach chair position before and during general anesthesia in patients with and without cardiovascular risk factors. J Clin Anesth 2015;27:457–62.
57. Li H, Fu Q, Wu Z, et al. Cerebral oxygen desaturation occurs frequently in patients with hypertension undergoing major abdominal surgery. J Clin Monit Comput 2018;32:285–93.
58. Lin R, Zhang F, Xue Q, et al. Accuracy of regional cerebral oxygen saturation in predicting postoperative cognitive dysfunction after total hip arthroplasty: regional cerebral oxygen saturation predicts POCD. J Arthroplasty 2013;28:494–7.

59. Robba C, Goffi A, Geeraerts T, et al. Brain ultrasonography: methodology, basic and advanced principles and clinical applications. A narrative review. Intensive Care Med 2019;45:913–27.

60. D'Andrea A, Conte M, Scarafile R, et al. Transcranial Doppler ultrasound: physical principles and principal applications in Neurocritical Care Unit. J Cardiovasc Echogr 2016;26:28–41.

61. Czosnyka M, Brady K, Reinhard M, et al. Monitoring of cerebrovascular autoregulation: facts, myths, and missing links. Neurocrit Care 2009;10:373–86.

62. Donnelly J, Aries MJ, Czosnyka M. Further understanding of cerebral autoregulation at the bedside: possible implications for future therapy. Expert Rev Neurother 2015;15:169–85.

63. Cardim D, Robba C, Matta B, et al. Cerebrovascular assessment of patients undergoing shoulder surgery in beach chair position using a multiparameter transcranial Doppler approach. J Clin Monit Comput 2019;33(4):615–25.

64. Robba C, Donnelly J, Bertuetti R, et al. Doppler non-invasive monitoring of ICP in an animal model of acute intracranial hypertension. Neurocrit Care 2015;23:419–26.

65. Moritz S, Kasprzak P, Arlt M, et al. Accuracy of cerebral monitoring in detecting cerebral ischemia during carotid endarterectomy: a comparison of transcranial Doppler sonography, near-infrared spectroscopy, stump pressure, and somatosensory evoked potentials. Anesthesiology 2007;107:563–9.

66. Lee CH, Jeon SH, Wang SJ, et al. Factors associated with temporal window failure in transcranial Doppler sonography. Neurol Sci 2020;41:3293–9.

67. Thudium M, Heinze I, Ellerkmann RK, et al. Cerebral function and perfusion during cardiopulmonary bypass: a plea for a multimodal monitoring approach. Heart Surg Forum 2018;21:E028–35.

68. Ghazy T, Darwisch A, Schmidt T, et al. Transcranial Doppler sonography for optimization of cerebral perfusion in aortic arch operation. Ann Thorac Surg 2016;101:e15–6.

69. Joshi B, Brady K, Lee J, et al. Impaired autoregulation of cerebral blood flow during rewarming from hypothermic cardiopulmonary bypass and its potential association with stroke. Anesth Analg 2010;110:321–8.

70. Okita Y, Miyata H, Motomura N, et al. Japan cardiovascular surgery database organization. A study of brain protection during total arch replacement comparing antegrade cerebral perfusion versus hypothermic circulatory arrest, with or without retrograde cerebral perfusion: analysis based on the Japan Adult Cardiovascular Surgery Database. J Thorac Cardiovasc Surg 2015;149:S65–73.

71. Halkos ME, Anderson A, Binongo JNG, et al. Operative strategies to reduce cerebral embolic events during on- and off-pump coronary artery bypass surgery: a stratified, prospective randomized trial. J Thorac Cardiovasc Surg 2017;154:1278–85.

72. Rodriguez RA, Rubens FD, Wozny D, et al. Cerebral emboli detected by transcranial Doppler during cardiopulmonary bypass are not correlated with postoperative cognitive deficits. Stroke 2010;41:2229–35.

73. Boodhwani M, Rubens F, Wozny D, et al. Effects of sustained mild hypothermia on neurocognitive function after coronary artery bypass surgery: a randomized, double-blind study. J Thorac Cardiovasc Surg 2007;134:1443–50.

74. Chung EM, Banahan C, Patel N, et al. Size distribution of air bubbles entering the brain during cardiac surgery. PLoS One 2015;10:e0122166.

75. Udesh R, Natarajan P, Thiagarajan K, et al. Transcranial Doppler monitoring in carotid endarterectomy: a systematic review and meta-analysis. J Ultrasound Med 2017;36:621–30.
76. Chongruksut W, Vaniyapong T, Rerkasem K. Routine or selective carotid artery shunting for carotid endarterectomy (and different methods of monitoring in selective shunting). Cochrane Database Syst Rev 2014;2014:CD000190.
77. McCulloch TJ, Liyanagama K, Petchell J. Relative hypotension in the beach-chair position: effects on middle cerebral artery blood velocity. Anaesth Intensive Care 2010;38:486–91.
78. Hanouz JL, Fiant AL, Gérard JL. Middle cerebral artery blood flow velocity during beach chair position for shoulder surgery under general anesthesia. J Clin Anesth 2016;33:31–6.
79. Demirgan S, Özcan FG, Gemici EK, et al. Reverse Trendelenburg position applied prior to pneumoperitoneum prevents excessive increase in optic nerve sheath diameter in laparoscopic cholecystectomy: randomized controlled trial. J Clin Monit Comput 2021;35:89–99.
80. Robba C, Bacigaluppi S, Cardim D, et al. Intraoperative non invasive intracranial pressure monitoring during pneumoperitoneum: a case report and a review of the published cases and case report series. J Clin Monit Comput 2016;30:527–38.
81. Kietaibl C, Engel A, Horvat Menih I, et al. Detection and differentiation of cerebral microemboli in patients undergoing major orthopaedic surgery using transcranial Doppler ultrasound. Br J Anaesth 2017;118:400–6.
82. Mojadidi MK, Winoker JS, Roberts SC, et al. Two-dimensional echocardiography using second harmonic imaging for the diagnosis of intracardiac right-to-left shunt: a meta-analysis of prospective studies. Int J Cardiovasc Imaging 2014; 30:911–23.
83. Stendel R, Gramm HJ, Schröder K, et al. Transcranial Doppler ultrasonography as a screening technique for detection of a patent foramen ovale before surgery in the sitting position. Anesthesiology 2000;93:971–5.
84. Rainov NG, Weise JB, Burkert W. Transcranial Doppler sonography in adult hydrocephalic patients. Neurosurg Rev 2000;23:34–8.

Perioperative Coagulation Monitoring

Christian Fenger-Eriksen, MD, PhD

KEYWORDS

- Bleeding management • Patient blood management • Bleeding
- Point-of-care testing • Platelet function test

KEY POINTS

- Coagulation disturbances in the perioperative setting are challenging due to multifactorial and complex causes.
- Conventional laboratory tests, such as prothrombin time/international normalized ratio and activated partial thromboplastin time, are unreliable predictors of perioperative bleeding, particularly in patients with normal liver function, without any known bleeding risk factors, and who are not on anticoagulant therapy.
- Point-of-care tests allow quick and clinically relevant coagulation monitoring in the perioperative setting. The results of these tests should be considered, however, in the context of current clinical conditions and patient history.
- Maximum clinical benefit from point-of-care monitoring requires evidence-based treatment algorithms tailored toward the specific analyzer.

INTRODUCTION

For decades, the need for a change in perioperative coagulation management had been growing. A proactive attitude, including frequent assessment and reassessment of bleeding and coagulation status, now is state of the art. Furthermore, goal-directed approach to administration of blood products based on point-of-care coagulation handling is becoming standard of care.[1–3] These strategies are part of a modern patient blood management strategy[4] and the reasons for this change are multifactorial. They may be attributed to a deeper understanding of issues related to perioperative coagulopathy; growing awareness of side effects from allogenic blood products; remarkable developments of point-of-care monitoring and evidence-based algorithms, including targeted administration of coagulation factors; and subsequent change in transfusion behavior.[5] Moreover, if major bleeding is aggravated by coagulopathy, the negative impact on outcome and survival is significant.[6]

Department of Anaesthesiology, Aarhus University Hospital, Palle Juul Jensens Boulevard, Aarhus N DK-8200, Denmark
E-mail address: chfen@dadlnet.dk

Anesthesiology Clin 39 (2021) 525–535
https://doi.org/10.1016/j.anclin.2021.03.010
1932-2275/21/© 2021 Elsevier Inc. All rights reserved.

The aim of perioperative coagulation monitoring is to identify possible and potential reversible coagulopathies. Point-of-care monitors, such as thromboelastometry/thromboelastography, are potent tools for this purpose. Weber and colleagues[7] randomized 100 patients undergoing complex cardiac surgery to hemostatic therapy guided by either conventional or point-of-care coagulation analyses. Improved outcome and reduced exposure to blood products were reported in the point-of-care group. In another study, including 111 trauma patients, massive transfusion was guided by point-of-care or conventional coagulation assays in a randomized study design. Fewer transfusion requirements and survival benefit were reported in the point-of-care group.[8] Moreover, there is a clear benefit using point-of-care monitoring because turnaround time from blood sample to the result is significantly shorter compared with the standard coagulation tests.[9]

In summary, increasing scientific evidence points toward reduced mortality and reduced transfusion requirements favoring clinical use of point-of-care coagulation monitoring.

PRINCIPLES OF PERIOPERATIVE COAGULOPATHY

During surgery and bleeding, the delicate balance between procoagulant and anticoagulant proteins and cells easily is disturbed, and hemostatic abnormalities are common, particularly in patients with major bleeding. These can lead to a further increase in blood loss, difficulties in achieving surgical hemostasis, increased risk for reoperation due to bleeding, and worse patient outcomes.[10]

The causes of cogulopathy during bleeding is multifaceted. Isolated major hemorrhage, surgical or following trauma, in a coagulation native patient does inevitably lead to a coagulopathy. The reasons are loss and consumption of coagulation factors and hemodilution from intravenous fluid given and can be further worsened by acidosis and hypothermia. Additionally, acute traumatic coagulopathy, hyperfibrinolysis, endotheliopathy, and coagulopathy from massive transfusion are factors with substantial negative effects on the coagulation system.[11] The clinical presentation often, but not always, is defined by low fibrinogen levels. Coagulopathy in a given patient, however, is case-specific and difficult to anticipate or diagnose without proper tools. Point-of-care monitoring is a crucial part of hemostatic optimization, which helps differentiate between platelet, thrombin generation, and fibrinogen deficiency and ascertains the presence of hyperfibrinolysis.

BENEFIT OF PREOPERATIVE COAGULATION SCREENING TEST

Prevention of unexpected bleeding remains a major goal during surgical procedures. Traditional plasma-based coagulation tests, such as prothrombin time (PT) and activated partial thromboplastin time (aPTT), together with measurement of platelet count, is used widely as screening tool before surgery. Such a strategy requires a close correlation between abnormal coagulation tests and increased bleeding tendency, which unfortunately is not the case. In a review, including 9 studies, positive predictive value of a prolonged PT for postoperative bleeding ranged from 0.03 to 0.22.[12] In another review by Levy and colleagues,[13] aPTT and PT were found poor predictors of bleeding complications based on a high number of studies included. Although routine preoperative testing may be beneficial to identify individuals without bleeding history but with coagulation factor deficiency (ie, mild hemophilia), its widespread use is not justified because unknown inherited coagulopathies are rare.

New modalities to precisely predict postoperative blood loss utilizing a novel machine learning approach are under development, as demonstrated by Stehrer and colleagues[14] among 950 patients. Positive predictive values of a family history and evidence of previous excessive postsurgical or postdental procedure bleeding and/or menorrhagia in general are poor.[15] A structured questionnaire may help, however, identifying patients with increased risk of bleeding and in whom preoperative coagulation tests can be advantageous.[16]

In summary, routine testing has no benefit in assessment of bleeding risk in standard patients with normal liver function and without any history of oral anticoagulant use.

COAGULATION TESTING IN THE PERIOPERATIVE SETTING
Standard Coagulation Tests

Standard coagulation tests include PT/international normalized ratio (INR), aPTT, platelet count, and fibrinogen levels. Although these tests are widely available, nonexpensive, and familiar to most physicians, they have significant shortcomings. First, the turnaround time from ordering the test until results are available can exceed 60 minutes, thus reducing their clinical utility. Second, hyperfibrinolysis is difficult to assess based on these tests. Third, sensitivity to detect the impact of non–vitamin k antagonist therapy is low. Fourth, platelet count only reflects the number of platelets available, not the function or the inhibition by antiplatelet drugs. Fifth, unlike the PT, aPTT results are not standardized across laboratories, whereby evaluation of results has to be individualized.[17]

Point-of-Care Coagulation Tests

The first viscoelastic test was described in 1948. Since then, there has been significant developments in techniques, software, and biochemical assays.[18] Some analyzers include platelet function measurement modules with automatic or semiautomatic equipment. This section provides an overview of the methodological principles behind the most used analyzers:

- ROTEM sigma/ROTEM delta (Instrumentation Laboratory, Bedford, Massachusetts)
- ClotPro, TEG 5000/TEG 6S Thromboelastograph Hemostasis Analyzers (Haemonetics, Massachusetts),
- Sonoclot analyzer (Sienco, Boulder, Colorado)
- Quantra Hemostasis Analyzer (HemoSonics Europe, Asnières-sur-Seine, France)

Analysis Principle

The classic viscoelastic test involves a small sample of patient blood placed into a cup. A pin is inserted into the cup and analysis begins by movement of cup and pin relative to each other. As the clotting process is ongoing, fibrin strands form between the cup and the pin as blood changes from a fluid phase into a clot. This change in viscosity is detected, via the pin, by an electronic sensor, and the signal is generated into a trace. Instead of a physical movement of the cup or the pin, some analyzers induce resonance by an ultrasound transducer.[19] **Table 1** represents an overview of some commercially available coagulation analyzers and their output results. Citrated blood and recalcification are recommended, although analyses on native whole blood also are an option. It is common to use an activator because this standardizes the test and speeds up the rate of clot formation. For research purposes, activation with low-dose tissue factor is well described, primarily employing ROTEM. This assay increases sensitivity in blood samples from from patients with for example mild haemophilia but

Table 1 Point-of-care coagulation devices				
	Clot Initiation	Clot Propagation	Clot Strength	Fibrinolysis
ROTEM	• CT (s)	• CFT (s) • Alpha-angle (°)	• MCF (mm)	• Maximum lysis (%) • Lysis index 30/60
TEG	• R	• K (s) • Alpha-angle (°)	• MA • Alpha-angle (°)	• Lysis 30/60
ClotPro	• CT (s)	• CFT (s)	• MCF (mm)	• Maximum lysis (%) • Lysis index 30
Quantra®	• CT (s) • Heparinase CT (s)	• None specific	• CS (hPa) • FCS (hPa) • Platelet part clot stiffness (hPa)	
Sonoclot	• ACT (s)	• Clot rate (U/min) • Time to peak (min)	• Platelet function (arbitrary 0–5)	—

Quick parameters are available for ROTEM, TEG, and ClotPro, given as amplitude of clot firmness at 5 minutes or 10 minutes (termed, A5 and A10, respectively). Likewise, values of amplitude at 30 minutes or 60 minutes (MCF lysis index, [LI]), termed, LI 30 and LI60) or MA (lysis termed Lysis 30/60) provides quick information.

the intrinsic system needs inhibition by corn trypsin inhibitor.[20] Multiple assays for analysis of various aspects of the coagulation cascade are available (**Table 2**).

Interpretation of Analysis

The results are displayed in both graphical format as well as various numerical measurements, with reference ranges, which can aid rapid diagnosis of specific coagulopathies. Intrinsic activated assays are, in principle, similar to the aPTT whereas extrinsic assays mimic the PT. A high degree of correlation between ROTEM and TEG is present but, in general, values obtained from different devices are not interchangeable. Thus, device-specific algorithms for interpretation of the results are mandatory.[21]

Evaluation of clot initiation

Prolonged clot initiation (like clotting time [CT], reaction time [R], and activated CT [ACT]) indicates reduced levels or inhibition of coagulation factors involved in the generation of thrombin burst. If both extrinsic and intrinsic clot initiation parameters are prolonged, a global lack of coagulation factors is likely, as seen during massive hemorrhage. If only intrinsic parameters of clot initiation are affected, heparin influence is likely and heparinase assays may be useful for the diagnosis. Shortened parameters are seen in hypercoagulable state.

Evaluation of clot propagation

Clot propagation parameters (like clot formation time [CFT], kinetic time [K], and clot rate) can be attributed to either low platelets, poor platelet function, low fibrinogen, or low coagulation factor activity. Thus, their clinical applicability is limited. Shortened parameters are seen in hypercoagulable state.

Evaluation of clot strength

Reduced clot strength (like maximum clot firmness [MCF], maximum amplitude [MA], and clot stiffness [CS]) demonstrates low platelet numbers and/or reduced fibrin polymerization. The different available fibrinogen assays (like FIBTEM, functional

Table 2
Assays and their contents

	Assay	Assay Contents
ROTEM	• EXTEM	Tissue factor
	• INTEM	Ellagic acid/phospholipids
	• FIBTEM	Cytochalasin D (platelet inhibitor) + TF
	• APTEM	Tranexamic acid + TF
	• HEPTEM	Heparinase + ellagic acid
TEG	• RapidTEG	TF + kaolin
	• Kaolin	Kaolin
	• Functional fibrinogen	Abciximab (platelet inhibitor) + TF
	• HTEG	Heparinase
	• Platelet Mapping	ADP/arachidonic acid
ClotPro	• EX-test	TF + heparin antagonist
	• FIB-test	Cytochalasin D + GPIIb/IIIa antagonist
	• AP-test	Aprotinin + TF
	• IN-test	Ellagic acid
	• HI-test	Ellagic acid + heparinase
Sonoclot	• kACT test	Kaolin
	• SonACT	Celite
	• gbACT/gbACT+	Glass bead
	• H-gbACT+	Glass bead + heparinase
	• aiACT	Celite + minerals
Quantra	• CT	Kaolin
	• Heparinase CT	Kaolin + heparinase
	• CS	Thromboplastin + heparin inhibitor
	• FCS	Thromboplastin + heparin inhibitor + abciximab
	• Platelet contribution to CS	Calculated value

Most assays contain $CaCl^2$ for recalcification of the citrated blood sample. More manufacturers provide additional, calculated parameters, that is, velocity of clot formation/thrombin generation. ClotPro provides additional assays: RVV-test (activation with Russell viper venom, an activator of factor X, thus sensitive to FX inhibitor therapy), ECA-test (activation with ecarin, a prothrombin activator thus sensitive to thrombin inhibitors ie, dabigatran), and TPA-test (recombinant tissue plasminogen activator, measure of fibrinolysis resistance). ROTEM provides an additional assay: ECATEM (activation with viper venom ecarin, with thrombin-like effect, thus sensitive to thrombin inhibitors [ie, dabigatran]).

fibrinogen, FIB-test, and fibrinogen contribution to clot stiffness [FCS]) contain potent platelet inhibitors, which block the platelet contribution to clot formation, leaving only the fibrin trace. This permits distinction between low platelet count and low fibrinogen levels as the fibrin trace correlates closely with and acts as a clinical meaningful marker of fibrinogen levels.[22]

Standard viscoelastic tests are insensitive to most pharmacologic inhibitors. Thus, a normal amplitude may be given despite significant platelet inhibition. Only glycoprotein (GP) IIb/IIIa inhibitors provide a reduction in amplitude detectable by viscoelastic testing. The reason is the complex activation pattern of platelets combined with strong activators, used during testing, which overcome the pharmacologic inhibition.[23] Factor XIII plays a pivotal role in stabilizing the fibrin clot at the site of injury and as such contributes to clot strength. Amplitudes at specific time points (A10, A30, and so forth) are available as surrogate marker of the final amplitude in an effort to speed up reporting.

Evaluation of fibrinolysis

The most commonly used fibrinolysis parameter is clot lysis at 30 minutes after maximum clot strength is achieved (measured as LY30 with TEG) or 30 minutes after

CT is detected (measured as LI30 with ROTEM). Both are given as percentage drops in amplitude from MA. Although a clear definition on hyperfibrinolysis is pending, a lysis percentage at/above 3% is associated with increased mortality and transfusion requirements during uncontrolled hemorrhage.[24] Assays containing tranexamic acid/aprotinin are available and are useful to verify the influence of hyperfibrinolysis.

Clinical Use and Pitfalls

Point-of-care coagulation tests provide rapid and useful information in the perioperative setting. An ideal test of blood coagulation, however, does not yet exist. As with other laboratory equipment, pre- and postanalytical errors are possible and, therefore, clinical conditions together with history always should be considered along with the results.[25]

Blood flow characteristics, endothelial cells, and their interaction with i.e. von Willebrand factors are not detected by point-of-care tests. Measurement runs at 37°, which is not reflective of the hemostatic pathology inside the hypothermic patient.

Furthermore, as discussed previously, sensitivity of all standard assays to detect non–vitamin k antagonist therapy and platelet inhibitors is low. Thus, a normal result may be reported despite significant anticoagulant effect.

For platelet analyzers, hemodilution and interference by thrombocytopenia are some of the limitations relevant to perioperative use.

Similar to standard coagulation tests, the ability to predict bleeding complications based on results from point-of-care testing is, in general, poor. Monitoring of patients without ongoing bleeding complications is questionable and may cause unnecessary treatment with coagulation active substances and increase both risk and cost.

Monitoring of Platelet Function

Platelet function during perioperative bleeding may be affected due to antiplatelet drugs, acquired qualitative platelet dysfunction, or combinations thereof. Clot amplitude/strength, as discussed previously, may not reliably indicate if a given patient is on antiplatelet medication.[26] Thus, a specific evaluation of platelet function can be advantageous in the perioperative setting if bleeding complications arise. Light transmission aggregometry is considered the gold standard assessment of platelet function. These tests are technically challenging and time consuming, which limit their applicability in bleeding.

Point-of-care assessment of platelet function is based on specific activators targeted at the receptor of interest. Drugs like clopidogrel, prasugrel, and cangrelor are P2Y12 antagonists with adenosine diphosphate (ADP) as the agonist. It follows that lack of platelet aggregation following ADP verifies platelet inhibition by this category of drugs. Similarly, arachidonic acid (AA) as activator reveals inhibition through cyclooxygenase inhibitors (aspirin), and thrombin receptor-activating peptide (TRAP) is used to verify GPIIb/IIIa antagonist (abciximab or tirofiban) affected platelets. Additional ristocetin and other specific agonist assays are accessible for diagnosing von Willebrand disease.

Numerous newer platelet function analyzers can aid clinicians in monitoring the platelet function in an attempt to ascertain whether a given patient is under the influence of antiplatelet drugs or not and to confirm recovery of function when they have been impaired. The following are among the more commonly available equipment:

- The PFA-100 (Siemens Medical Solutions, Malvern, Pennsylvania) stands out as the methodology includes shear stress. Citrated whole blood is aspirated at high shear rates through disposable cartridges containing an aperture within a membrane coated with 1 of the following substances: collagen, epinephrine, collagen plus ADP or ADP plus prostaglandin E1. Upon platelet adhesion and aggregation, a plug is formed that closes the tiny aperture and flow stops whereby the output—closure time—is defined.

- VerifyNow (Accriva, San Diego, California) is based on the capacity of activated platelets to bind to fibrinogen-coated beads within the cartridge detected by optical light transduction and transformed to an arbitrary scale. The test uses ADP to stimulate platelets in the presence of prostaglandin E1 (thus sensitive to P2Y12 inhibitors) or AA (sensitive to aspirin). Results are reported as P2Y12 reaction units and/or aspirin reaction units.

- The Multiplate Analyzer (Roche Diagnostics, Mannheim, Germany) is a semiautomated point-of-care device that measures platelet aggregation by detecting change in electrical impedance as platelets adhere to metal sensor wires immersed in a whole-blood sample. Aggregation (AU), velocity (AU/min), and area under the curve are output parameters. Available agonists are ADP, AA, TRAP, and ristocetin.

- TEG platelet mapping is available without any additional equipment because the method originates from a standard TEG trace and as such includes a low shear stress model. Quantification of platelet aggregation is based on subtraction of MA analysis comparing the fibrin and kaolin trace with a sample, including platelet activation with AA or ADP.

- PAP-8E (Bio/Data, Horsham, Pennsylvania) evaluates platelet aggregation through light transmission using platelet rich plasma as test medium. Results include area under the curve and area under the slope, with more assays accessible like AA, ADP, and collagen.

CLINICAL IMPLICATIONS
Major Hemorrhage

Point-of-care monitoring during major hemorrhage enables bedside rapid diagnosis of any coagulopathy present and the possibility to distinguish between fibrinogen/platelet deficiency, hyperfibrinolysis, and lack of thrombin generation. This allows a targeted approach, including individualized hemostatic intervention and transfusion guidance. Application of such a strategy, which includes intervention algorithms with predefined triggers, has been shown to reduce transfusion requirement, improve outcome and is recommended by European Society of Anesthesiology and Intensive Care and National Institute for Health and Care Excellence guidelines.[27]

Cardiac Surgery

Coagulation disturbance in cardiac surgery is common due to the extent of surgery and the use of anticoagulants before and during the operation occasionally combined with cardiopulmonary support devices. The ability to diagnose residual heparin effects despite protamine administration, hyperfibrinolysis, and specific coagulation factor deficiency, such as low fibrinogen levels, represents a major benefit of point-of-care monitoring in this setting. Moreover, platelet function tests are of particular benefit for the timing of discontinuation of platelet inhibitors in subacute cardiac surgery.[28]

Emergency surgery in patients on antiplatelet/anticoagulant therapy:
Anticoagulants cause prolongation of CT/clot initiation detectible by point-of-care monitoring and can be useful in the clinical setting of trauma. The correlation between anticoagulant levels and the point-of-care trace is poor, especially for factor Xa

inhibitors, and clinical cutoff levels still need to be defined properly in clinical trials. Assay developments are under way, however, and some manufacturer already provide more specific assays (ie, ClotPro; RVV/ECA test or ROTEM; and ECATEM), although further validation is required.[29]

DISCUSSION

The diversity of etiology affecting the hemostatic system during surgery and bleeding calls for a tailor-made and targeted response. Point-of-care devices provide a rapid and unique opportunity to assess coagulopathy and to target intervention precisely.

Point-of-care guided hemostatic resuscitation with blood products and coagulation factor concentrates is considered gold standard in bleeding patients and recommended in several guidelines.[27]

Commercially available devices differ in methodology because some use the traditional viscoelastic method whereas others implemented ultrasound. Additionally, assays are very different in composition and concentration of activation substances, whereby values are not comparable, and each device needs a separate treatment algorithm.

Platelet function devices are developed to monitor the use of antiplatelet drugs precisely and not to monitor a more diffuse and often multifactorial platelet inhibition observed in a bleeding situation in patients not receiving antiplatelet drugs. Nevertheless, the information on platelet function can be relevant in the perioperative setting, especially if influence from antiplatelet drugs is present or suspected.

Maximum clinical benefit from point-of-care monitoring requires evidence-based treatment algorithms tailored toward the specific analyzer. So far, algorithms based on ROTEM and TEG are the most scientifically robust. In general, these bleeding management algorithms are effective in reducing blood loss, transfusion requirements, and health care costs and improving outcomes, including perioperative morbidity and mortality.[30,31]

Implementation of patient blood management strategies, however, often requires enthusiasm to change current practice and an agile organization.

The predictive value of a preoperative point-of-care measurement is poor and could, in cases of an abnormal result, cause unnecessary treatment or concerns that may harm the patient or increase costs. It general, it is recommended to initiate testing when bleeding problems occur. Standard coagulation tests like aPTT, INR, PT, platelet count, and fibrinogen are possible alternatives to point-of-care measurements. These assays, however, are based on plasma only, take significantly longer time, and are not developed to monitor coagulopathy in the perioperative setting and, therefore, are of limited benefit. So far, the most robust evidence originates from cardiac surgery and trauma settings. Future large trials are needed to expand knowledge in other clinical scenarios.[32] In addition to the direct measurement of clot formation potential, repeated evaluation of temperature, pH, and calcium levels is necessary, because these factors may lead to significant coagulopathy.[11]

SUMMARY

Optimizing hemostasis, avoidance of transfusion, and proper coagulation support all are part of a modern perioperative approach to improve patient outcome. Point-of-care devices are an essential and necessary part of this strategy. Correct application is crucial, and predefined, evidence-based algorithms are important alongside a quick and comprehensive test strategy.

CLINICS CARE POINTS

- Point-of-care tests can provide a global picture of a patient's hemostatic capacity within 15 minutes to 20 minutes.

- Point-of-care tests are indicated during major hemorrhage and are essential to guide the correct transfusion component strategy and diagnose any coagulopathy.

- Major hemorrhage in the presence of normal point-of-care coagulation parameters indicates that coagulopathy is unlikely and surgical reasons should be sought.

- Impaired primary hemostasis caused by von Willebrand disease/antiplatelet von Willebrand disease/antiplatelet drugs cannot be detected by standard point-of-care tests alone; additional platelet function analysis is useful.

- Evidence-based treatment algorithms, tailored toward local practice, are an important part of point-of-care testing.

DISCLOSURE

Author received unrestricted grants/travel support from Instrumentation Laboratory, Tem Innovations, CSL Behring, and Portola.

REFERENCES

1. Innerhofer P, Fries D, Mittermayr M, et al. Reversal of trauma-induced coagulopathy using first-line coagulation factor concentrates or fresh frozen plasma (RETIC): a single-centre, parallel-group, open-label, randomised trial. Lancet Haematol 2017;4(6):e258–71.

2. Ganter MT, Spahn DR. Active, personalized, and balanced coagulation management saves lives in patients with massive bleeding. Anesthesiology 2010;113(5): 1016–8.

3. Schöchl H, Nienaber U, Hofer G, et al. Goal-directed coagulation management of major trauma patients using thromboelastometry (ROTEM)-guided administration of fibrinogen concentrate and prothrombin complex concentrate. Crit Care 2010; 14(2):R55.

4. Franchini M, Marano G, Veropalumbo E, et al. Patient blood management: a revolutionary approach to transfusion medicine. Blood Transfus 2019;17(3):191–5.

5. Stein P, Kaserer A, Sprengel K, et al. Change of transfusion and treatment paradigm in major trauma patients. Anaesthesia 2017;72(11):1317–26.

6. MacLeod JBA, Lynn M, McKenney MG, et al. Early coagulopathy predicts mortality in trauma. J Trauma 2003;55(1):39–44.

7. Weber CF, Görlinger K, Meininger D, et al. Point-of-care testing: a prospective, randomized clinical trial of efficacy in coagulopathic cardiac surgery patients. Anesthesiology 2012;117(3):531–47.

8. Gonzalez E, Moore EE, Moore HB, et al. Goal-directed hemostatic resuscitation of trauma-induced coagulopathy. A pragmatic randomized clinical trial comparing a viscoelastic assay to conventional coagulation assays). Ann Surg Ann Surg 2016; 263(6):1051–9.

9. Haas T, Spielmann N, Mauch J, et al. Comparison of thromboelastometry (ROTEM) with standard plasmatic coagulation testing in paediatric surgery. Br J Anaesth 2012;108(1):36–41.

10. Brohi K, Singh J, Heron M, et al. Acute traumatic coagulopathy. J Trauma 2003; 54(6):1127–30.

11. Fenger-Eriksen C, Haas T, Fries D. Coagulation disturbances during major perioperative or traumatic bleeding. Trends Anaesth Crit Care 2019;(28):6–13.

12. Chee YL, Crawford JC, Watson HG, et al. Guidelines on the assessment of bleeding risk prior to surgery or invasive procedures. British Committee for Standards in Haematology. Br J Haematol 2008;140(5):496–504.

13. Levy JH, F Szlam F, Wolberg AS, et al. Clinical use of the activated partial thromboplastin time and prothrombin time for screening: a review of the literature and current guidelines for testing. Clin Lab Med 2014;34(3):453–77.

14. Stehrer R, Hingsammer L, Staudigl C, et al. Machine learning based prediction of perioperative blood loss in orthognathic surgery. J Craniomaxillofac Surg 2019; 47(11):1676–81.

15. Guay J, Faraoni D, Bonhomme F, et al. Ability of hemostatic assessment to detect bleeding disorders and to predict abnormal surgical blood loss in children: a systematic review and meta-analysis. Paediatr Anaesth 2015;25(12):1216–26.

16. Deutsche Gesellschaft für Anästhesiologie und Intensivmedizin (DGAI), Deutsche Gesellschaft für Innere Medizin (DGIM), Deutsche Gesellschaft für Chirurgie (DGCH), et al. Preoperative evaluation of adult patients before elective, noncardiothoracic surgery. Anaesthesist 2019;68:25–39.

17. Haas T, Fries D, Tanaka KA, et al. Usefulness of standard plasma coagulation tests in the management of perioperative coagulopathic bleeding: is there any evidence? Br J Anaesth 2015;114(2):217–24.

18. Whiting D, DiNardo JA. TEG and ROTEM: technology and clinical applications. Am J Hematol 2014;89(2):228–32.

19. Sahli SD, Rössler J, Tscholl DW, et al. Point-of-care diagnostics in coagulation management. Sensors (Basel) 2020;20(15):4254.

20. Young G, Sørensen B, Dargaud Y, et al. Thrombin generation and whole blood viscoelastic assays in the management of hemophilia: current state of art and future perspectives. Blood 2013;121(11):1944–50.

21. Ziegler B, Voelckel W, Zipperle J, et al. Comparison between the new fully automated viscoelastic coagulation analysers teg 6s and rotem sigma in trauma patients: A prospective observational study. Eur J Anaesthesiol 2019;36:834–42.

22. Schlimp CJ, Solomon R, Hochleitner G, et al. The effectiveness of different functional fibrinogen polymerization assays in eliminating platelet contribution to clot strength in thromboelastometry. Anesth Analg 2014;118(2):269–76.

23. Ranucci M, Baryshnikova E. Sensitivity of viscoelastic tests to platelet function. J Clin Med 2020;9(1):189.

24. Chapman MP, Moore EE, Ramos CR, et al. Fibrinolysis greater than 3% is the critical value for initiation of antifibrinolytic therapy. J Trauma Acute Care Surg 2013; 75(6):961–7 [discussion 967].

25. Mukhopadhyaya T, Subramanianb A. An overview of the potential sources of diagnostic errors in (classic) thromboelastography curve interpretation and preventive measures. Pract Lab Med 2020;22:e00193.

26. Connelly CR, Yonge JD, McCully SP, et al. Assessment of three point-of-care platelet function assays in adult trauma patients. J Surg Res 2017;212:260–9.

27. Spahn DR, Bouillon B, Cerny V, et al. The European guideline on management of major bleeding and coagulopathy following trauma: fifth edition. Crit Care 2019; 23(1):98.

28. Bolliger D, Lancé MD, Siegemund M. Point-of-care platelet function monitoring: implications for patients with platelet inhibitors in cardiac surgery. J Cardiothorac Vasc Anesth 2021;35(4):1049–59.

29. Lapichino GE, Bianchi P, Ranucci M, et al. Point-of-care coagulation tests monitoring of direct oral anticoagulants and their reversal therapy: state of the art. Semin Thromb Hemost 2017;43(04):423–32.
30. Cochrane C, Chinna S, Young Um J, et al. Site-of-care viscoelastic assay in major trauma improves outcomes and is cost neutral compared with standard coagulation tests. Diagnostics (Basel) 2020;10(7):486.
31. Deppe AC, Weber C, Zimmermann J, et al. Point-of-care thromboelastography/thromboelastometry based coagulation management in cardiac surgery: a meta-analysis of 8332 patients. J Surg Res 2016;203:424–33.
32. Wikkelso A, Wetterslev J, Moller AM, et al. Thromboelastography (TEG) or thromboelastometry (ROTEM) to monitor haemostatic treatment versus usual care in adults or children with bleeding. Cochrane Database Syst Rev 2016;8: CD007871.

Ultrasound
The New Stethoscope (Point-of-Care Ultrasound)

Amber Bledsoe, MD*, Josh Zimmerman, MD

KEYWORDS

- Gastric ultrasound • Lung ultrasound • Point of care ultrasound (POCUS)
- Chest sonography • Emergency ultrasound • Abdominal ultrasound

KEY POINTS

- Gastric and lung point-of-care ultrasound have proven to be user friendly and quickly performed with recognizable, real-time findings.
- Lung ultrasound examination is particularly useful in urgent settings, when a rapid diagnosis is critical and can identify multiple pathologies, including pneumothorax, pleural effusion, and increased lung density.
- Gastric ultrasound examination can applied to various scenarios, including elective procedures when nil per os guidelines were not followed, urgent/emergent procedures, and questionable nil per os status and can be used to identify stomach contents and quantify gastric volume.

 Video content accompanies this article at http://www.anesthesiology. theclinics.com.

For decades, clinical ultrasound examinations were performed by sonographers on cumbersome machines and interpreted by radiologists and cardiologists in dark rooms. In recent years, there has been both an expansion and a shrinking in the application of ultrasound examinations. The shrinking comes in the form of dramatic decreases in the size and cost of ultrasound technology. A machine that once would have weighed 400 lbs. and occupied 10 square feet of space can now fit into a pocket at 1% the cost. With this development has come an explosion in the breadth and depth of the application of point-of-care ultrasound examination. This is ultrasound examination performed and interpreted by the clinician at the bedside, in physicians' offices, in emergency rooms, in critical care units, and in every imaginable perioperative setting.[1] In anesthesiology, cardiac ultrasound examination was the initial focus of point-of-care diagnostic imaging, but there has subsequently been rapid growth in

Department of Anesthesiology, University of Utah, 30 North 1900 East, Room 3C444 SOM, Salt Lake City, UT 84132, USA
* Corresponding author.
E-mail address: amber.bledsoe@hsc.utah.edu

Anesthesiology Clin 39 (2021) 537–553
https://doi.org/10.1016/j.anclin.2021.03.011
1932-2275/21/© 2021 Elsevier Inc. All rights reserved.

lung and gastric applications. Point-of-care ultrasound examination has proven to be user friendly and quickly performed with recognizable, real-time findings.[2] This review covers the basics of perioperative point-of-care gastric and lung ultrasound examinations, with a focus on the indications, procedural description, and clinical findings with the goal of building confidence and expanding the knowledge base of those wanting to incorporate these techniques into their everyday practice.

POINT-OF-CARE LUNG ULTRASOUND

Although the lungs have often been considered "in the way" of traditional cardiac ultrasound examination, the clinical application of lung ultrasound examination was originally described more than 20 years ago.[3] The International Consensus Conference on Lung Ultrasound met in 2009 to produce a unified lung ultrasound approach with common terminology based on a review of evidence.[4] Several different protocols/approaches have been described, including bedside lung ultrasound in an emergency and indication, acquisition, interpretation, and medical decision-making. Selecting a systematic approach allows the practitioner to apply the technology, identify the pertinent findings, and avoid the omission of relevant findings.[2,5]

Lung ultrasound examination is an imaging modality with both a steep learning curve and a high level of diagnostic accuracy. A recent study showed that even 25 supervised examinations were adequate to allow trainees to distinguish among normal lung, interstitial–alveolar syndrome, or lung consolidation.[6] Lung ultrasound has been shown superior to chest radiographs in the identification of pneumothorax, consolidation, pleural effusion, and pulmonary edema and, in many cases, on par with a chest computed tomography scan in diagnosing significant lung and pleural pathologies, with the added benefit of less radiation exposure.[7–12] Lung ultrasound examination is particularly useful in urgent settings when a rapid diagnosis is critical and obtaining a chest radiograph can cause unacceptable delays.

Indications

Indications for lung ultrasound examination continue to expand and can be divided into 2 distinct categories: diagnostic and monitoring. Common indications for diagnostic lung ultrasound examination include signs and symptoms of acute respiratory distress, including dyspnea, pleuritic chest pain, hypoxia, and tachypnea. The pathologies identified may include pneumothorax, cardiogenic pulmonary edema, pleural effusion, pneumonia, pulmonary embolus, and asthma or chronic obstructive pulmonary disease exacerbation. Monitoring indications typically include an assessment after a focused intervention, such as recruitment strategies, treatment of pneumothorax, or response to diuresis in cardiogenic pulmonary edema.[13]

Ultrasound Machine and Probe

The type of ultrasound probe used for a lung ultrasound examination should be selected based on the structure(s) of interest being evaluated.[4] The performance of different probes for lung ultrasound imaging relates to both their frequency response as well as their footprint. A high-frequency linear probe will have excellent resolution but poor tissue penetration and will be best for imaging structures near the probe. High-frequency probes are good at visualizing the pleura for lung sliding or small peripheral consolidations, but will rarely be adequate to characterize a pleural effusion. A lower frequency probe (phased array or curvilinear) will have better tissue penetration but a lower resolution. These probes may be best for identifying pleural effusions and interstitial syndrome. The large footprint of curvilinear probes allows the simultaneous scanning of multiple interspaces and a broad swath of lung, whereas a smaller phased array or microconvex probe will allow manipulation within more limited spaces (dependent areas in supine patients and imaging within single interspaces.) Probe selection will naturally be determined by what is available to the user and what interfaces with a portable, lightweight ultrasound machine with the ability to capture and store images. Ultimately, valuable lung ultrasound examinations can be performed with almost any available probe and technology should not represent a barrier to entry.

Technique

The first step before probe placement is patient positioning. The position will depend on the structures of interest and the suspected pathology. Position matters most when looking for dependent findings and less when assessing nondependent pathologies. With rare exception (eg, loculated effusions/air), pleural air will be nondependent, whereas pleural fluid collects in dependent areas. The evaluation of lung consolidation and interstitial syndrome are less position dependent and can be evaluated in either the semisitting or supine position. It is important to note that, when lung ultrasound imaging is being used for monitoring, the patient should be in the same position during each serial examination to facilitate accurate comparisons.

Many imaging techniques have been described and there is no "best" way to perform an examination; rather, it varies with the degree of urgency and the clinical question. Approaches that image up to 28 sites per hemithorax have been described, although in some cases a single image may be adequate to answer a simple question. Focusing on 3 zones (anterior, lateral, and posterior) in each hemithorax is a fast, user-friendly approach that will identify the cause of most acute respiratory failure pathologies (**Fig. 1**).

Anterior

Place the probe in the third or fourth intercostal space between the midclavicular and anterior axillary line with the probe aligned with the long axis of the body (parasagittal). Identify at least 1 rib on the screen, which helps to define the location of the pleura. Adjust the screen depth to approximately 2.5 times the depth of the pleural line. Rock the probe so that the pleura seems to be "horizontal" on the screen, then tilt the probe until an A-line is visualized. This practice ensures that the beam is perpendicular to the pleura.

Lateral

Place the probe in the midaxillary line with the probe aligned with the long-axis of the body as described and create an image as described for anterior imaging.

Posterior

Place the probe between the mid and posterior axillary lines with the probe aligned with the long axis of the body and with the beam directed toward the spine itself. These images should be at the level of the diaphragm and should demonstrate the liver or the spleen as well as the spine.

Lung Anatomy and Normal Findings

Findings seen on lung ultrasound examinations can be divided into 2 categories: nonanatomic (artifacts) and anatomic (visualized lung anatomy) (**Table 1**). When an ultrasound probe is placed cephalad to caudad over the intercostal space, the following structures can be identified: subcutaneous tissues and intercostal muscles, ribs, hyperechoic horizontal line at the interface between the visceral pleura

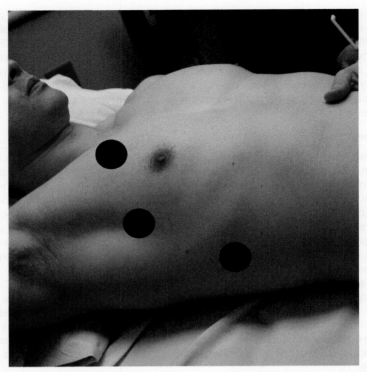

Fig. 1. Patient positioning and imaging location for lung ultrasound examination. The patient is in the supine position with the upper arm abducted to allow access to the chest. Suggested anterior, lateral, and posterior imaging locations are identified with black dots.

and aerated lung (referred to as the pleural line), and hyperechoic horizontal lines below the pleural line that are regularly spaced at multiples from the distance of the probe to the pleural line (referred to as A-lines) (**Figs. 2** and **3**, Videos 1 and 2). A-lines are present when air is homogenously distributed below the pleural line, as in normal aerated lung and pneumothorax. Hyperechoic vertical lines that originate from and move with the pleural line may also be seen (referred to as B-lines). They are only considered pathological if they traverse the entire screen (eg, from the pleural line to the end of the ultrasound imaging window) and are numerous (≥ 3 seen in an intercostal space). Pathological B-lines are discussed in greater detail in the Lung Pathologies Section.[14]

Two key points in lung ultrasound are that (1) aerated lung cannot be visualized on ultrasound examination; however, the loss of aerated lung (eg, consolidation, edema, atelectasis) results in improved beam penetration and the visualization of lung tissue. Another way to state that is, "You cannot 'see' normal lung, and if you can see lung it's not normal." (2) High acoustic impendence (as seen between tissue and lung) results in significant reflection of the ultrasound beam, producing a bright, echodense structure (eg, the pleural line).

It is important to discuss 2 other concepts involving the pleural line: lung sliding and lung pulsation. Lung sliding is movement between the lung surface (visceral pleura) and the chest wall (parietal pleural) and is an indication of ventilated lung with no pneumothorax.[3] Lung pulse is the movement of the visceral pleura secondary to

Table 1
Description of anatomical and artifactual findings on lung ultrasound

Finding on Ultrasound	Anatomic or Artifact	Cause of Artifact	Significance
Subcutaneous tissue	Anatomic	—	—
Intercostal muscles	Anatomic	—	—
Ribs	Anatomic	—	Aim to show 2 in each image
Pleural line	Artifact	Near complete reflection of ultrasound beam at aerated lung	Interface between visceral pleura and aerated lung
A line	Artifact	Reverberation from the strong reflectivity of the pleural line	Present when air is homogenously distributed below the pleural line
B line	Artifact	Reverberation artifacts from alveolar interstitial abnormalities at the visceral pleural surface	Only pathological if they extend to the bottom of the imaging window and are numerous (3 or more in an intercostal space)
Z line or comet tail artifact	Artifact	Focal lung densities at the level of the pleural line	Present in normal lungs

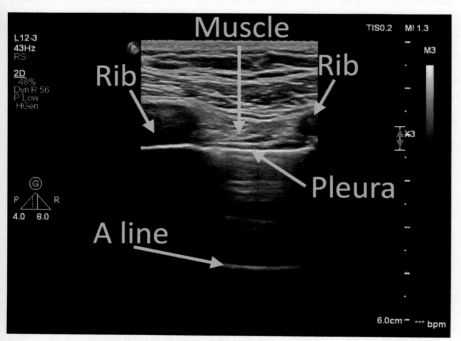

Fig. 2. Anatomy of a normal lung ultrasound image, in this example made with a high-frequency linear ultrasound probe. It is important to demonstrate at least one rib to ensure that the pleura is correctly identified. An A-line is seen, representing a reverberation artifact from the level of the pleura. Although A-lines are a normal finding and suggests that the beam is correctly oriented perpendicular to the pleura, it does not exclude pneumothorax.

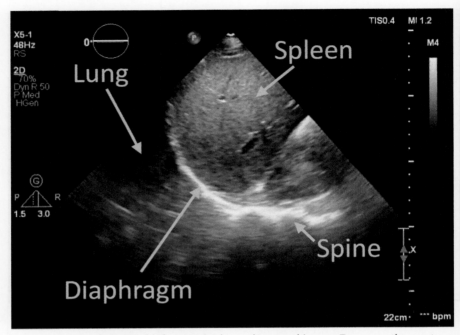

Fig. 3. Anatomy of a normal left posterior lung ultrasound image. To ensure the most posterior portion of the hemithorax is visualized, allowing identification of small pleural effusions, the spine should be seen. Note that normal, aerated lung cannot be "seen" on ultrasound imaging.

transmitted cardiac activity and not ventilation (Video 3).[15] Neither of these findings is seen when fluid or air is interposed between the pleura.

PUTTING IT TOGETHER

1. Positioning and probe selection
   a. Supine or recumbent position (see **Fig. 1**)
   b. High-frequency probe preferred for higher resolution when imaging shallow structures, lower frequency probe preferred for sufficient depth penetration when imaging deeper structures
2. Optimization of machine settings
   a. Set the acquisition time (beats or seconds) to capture 2 full respiratory cycles (at least 6–8 seconds)
3. Probe placement
   a. Place the probe in a cephalad to caudad orientation over 3 (anterior, lateral, and posterior) locations of the right and left hemithorax
4. Image creation, anterior and lateral (see **Fig. 2**, Video 1)
   a. Make sure that at least 1 rib is visible to ensure the pleural line is correctly identified
   b. Angle the probe and adjust the gain to maximize pleural line definition
   c. Set depth to visualize the pleural line and 1 associated A line
5. Image creation, posterior
   a. Probe oriented parasagittal, at the level of the diaphragm
   b. Demonstrate the spleen or liver with the spine in the far field (see **Fig. 3**, Video 2)

LUNG PATHOLOGIES
Pneumothorax

When a pneumothorax is present, there is a separation between the parietal and visceral pleura by intrapleural air. The intrapleural air reflects and attenuates the ultrasound waves at the interface of the parietal pleura, thus underlying lung movements and vertical artifacts that originate at the visceral pleura (eg, lung sliding and B-lines) are not appreciated.[3,16] With this principle in mind, the approach to pneumothorax includes several key diagnostic features: lung sliding, lung pulse, vertical artifacts, and lung point. The absence of lung sliding alone has a poor positive predictive value, stressing the importance of other diagnostic criteria. In contrast, a high positive predictive value for pneumothorax is seen with a lung point.[17] A lung point can be identified when a partially collapsed lung comes into contact with the parietal pleura during respiration. To evaluate for a lung point, the ultrasound probe is placed parallel to an intercostal space anteriorly, then slowly moved posteriorly seeing the "point" where lung sliding is visualized in only a portion of the image. This phenomenon is only visible in a noncomplete pneumothorax (Video 4).

Putting it together
Step 1: Do you see lung sliding, lung pulse, or vertical artifacts (B-lines)? If so, pneumothorax at the location of the probe is very unlikely.
Step 2: If the above are not seen, a lung point should be sought. The presence of a lung point creates a VERY HIGH suspicion for pneumothorax with a near-100% specificity.

False positives
Endobronchial intubation, pleural adhesion, large emphysematous bullae, airway obstruction, and apnea may all result in the absence of lung sliding, although a lung pulse and vertical artifacts may still be present. Keep in mind that a false-positive lung point can be seen at the level of the diaphragm.

Pleural Effusion

A pleural effusion is a fluid collection between the parietal and visceral pleura and is typically seen in the dependent portion of the lung. A lower frequency probe is preferred for sufficient depth penetration. With the probe positioned in the mid to posterior axillary line, the following structures should be visualized: left of the screen—lung artifact and diaphragm; right of the screen—liver/spleen, spine, and possibly kidney (see **Fig. 3**). In the absence of a pleural effusion, an aerated lung will slide across the image and obscure the diaphragm, liver/spleen, and spine during inspiration and is referred to as a "curtain sign" (see Video 2). The "spine sign" is seen when the spine is visualized both above and below the diaphragm (Video 5). The spine is not seen above the diaphragm in the absence of pleural fluid, because the aerated lung does not allow penetration of the ultrasound beam past the diaphragm.

Putting it together
Step 1: Place the probe in the eighth or ninth intercostal space between the mid and posterior axillary lines (see **Fig. 1**) in a cephalad caudad orientation with slight counterclockwise rotation and the beam angulated toward the spine.
Step 2: Hold the probe in a steady position while the patient inspires:

- Is there a curtain sign? If not, there is greater suspicion for pleural effusion.
- Is there a spine sign? If so, there is greater suspicion for pleural effusion.

- Significant effusions are typically easily visualized cephalad to the diaphragm as hypoechoic areas surrounding consolidated lung.

Step 3: Further evaluate the size of the pleural effusion by sliding the probe cranially and angulate anteriorly.[18]

False positives
Peritoneal fluid, pericardial effusion, and hemidiaphragmatic paralysis (lack of curtain sign) may lead to false-positive results.

Increased Lung Density (Pulmonary Edema and Pneumonia)

Increased lung density can be divided into 2 categories: increased lung weight (eg, water, pus, protein, blood, connective tissue, lipids) and lung de-aeration (eg, atelectasis). In these circumstances, the acoustic impedance is altered as the normal homogenous air interface changes into a heterogenous air–tissue interface. Variations in the visceral pleura result in B-line formation. Lower frequency probes are preferred for increased penetration depth. Each hemithorax should be interrogated in the anterior and lateral regions, with a focus on the presence of B-lines[14,19] (Video 6). The number of B-lines correlates with the severity of disease.

Putting it together
Step 1: Are B-lines present? If present, consider increased lung density.
Step 2: How many B-lines are present per intercostal space? If greater than or equal to 3, there is high suspicion for increased lung density.
Step 3: Are B-lines discrete or coalesced?

- Discrete, well-defined B-lines suggesting moderate loss of aeration with primarily interstitial edema.
- Coalesced B-lines suggest severe loss of aeration.

False positives
Misinterpretation of the Z-line (short vertical artifact that does not extend to the bottom of the imaging window), elderly patients (have higher prevalence of B lines without associated pathology), and misinterpretation of E-lines (vertical lines that originate from the subcutaneous tissue, not the visceral pleura) can produce false-positive results.

Summary
Do not let obstacles such as not having the right probe or a lack of knowledge limit your ability to implement this technology. It is a reliable, user friendly technique that can be learned in a short amount of time with appropriate training. Take the time to familiarize yourself with the principles, identify a preceptor to help refine your technique, and then start looking to see what you uncover. As has been said many times before: "If you do not look you do not know!"

CLINICS CARE POINTS

- No probe or technique has been proven superior to another. Use the equipment that you have available and a reproducible technique that is performed in the same fashion every time.
- Aerated lung is poorly visible on ultrasound examination, does not allow for significant penetration of the ultrasound beam, and therefore will create artifacts such as the pleural line and A-lines.

- Lung sliding is the interactive counter motion between the parietal and visceral pleura.
- Classic findings in pneumothorax include a lack of lung sliding, lung pulse, and B-lines. There is a high specificity for pneumothorax if a lung point also identified.
- Classic findings in pleural effusion include a negative curtain sign and positive spine sign.
- Classic findings in increased lung density include greater than or equal to 3 B-lines (interstitial B1 pattern) or coalesced B-lines (consolidated B2 pattern). B-lines are vertical reverberation artifacts that arise from the visceral pleura and extend longitudinally to the bottom of the imaging screen.

POINT-OF-CARE GASTRIC ULTRASOUND

Although gastric ultrasound examination has been described for more than 40 years, its application as a perioperative point-of-care technique has expanded dramatically in the past decade.[20] Preoperative fasting guidelines exist to decrease the risk of aspiration, and the nil per os (NPO) recommendations are designed as educated best guesses of when patients' stomachs may be empty.[21] Although the NPO recommendations are based on a rigorous review of the available literature, their applicability to an individual can always be questioned. Gastric ultrasound examination provides valuable additional information about what is (or is not) actually in a patient's stomach, taking away some of that guesswork. Although clinically significant perioperative aspiration is uncommon, and fatal aspiration even more rare (<1/70,000 anesthetics), it is nonetheless a much-feared complication of anesthesia.[22] Gastric ultrasound imaging, applied with an understanding of established NPO recommendations, can further stratify aspiration risk in individual patients and has been shown to affect clinical decision making when applied preoperatively.[23]

When performing a gastric ultrasound examination, there are 2 objectives: (1) characterize the contents of the stomach (empty, clear fluid, thick fluid, or solid) and (2) assess the volume.[24] The first triage point is to identify what is in the stomach. If the stomach is empty, the aspiration risk is low; if the stomach contains solid contents, the aspiration risk is high. If fluid is identified, it is then important to quantify the volume of gastric contents to further evaluate the aspiration risk (**Fig. 4**).

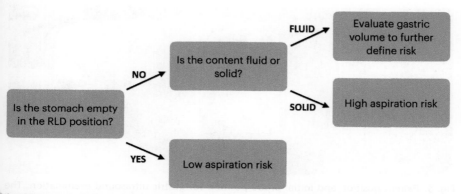

Fig. 4. Proposed approach to gastric ultrasound examination in the assessment of potential aspiration risk.

Indications

The primary indication for gastric ultrasound examination is to further stratify aspiration risk and may include possible scenarios such as elective procedures when NPO recommendations were not followed, urgent/emergent procedures, and questionable NPO status. Knowing the risk of aspiration may then lead to changes in airway management and anesthetic approach. It is important to recognize that these techniques have not been thoroughly studied in those with prior gastric or lower esophageal surgery and, therefore, caution must be taken when assessing for gastric volume in that patient population.

Ultrasound Machine and Probe

Although it is possible to perform gastric ultrasound with a low-frequency phased array probe (a "cardiac probe"), a low-frequency (2–5 MHz) curvilinear probe and a machine with abdominal presets is preferred. A linear probe, with a higher frequency, can be used in patients with minimal abdominal subcutaneous tissue and pediatric patients, when deeper ultrasound penetration is not necessary.

Technique

The examination is performed first in the supine then in the lateral position. Starting supine allows for initial visualization of the stomach with further interrogation when rotating into the right lateral decubitus (RLD) position. The RLD position puts gastric contents in a dependent location against the pylorus, allowing for better visualization of lower volumes of gastric content in the gastric antrum.[25] The probe should be aligned in the sagittal/parasagittal direction with the indicator pointed cephalad (**Fig. 5**).

Gastric Anatomy and Findings

It is important to distinguish the stomach from other hollow viscus structures seen in the abdomen (eg, colon, small bowel). Notable landmarks in proximity to the stomach include the liver anteriorly and the pancreas posteriorly (**Fig. 6**). The stomach can be divided into the cardia, fundus, body, and pyloric antrum. The antrum is typically seen when the long axis of the aorta comes into view. The antrum has been described as the most amenable to ultrasound examination and accurately reflects the contents of the entire stomach.[25] The body and fundus are often difficult to visualize owing to

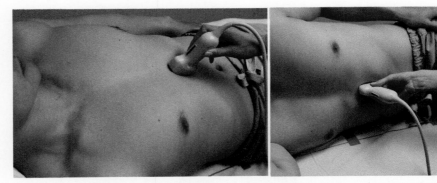

Fig. 5. Patient position and initial probe position for gastric ultrasound examination. The patient is initially in the supine position then turns to the RLD position. The curvilinear probe is placed below the diploid process and oriented in the sagittal plane.

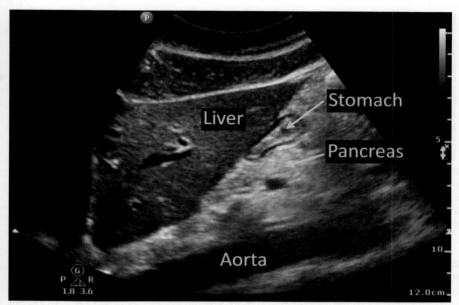

Fig. 6. Normal anatomy of a gastric ultrasound image. It is important to locate the abdominal aorta, as an additional indicator that the antrum of the stomach is being evaluated rather than the pylorus.

poor ultrasound penetration from the presence of air. The stomach wall is 4 to 6 mm thick and comprises 5 layers. From the inner surface of the stomach outward, these layers include the mucosal–air interface, muscularis mucosa, submucosa, muscularis propria, and serosa. The most notable layer on ultrasound imaging is the thick, hyperechoic muscularis propria.

Perlas and colleagues[26] described a qualitative antral classification system to describe the fluid contents of the stomach. When the stomach is empty, the antrum will appear flattened or oval shaped with a thick muscular wall. This is often described as a bullseye or target pattern and is classified as grade 0 if the stomach seems to be empty in both the supine and RLD positions (**Fig. 7**). When the stomach contains clear fluid with low gastric volume, it is classified as grade 1 if the stomach seems to be empty in the supine position with liquid seen in the RLD position (**Fig. 8**). When fluid is seen in both supine and RLD positions, it is classified as grade 2 and suggests significant gastric volume (**Fig. 9**).

When liquid is consumed, the antrum seems to be round and distended with a thin muscular wall and hypoechoic content. When gastric fluid contains air particles, the characteristic pattern has been described as a starry night (air bubbles within hypoechoic fluid) (**Fig. 10**). If the antrum is interrogated shortly after the consumption of solids, the stomach is filled with particulate matter and air. Air and solids layered along the anterior stomach wall prevent further penetration of the ultrasound beam, thus blurring the posterior wall and deeper structures. This has been described as a frosted glass appearance (**Fig. 11**). Solids in a later stage of digestion, will appear as heterogeneous, hyperechoic material (**Fig. 12**).

When gastric fluid is seen in the antrum and further quantification of gastric volume is warranted, the antral cross-sectional area (CSA) is measured using the free tracing

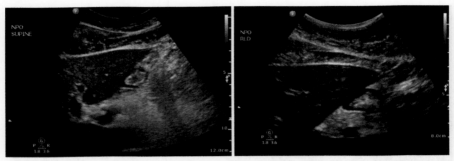

Fig. 7. In a grade 0 antrum, there is no fluid visible in either the supine or RLD position. In the left image the patient is supine, and no contents can be visualized in the stomach. In the right image the patient has now been turned to the RLD position. No contents are visualized in the gastric antrum. This patient is likely at extremely low risk of pulmonary aspiration as the stomach is completely empty.

application on the ultrasound machine. The antrum is identified in the RLD position at the level of the aorta (where it seems to be the largest) and a still image is captured for easier tracing. The CSA of the antrum is then traced (including the muscular gastric wall) and applied to the following equation: volume (mL) = 27.0 + 14.6 × RLD CSA − 1.28 × age. This equation has been validated in nonpregnant subjects with a

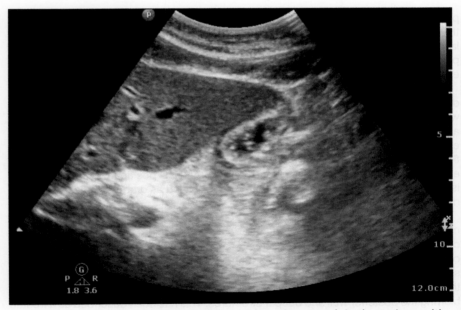

Fig. 8. In a grade 1 antrum, there is no fluid visible in the stomach in the supine position. When the patient is turned to the RLD position; however, fluid is seen in the gastric antrum. This image shows a small amount of fluid in a patient in the RLD position. This is consistent with normal gastric fluid in a patient who is appropriately NPO. This patient is likely at very low risk of pulmonary aspiration.

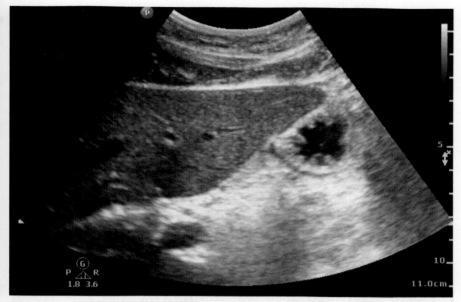

Fig. 9. In a grade 2 antrum, there is fluid visible in the stomach even in the supine position (shown here.) This patient may be at higher risk of aspiration owing to the large volume of liquid visualized in the stomach.

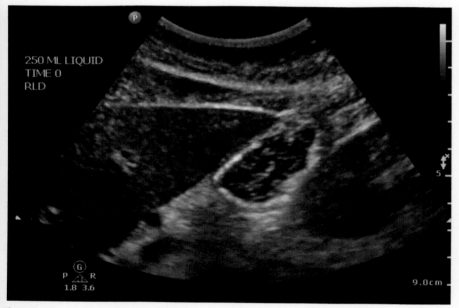

Fig. 10. The "starry night" pattern. This patient has recently consumed liquids, and the stomach is filled with a combination of anechoic fluid and bright air bubbles.

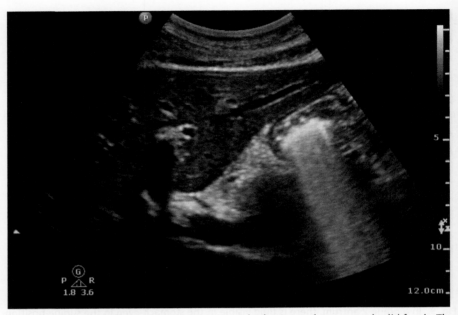

Fig. 11. The "frosted glass" pattern in a patient who has recently consumed solid foods. The combination of these solids with air creates a reverberation artifact originating at the anterior wall of the stomach.

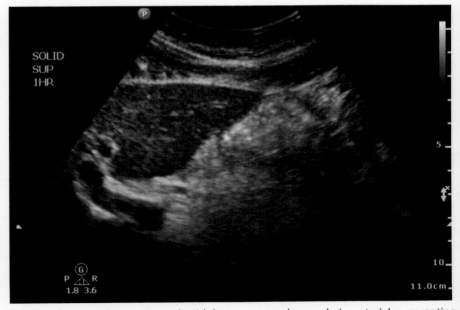

Fig. 12. This image shows a stomach with heterogenous, hyperechoic material representing a large amount of solids.

body mass index of less than 40 kg/m². Volumes greater than 1.5 mL/kg are abnormal in fasted patients and may carry concern for a greater risk of aspiration.[27]

Putting It Together

1. Positioning and probe selection
   a. Supine then RLD position
   b. Low-frequency curvilinear probe preferred for sufficient depth penetration
2. Optimization of machine settings
   a. Abdominal presets, if available
   b. Adjust gain, depth, focus, and tissue harmonics as necessary
3. Probe placement
   a. Place probe in a sagittal/parasagittal direction with the indicator pointed cephalad
   b. Sweep from the right to left subcostal margin to identify the stomach
   c. Look for a hollow viscus with a prominent dark band representing the muscularis propria
   d. Identify the antrum at the level of the aorta (a thick-walled vessel with pulsation only in systole)
4. Gastric content and volume identification
   a. What is in the stomach (empty, clear fluid, thick fluid/solid)
      1. Empty—bullseye pattern
         a. Grade 0 antrum—flattened antrum in the supine and RLD position
      2. Clear fluid—starry night pattern (distended antrum with air bubbles in hypoechoic content)
         a. Grade 1 antrum—fluid visible only in the RLD position (low gastric volume)
         b. Grade 2 antrum—fluid visible in both the RLD and supine position (higher gastric volume)
      3. Thick fluid/solid—frosted glass pattern (distended antrum with hyperechoic/heterogenous content)
   b. If the content is fluid, quantify the volume
      1. Trace the CSA of the antrum (including the gastric wall)
      2. Calculate the volume using the following equation:
         a. Volume (mL) = 27.0 + 14.6 × RLD CSA – 1.28 × age
      3. A volume of 1.5 mL/kg is considered abnormal in fasting patients

SUMMARY

Gastric ultrasound examination can improve the understanding of aspiration risk and may be most useful in scenarios such as lack of compliance, unclear fasting history, and comorbid conditions in which gastric emptying may be delayed.

CLINICS CARE POINTS

- Gastric ultrasound examination can be used as an adjunct to NPO fasting guidelines to better assess risk of aspiration based on gastric contents (empty, clear fluid, thick fluid/solid).
- A curvilinear, low-frequency probe is preferred owing to increased penetration for deeper structures.
- The gastric antrum should be assessed in both the supine and RLD position. Gastric contents are best seen in the RLD position.

- Gastric contents can be graded according to the antral grading system: grade 0 (no fluid seen in supine and RLD position—low aspiration risk), grade 1 (no fluid seen in supine position but visualized in RLD position—low gastric volume with low aspiration risk), and grade 2 (fluid seen in supine and RLD position—high gastric volume with higher aspiration risk).
- The antral CSA can be used to further quantify the volume of gastric contents.
- More information with images and examples can be found at Gastricultrasound.org.

DISCLOSURE

The authors have nothing to disclose.

SUPPLEMENTARY DATA

Supplementary data to this article can be found online at https://doi.org/10.1016/j.anclin.2021.03.011.

REFERENCES

1. Goffi A, Kruisselbrink R, Volpicelli G. The sound of air: point-of-care lung ultrasound in perioperative medicine Le bruit de l'air: e chographie pulmonaire au point d'intervention en me decine pe riope ratoire. Can J Anesth 2018;65:399–416.
2. Kruisselbrink R, Chan V, Cibinel GA, et al. I-AIM (Indication, Acquisition, Interpretation, Medical Decision-making) framework for point of care lung ultrasound. Anesthesiology 2017;127:568–82.
3. Lichtenstein DA, Menu Y. A bedside ultrasound sign ruling out pneumothorax in the critically ill. Lung sliding. Chest 1995;108:1345–8.
4. International Liaison Committee on Lung Ultrasound (ILC-LUS) for the International Consensus Conference on Lung Ultrasound (ICC-LUS), Volpicelli G, ElBarbary M, Blaivas M, et al. International evidence-based recommendations for point-of-care lung ultrasound. Intensive Care Med 2012;38:577–91.
5. Lichtenstein DA, Mezière GA. Relevance lung ultrasound in the diagnosis of acute respiratory failure: the BLUE protocol. Chest 2008;134:117–25.
6. Arbelot C, Dexheimer Neto FL, Gao Y, et al. Lung ultrasound in emergency and critically ill patients: number of supervised exams to reach basic competence. Anesthesiology 2020;132:899–907.
7. Lichtenstein D, Goldstein I, Mourgeon E, et al. Comparative diagnostic performances of auscultation, chest radiography, and lung ultrasonography in acute respiratory distress syndrome. Anesthesiology 2004;100:9–15.
8. Pivetta E, Goffi A, Nazerian P, et al. Lung ultrasound integrated with clinical assessment for the diagnosis of acute decompensated heart failure in the emergency department: a randomized controlled trial. Eur J Heart Fail 2019;21:754–66.
9. Xirouchaki N, Magkanas E, Vaporidi K, et al. Lung ultrasound in critically ill patients: comparison with bedside chest radiography. Intensive Care Med 2011;37:1488–93.
10. Blaivas M, Lyon M, Duggal S. A prospective comparison of supine chest radiography and bedside ultrasound for the diagnosis of traumatic pneumothorax. Acad Emerg Med 2005;12:844–9.

11. Soldati G, Testa A, Sher S, et al. Occult traumatic pneumothorax: diagnostic accuracy of lung ultrasonography in the emergency department. Chest 2008;133: 204–11.
12. Nazerian P, Volpicelli G, Vanni S, et al. Accuracy of lung ultrasound for the diagnosis of consolidations when compared to chest computed tomography. Am J Emerg Med 2015;33:620–5.
13. Bouhemad B, Mongodi S, Via G, et al. Ultrasound for "Lung Monitoring" of Ventilated Patients. Anesthesiology 2015;122:437–47.
14. Lichtenstein D, Mezière G, Biderman P, et al. The comet-tail artifact. An ultrasound sign of alveolar-interstitial syndrome. Am J Respir Crit Care Med 1997; 156:1640–6.
15. Lichtenstein DA. Lung ultrasound in the critically ill. Ann Intensive Care 2014; 4(1):1.
16. Lichtenstein D, Mezière G, Biderman P, et al. The comet-tail artifact: an ultrasound sign ruling out pneumothorax. Intensive Care Med 1999;25:383–8.
17. Lichtenstein D, Mezière G, Biderman P, et al. The "lung point": an ultrasound sign specific to pneumothorax. Intensive Care Med 2000;26:1434–40.
18. Balik M, Plasil P, Waldauf P, et al. Ultrasound estimation of volume of pleural fluid in mechanically ventilated patients. Intensive Care Med 2006;32:318.
19. Volpicelli G, Mussa A, Garofalo G, et al. Bedside lung ultrasound in the assessment of alveolar-interstitial syndrome. The Am J Emerg Med 2006;24:689–96.
20. Holt S, McDicken WN, Anderson T, et al. Dynamic imaging of the stomach by real-time ultrasound–a method for the study of gastric motility. Gut 1980;21: 597–601.
21. Practice guidelines for preoperative fasting and the use of pharmacologic agents to reduce the risk of pulmonary aspiration: application to healthy patients undergoing elective procedures: an updated report by the American Society of Anesthesiologists Task Force on preoperative fasting and the use of pharmacologic agents to reduce the risk of pulmonary aspiration. Anesthesiology 2017;126: 376–93.
22. Warner MA. Clinical significance of pulmonary aspiration. Anesthesiology 2006; 78:56–62.
23. Alakkad H, Kruisselbrink R, Chin KJ, et al. Point-of-care ultrasound defines gastric content and changes the anesthetic management of elective surgical patients who have not followed fasting instructions: a prospective case series. Can J Anesth 2015;62:1188–95.
24. Perlas A, Van de Putte P, Van Houwe P, et al. I-AIM framework for point-of-care gastric ultrasound. Br J Anaesth 2016;116:7–11.
25. Van de Putte P, Perlas A. Ultrasound assessment of gastric content and volume. Br J Anaesth 2014;113:12–22.
26. Perlas A, Davis L, Khan M, et al. Gastric sonography in the fasted surgical patient: a prospective descriptive study. Anesth Analg 2011;113:93–7.
27. Perlas A, Mitsakakis N, Liu L, et al. Validation of a mathematical model for ultrasound assessment of gastric volume by gastroscopic examination. Anesth Analg 2013;116:357–63.

Toward Smart Monitoring with Phones, Watches, and Wearable Sensors

Frederic Michard, MD, PhD

KEYWORDS

- Smartphone • Smartwatch • Wearable • Digital health • Mobile monitoring
- Home monitoring • Self-monitoring • Perioperative medicine

KEY POINTS

- Smartphones, smartwatches, and wireless wearables are increasingly used by patients and clinicians to gather physiologic information.
- They may help to involve patients in their surgical journey, unmask comorbidities, optimize prehabilitation programs, and individualize perioperative care.
- Ultrasound probes, connectable to smartphones, may soon replace the stethoscope in the pocket of many perioperative clinicians. They may be used in the operating room to guide regional anesthesia and central venous catheter insertion, and in the ICU and on surgical wards for echocardiographic evaluations in hemodynamically unstable patients.
- Wireless wearables will be increasingly used for the continuous monitoring of vital signs on hospital wards, and clinicians will have the option to be informed without any delay on their smartphone in case of clinical deterioration.
- Smartphone applications (Apps) may help to optimize the adherence to enhanced recovery after surgery programs and to follow patients during the rehabilitation phase.

Smartphones are increasingly powerful computers that fit in our pocket. Thanks to dedicated applications or Apps, they can connect with external sensors to record, analyze, display, store, and share multiple physiologic signals and data.[1] In addition, because modern smartphones are equipped with accelerometers, gyroscopes, cameras, and pressure sensors, they can also be used to directly gather physiologic information.[2] In this respect, smartphones and connected sensors are creating opportunities to empower patients, facilitate the diagnosis of disease states, individualize perioperative care, and simplify clinicians' life.[3]

In this article, main opportunities for patient self-monitoring are first discussed. The next section describes how health care workers, and perioperative clinicians in particular, could use more often and more efficiently in their professional life the smartphone they have in their pocket.

MiCo, Chemin de Chapallaz 4, Denens 1135, Switzerland
E-mail address: frederic.michard@bluewin.ch

Anesthesiology Clin 39 (2021) 555–564
https://doi.org/10.1016/j.anclin.2021.04.005
1932-2275/21/© 2021 Elsevier Inc. All rights reserved.

SELF-MONITORING WITH SMARTPHONES AND CONNECTED DEVICES
Detection of Cardiac Rhythm and Electrocardiographic Abnormalities

In case of chest pain or palpitations, patients can use their smartphone for measuring their heart rate and detect irregular patterns, suggestive of cardiac arrhythmia. To do so, they just need to cover with their finger the flashlight and camera of their smartphone. Assuming they have installed the appropriate App, the camera will record a peripheral pulse waveform, similar to the signal that would be recorded by a pulse oximeter. From this easy-to-record signal, several Apps have been shown to be able to detect cardiac arrhythmia with fair sensitivity and specificity.[4–6] Heart rate and heart rate variability can also be computed from selfie videos. The user simply needs to look at the smartphone camera, and the App software will track and analyze subtle changes in skin color induced by heart beats, which are not visible to the human eye.[7]

Many smartwatches now integrate a photoplethysmographic sensor (with red or green light) on their rear side that can be used to record (on demand or continuously) a peripheral pulse waveform. Specific App algorithms can derive pulse rate and abnormalities in pulse intervals (suggesting cardiac arrhythmia) from this waveform. Notably, the large Apple heart study,[8] done in collaboration with Stanford University and published in the New England Journal of Medicine, showed that we may reasonably envisage to use smartwatches to unmask asymptomatic episodes of atrial fibrillation. The Apple algorithm was designed to favor specificity over sensitivity, to minimize false alerts and unjustified medical visits. In this large study,[8] notifications for irregular pulse reached 0.5% in the study population and dramatically increased in patients older than 65 years. A large study is currently ongoing to investigate whether the detection of atrial fibrillation with a smartwatch could help reduce the risk of stroke.

Once an abnormal cardiac rhythm has been detected, the logical next step is to record an electrocardiogram (ECG). This recording is now possible from a smartwatch (**Fig. 1**). Initially, a specific bracelet integrating a surface electrode was necessary.

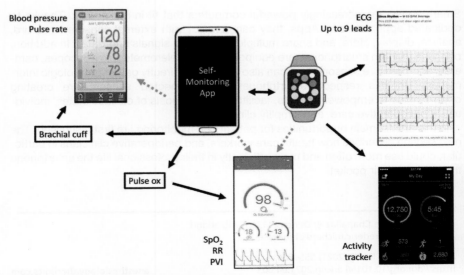

Fig. 1. Self-monitoring with a smartphone and connected devices.

When wearing the watch on the left wrist, it was possible to record a D1 lead by putting any right finger on the bracelet electrode (and then closing the electric loop). Several studies have shown that this method was accurate to detect atrial fibrillation or an ST segment elevation, as well as to measure the QT interval.[9–12] Today, it is no longer necessary to use a dedicated bracelet. Assuming the watch is worn on the left wrist, the electric loop can be closed by putting any right finger on the watch crown. In addition, when placing the watch on the ankle or on the chest, it becomes possible to record up to 9 ECG leads.[13]

Blood Pressure Self-Monitoring

Self-monitoring of blood pressure (BP) may be useful to unmask hypertension and to prevent false-positive diagnoses related to the white coat effect; it may also help to titrate antihypertensive medication in individuals with poorly controlled BP.[14] Blood pressure is easy to self-measure with a classic medical-grade oscillometric brachial cuff. Some are wireless, and most enable to record, store, and visualize BP values and trends on a smartphone (see **Fig. 1**). Brachial cuffs remain bulky, therefore watches have been modified to integrate an inflatable cuff in their bracelet, enabling radial BP measurements anywhere and at any time.

Several methods have been proposed to monitor BP directly from a smartphone, without the need for any external sensor. The InstantApp was initially developed to estimate the pulse wave transit time (PWTT) from the simultaneous recording of a ballistocardiogram and a peripheral pulse waveform. The ballistocardiogram was recorded by the smartphone built-in accelerometers when applying it on the thorax, close to the heart apex. The peripheral pulse was obtained, as previously described, by covering the smartphone camera with a finger. The PWTT is highly dependent on blood flow and vascular tone, and several studies have shown that changes in PWTT are useful to track changes in BP.[15] Unfortunately, clinical evaluations have concluded that the InstantApp was not accurate, leading to a possible underestimation of BP and hence to the under-treatment of patients with chronic hypertension.[16,17] As a result, this App is no longer available.

More recently, the oscillometric finger pressing method has been proposed to measure blood pressure directly from a smartphone, using the pressure sensitivity of modern screens.[18] The user presses his or her fingertip on both the front camera and screen to increase the external pressure of the underlying artery, while the App measures the resulting variable-amplitude blood volume oscillations via the camera and applied pressure via the strain gauge array under the screen. The App visually guides the fingertip placement and actuation and then computes BP from the measurements just like automatic cuff devices. Initial evaluations yielded bias and precision errors that did not meet yet international standards.[18]

A transdermal optical method, based on selfie videos, has also been proposed. This method has been tested in healthy volunteers[19] and a correlation has been observed between reference systolic BP measurements and values predicted by the optical method. Although the correlation was statistically significant, it was weak, and the study was conducted in volunteers who had a normal systolic BP. Studies are therefore needed to investigate whether this video-based method may detect low or high BP numbers.

Other methods based on peripheral pulse wave analysis look promising.[20–22] These methods are based on the recording of a peripheral pulse waveform from a pulse oximeter,[20] from a dedicated bracelet integrating a photoplethysmographic sensor,[21] or directly from a smartphone camera.[22] Then, machine learning algorithms, which have been trained to detect specific patterns or signatures associated with BP deviations from an initial calibration, are used to monitor BP continuously. A proof-of-concept study,[20] recently published in Anesthesia & Analgesia, showed that the mere analysis of a pulse oximetry waveform can be used to track acute changes in BP during anesthesia induction. A more recent study[22] suggested interchangeability between auscultatory reference measurements and measurements done directly with a smartphone over a short period. Studies are now required to clarify how long these methods can provide reliable BP measures after initial calibration.

Self-Monitoring of Respiratory Variables

Today, medical-grade wireless pulse oximeters are easy to buy from online stores. These devices enable the recording of not only oxygen saturation (oxygen saturation as measured by pulse oximetry [Spo_2]) but also the pulse rate and the peripheral perfusion index, which may have value to assess tissue perfusion.[23] Modern pulse oximeters may also provide an estimation of respiratory rate (from the respiratory oscillations of the pulse oximetry waveform) and of the pleth variability index (PVI) (see **Fig. 1**). PVI is a quantification of the magnitude of the respiratory swings in the pulse oximetry waveform. In mechanically ventilated patients, it is known as a surrogate for the arterial pulse pressure variation (PPV) in patients who do not have an arterial catheter in place. As such, it may be used to predict fluid responsiveness, a now-established clinical practice with demonstrated outcome benefits in surgical patients.[24] In spontaneously breathing patients, respiratory changes in pulse oximetry waveform reflect the cyclic changes in intrathoracic pressure rather than volume status. These changes are correlated with the magnitude of respiratory efforts and may help to assess the severity of patients with acute respiratory failure, such as those with the coronavirus disease 2019 (COVID-19).[25]

As they integrate photoplethysmographic sensors, several recent smartwatches measure and display Spo_2 estimations. It is important to bear in mind that reflective photoplethysmography is known to be less accurate than the classic transmissive technique based on the transillumination of a finger. In this respect, smartwatch-derived Spo_2 measurements have not yet been approved for medical use.

Self-monitoring of Spo_2 and other respiratory variables (mainly respiratory rate and PVI) has been extensively promoted since the beginning of the COVID-19 pandemic.[25,26] Indeed, the self-detection of hypoxemia may lead to timely hospital admission and ultimately better outcome. For patients in whom self-monitoring is not an option (because either they do not know how or they do not want to do it themselves) command centers have been created to monitor patients remotely and inform them in case of clinical deterioration requiring a medical consultation. In practice, patients wear a finger pulse oximeter, and their smartphone is used as a gateway to transmit physiologic signals and measurements to the command center. This strategy has potential, not only to trigger hospital admissions as soon as necessary but also to discharge patients earlier from the hospital, knowing we can keep an eye on them until full recovery.[26] It is obviously too soon to fully appreciate the pros and cons of these new strategies, but the pandemic has been a catalyst for the implementation of remote monitoring solutions. Several programs and initiatives are currently going on, and evaluations should be published within the next months and years.

The use of connected sensors has also been proposed to detect patients with COVID-19 at an early stage, before patients become symptomatic, or, once they have symptoms, to predict the need for hospitalization. Indeed, the close monitoring of heart rate, heart rate variability, and respiratory rate may reveal specific patterns and trends enabling the early detection of infection and/or the prediction of clinical trajectories.[27]

In summary, many Apps and connected devices are now available for patient's self-monitoring. These Apps may help clinicians, and in particular anesthesiologists, during the preoperative visit, to better detect co-morbidities in their patients and also to individualize physiologic targets to be used during the perioperative period. As an example, it has been shown that both intraoperative and postoperative hypotension are associated with postoperative complications and death, but the optimal BP for any given patient remains unclear. It has been established that the BP measured during the preoperative visit or right before anesthesia induction may not reflect the usual BP of any given patient.[28] The BP may significantly vary during daytime and usually reaches a minimum during the night. It has recently been suggested that this minimal BP value may be considered as the lower acceptable limit during anesthesia for the individual patient.[28] In other words, a better identification of personal physiologic values may help to individualize perioperative management. Finally, many Apps have been developed to invite people increase their physical activity, lose weight, and stop smoking.[29,30] These Apps may help during the prehabilitation period to improve the physiologic status of high-risk surgical patients and ultimately postoperative outcomes.

SMARTPHONES APPLICATIONS FOR PERIOPERATIVE CLINICIANS

Digital Auscultation

Smartphones can help with physical examination. Digital auscultation is a new reality, and several stethoscopes are now designed to connect to and display the recorded information on a smartphone.[1,2] A phone case integrating a stethoscope membrane has also been developed.[2,31] The digitization of auscultation enables not only the amplification of sounds and their recording but also the automatic detection of abnormalities. Indeed, like the well-known Shazam App able to put a name on any song in a few seconds, smart algorithms have been developed to detect valve and lung disease from digital auscultation.[31] The digitization of acoustic signals also enables the visualization of heart sounds, as done in the past with phonocardiograms.[2] These digital stethoscopes may help the nonexpert in cardiac auscultation to suspect a valve disease and trigger an ultrasound evaluation that, as explained in the next paragraph, can also be done with a smartphone.

Pocket Ultrasonography

Pocket ultrasound devices are on the rise, and some are simply probes that can be connected to a smartphone or an electronic tablet (**Fig. 2**). These probes are usually much less expensive than classic ultrasound devices, and this may explain, at least in part, their increasing adoption by clinicians. Some predict they may soon replace the stethoscope (even digital) in the pocket of most clinicians, particularly if they belong to the generation who grew up surrounded by digital tools. The only remaining limitation to wide clinical adoption is the lack of skills to record and analyze echo images. The increasing number of training programs is, however, progressively closing that knowledge gap.

Pocket ultrasound devices are everything but gizmos; they are useful to detect cardiac abnormalities with high sensitivity and specificity, as well as to assess ventricular dimension and function.[32,33] In deteriorating ward patients, a recent study[34] showed that a quick cardiac and lung evaluation with a pocket echo device enabled early diagnosis, early intervention, and improvement in patient outcome. Pocket echo devices can also help to guide the insertion of central venous catheters and facilitate regional anesthesia.[35,36]

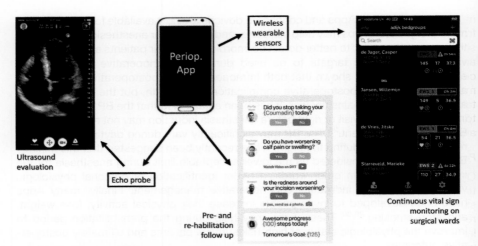

Fig. 2. Examples of smartphone applications in perioperative medicine.

Apps for Enhanced Recovery after Surgery Programs

Apps have been developed for hospitals implementing enhanced recovery after surgery (ERAS) programs. These Apps are electronic checklists designed to improve the compliance to ERAS programs and ensure all key elements of these programs are effectively implemented (see **Fig. 2**). Most of these Apps also allow direct communication with patients and may help to ensure they follow preoperative recommendations (eg, for anticoagulation medications) and, after surgery and hospital discharge, to check if they develop any postoperative complications. For example, a patient developing a wound infection would have the opportunity to describe his symptoms and send a picture of the wound to the surgeon; this may seem trivial, but it may actually considerably facilitate and speed up care processes and help both patients and hospitals to save time and money.

Intraoperative Monitoring

The pulse decomposition method is part of new techniques that have been developed for the continuous and noninvasive monitoring of BP.[37] A finger cuff inflated at a low (40 mm Hg) and constant pressure, coupled with a piezoelectric sensor, enables the continuous recording of a finger pressure waveform, which is ultimately converted into a BP waveform by a proprietary algorithm. When compared with invasive reference measurements, this method has been shown to be accurate and precise to monitor BP during surgery.[38] In contrast to existing bulky volume clamp monitoring systems, the pulse decomposition system has the advantage to be light and wireless, and it does not require any stand-alone monitor: the BP waveform and numerical values are displayed on an electronic tablet or a smartphone.[37,38]

In patients monitored with an arterial radial catheter for continuous BP monitoring, pulse contour methods are increasingly used for intraoperative fluid and hemodynamic management. Pulse contour algorithms are able to compute stroke volume and cardiac output from a BP waveform. However, their cost may be a significant obstacle to hospital adoption. A hemodynamic App has been developed to offer a solution to anesthesiologists who do not have access to pulse contour techniques. The App is used to take a picture of the BP waveform (displayed on a multiparameter monitor or anesthesia machine), then an algorithm computes PPV and stroke volume from the waveform, as any pulse contour monitor would do. Several studies have shown the App to be reliable enough to assess PPV (ie, to predict fluid responsiveness and guide fluid therapy).[39,40] Unfortunately, the pulse contour algorithm of the App is currently too basic to provide reliable stroke volume and cardiac output measurements. However, the concept of extracting physiologic information from pictures taken by a smartphone may be here to stay. Indeed, another App has been designed to quantify intraoperative blood loss from the picture of a surgical sponge or cannister, and a few studies have suggested that it provides quick and accurate estimations.[41,42]

Postoperative Monitoring

Over the last decade, multiple solutions emerged to transform the way we monitor patients on surgical wards.[43] This development was fueled by the increasing number of studies demonstrating that the intermittent nature of vital sign spot-checks may be responsible for delayed detection of clinical deterioration.[44] Several prospective and large before-after studies have suggested that continuous monitoring of vital signs, with tethered or untethered monitoring systems, enables a decrease in the number of rescue interventions, intensive care unit (ICU) admissions, and calls for cardiac arrest.[45] Several of these new monitoring solutions, often based on wireless wearable sensors stuck to the skin or attached to the finger, use smartphones (or smartphone-like dedicated pocket devices) to display vital signs, early warning scores, or their trends over time and to alert ward nurses in case of deterioration[46] (see **Fig. 2**).

Rehabilitation

Early mobilization and physiotherapy are key elements of ERAS programs. Multiple Apps have been designed to track physical activity from external skin sensors, smartwatches, or simply from the smartphone built-in accelerometers and gyroscopes (see **Fig. 1**). An increasing number of studies report the use of activity trackers during the postoperative period, particularly after orthopedic surgery.[47–49] Multiple Apps are available to set physical activity goals (eg, minimum number of steps, minimum distance per day) as well as for the objective quantification of progress made during the recovery phase. Whether they really help to increase the efficiency of rehabilitation programs remains to be demonstrated by large trials.

SUMMARY

Smartphones, smartwatches, and wireless wearables are increasingly used by patients and clinicians. These devices may help to empower patients, to optimize prehabilitation programs, and to individualize perioperative care by determining personal physiologic targets (eg, personal BP to be maintained during and after surgery). These devices may also simplify clinicians' life. In case of postoperative cardiorespiratory deterioration, in the ICU or on the wards, physicians can simply connect an echo probe to their smartphone to quickly understand the underlying mechanisms and select the most appropriate treatment. On surgical wards, nurses can be automatically and immediately alerted on their smartphone in case of patient deterioration. Smartphone Apps may also have value to optimize the adherence to ERAS programs and to follow patients during the rehabilitation phase.

In this article, we briefly described the main existing medical grade applications of smartphones and smartwatches, and there is no doubt that many more will soon become available. As clinicians, our responsibility is not only to embrace technical innovations that may improve quality of care but also to stay away from novelty blindness.[50,51] In this regard, we need to conduct well-designed studies to assess the real impact of digital innovations on patient outcome and health care costs.

CLINICS CARE POINTS

- Smartphones can connect to medical-grade oscillometric brachial cuffs and pulse oximeters for self-measurement of blood pressure and oxygen saturation, respectively.
- Smartwatches can be used to record up to 9 ECG leads.
- Smartphones can connect to ultrasound probes for Point Of Care UltraSound (POCUS) evaluations.
- Smartphones can connect to wireless wearable sensors for continuous and remote monitoring of patient vital signs on hospital wards.

DISCLOSURE

F. Michard is the founder and managing director of MiCo, a Swiss consulting and research firm. MiCo does not sell any medical product, and F. Michard neither owns shares nor receives royalties from any medical device company.

REFERENCES

1. Michard F, Barrachina B, Schoetkker P. Is your smartphone the future of physiologic monitoring? Intensive Care Med 2019;45:869–71.
2. Michard F. A sneak peek into digital innovations and wearable sensors for cardiac monitoring. J Clin Monit Comput 2017;31:253–9.
3. Michard F. Smartphones and e-tablets in perioperative medicine. Korean J Anesthesiol 2017;70:493–9.
4. Matsumura K, Yamakoshi T. iPhysioMeter: a new approach for measuring heart rate and normalized pulse volume using only a smartphone. Behav Res 2013; 45:1272–8.
5. Chan PH, Wong CK, Poh YC, et al. Diagnostic performance of a smartphone-based photoplethysmographic application for atrial fibrillation screening in a primary care setting. J Am Heart Assoc 2016;5:e003428.
6. Huang RY, Dung LR. Measurement of heart rate variability using off-the-shelf smartphones. Biomed Eng Online 2016;15:11.
7. Nam Y, Kong Y, Reyes B, et al. Monitoring of heart and breathing rates using dual cameras on a smartphone. PLoS One 2016;11:e0151013.
8. Perez MV, Mahaffey KW, Hedlin H, et al. Large-scale assessment of a smartwatch to identify atrial fibrillation. N Engl J Med 2019;381:1909–17.
9. Saxon LE. Ubiquitous wireless ECG recording: a powerful tool physicians should embrace. J Cardiovasc Electrophysiol 2013;24:480–3.
10. Halcox JPJ, Wareham K, Cardew A, et al. Assessment of remote heart rhythm sampling using the AliveCor heart monitor to screen for atrial fibrillation: the REHEARSE-AF study. Circulation 2017;136:1784–94.
11. Garabelli P, Stavrakis S, Albert M, et al. Comparison of QT interval readings in normal sinus rhythm between a smartphone heart monitor and a 12-lead ECG for healthy volunteers and in patients receiving sotalol or dofetilide. J Cardiovasc Electrophysiol 2016;27:827–32.
12. Muhlestein JB, Le V, Albert D, et al. Smartphone ECG for evaluation of STEMI: results of the ST LEUIS pilot study. J Electrocardiol 2015;48:249–59.

13. Cobos Gil MA. Standard and precordial leads obtained with an Apple watch. Ann Intern Med 2020;172:436–7.

14. McManus RJ, Mant J, Franssen M, et al. Efficacy of self-monitored blood pressure, with or without telemonitoring, for titration of anti-hypertensive medication (TASMINH4): an unmasked randomized controlled trial. Lancet 2018;391:949–59.

15. Kim SH, Song JG, Park JH, et al. Beat-to-beat tracking of systolic blood pressure using noninvasive pulse transit time during anesthesia induction in hypertensive patients. Anesth Analg 2013;116:94–100.

16. Plante TB, Urrea B, MacFarlane ZT, et al. Validation of the Instant Blood Pressure Smartphone App. JAMA Intern Med 2016;176:700–2.

17. Alexander JC, Minhajuddin A, Joshi G. Comparison of smartphone application-based vital signs monitors without external hardware versus those used in clinical practice: a prospective trial. J Clin Monit Comput 2017;31:825–31.

18. Chandrasekhar A, Natarajan K, Yavarimanesh M, et al. An iPhone application for blood pressure monitoring via the oscillometric finger pressing method. Sci Rep 2018;8:13136.

19. Luo H, Yang D, Barszczyk A, et al. Smartphone-based blood pressure measurement using transdermal optical imaging technology. Circ Cardiovasc Imaging 2019;12:e008857.

20. Ghamri Y, Proença M, Hofmann G, et al. Automated pulse oximeter waveform analysis to track changes in blood pressure during anesthesia induction: a proof-of-concept study. Anesth Analg 2020;130:1222–33.

21. Pellaton C, Vybornova A, Fallet S, et al. Accuracy testing of a new optical device for noninvasive estimation of systolic and diastolic blood pressure compared to intra-arterial measurements. Blood Press Monit 2020;25:105–9.

22. Schoettker P, Degott J, Hofmann G, et al. Blood pressure measurements with the OptiBP smartphone app validated against reference auscultatory measurements. Sci Rep 2020;10:17827.

23. Michard F. Hemodynamic monitoring: would a pulse oximeter do the job? Crit Care Med 2021;49:383–6.

24. Benes J, Giglio M, Brienza N, et al. The effects of goal-directed fluid therapy based on dynamic parameters on post-surgical outcome: a meta-analysis of randomized controlled trials. Crit Care 2014;18:584.

25. Michard F, Shelley K. Should we monitor pulsus paradoxus via pulse oximetry in patients with COVID-19 and acute respiratory failure. Am J Respir Crit Care Med 2020;202:770–1.

26. Shah S, Majmudar K, Stein A, et al. Novel use of home pulse oximetry monitoring in COVID-19 patients discharged from the emergency department identifies need for hospitalization. Acad Emerg Med 2020;27:681–92.

27. Natarajan A, Su HW, Heneghan C. Assessment of physiological signs associated with COVID-19 measured using wearable devices. NPJ Digit Med 2020;3:156.

28. Saugel B, Reese PC, Sessler DI, et al. Automated ambulatory blood pressure measurements and intraoperative hypotension in patients having non cardiac surgery with general anesthesia: a prospective observational study. Anesthesiology 2019;131:74–83.

29. Stephens J, Allen J. Mobile phone interventions to increase physical activity and reduce weight: a systematic review. J Cardiovasc Nurs 2013;28:320–9.

30. Whittaker R, McRobbie H, Bullen C, et al. Mobile phone-based interventions for smoking cessation. Cochrane Database Syst Rev 2016;4:CD006611.

31. Michard F, Badheka A. Toward the Shazam-like identification of valve diseases with digital auscultation. Am J Med 2019;132:e595–6.

32. Liebo MJ, Israel RL, Lillie EO, et al. Is pocket mobile echocardiography the next-generation stethoscope? A cross-sectional comparison of rapidly acquired images with standard transthoracic echocardiography. Ann Intern Med 2011;155:33–8.

33. Biais M, Carrie C, Delaunay F, et al. Evaluation of a new pocket echoscopic device for focused cardiac ultrasonography in an emergency setting. Crit Care 2012;16:R82.

34. Zieleskiewicz L, Lopez A, Hraiech S, et al. Bedside POCUS during ward emergencies is associated with improved diagnosis and outcome: an observational, prospective, controlled study. Crit Care 2021;25:34.

35. Brass P, Hellmich M, Kolodziej L, et al. Ultrasound guidance versus anatomical landmarks for internal jugular vein catheterization. Cochrane Database Syst Rev 2015;1:CD006962.

36. Lewis SR, Price A, Wlaker KJ, et al. Ultrasound guidance for upper and lower limb blocks. Cochrane Database Syst Rev 2015;9:CD006459.

37. Michard F, Sessler DI, Saugel B. Non-invasive arterial pressure monitoring revisited. Intensive Care Med 2018;44:2213–5.

38. Gratz I, Spitz F, Baruch M, et al. Continuous non-invasive finger cuff CareTaker comparable to invasive intra-arterial pressure in patients undergoing major intra-abdominal surgery. BMC Anesthesiol 2017;17:48.

39. Barrachina B, Cobos R, Mardones N, et al. Assessment of a smartphone app (Capstesia) for measuring pulse pressure variation: agreement between two methods. Eur J Anaesthesiol 2016;33:1–6.

40. Desebbe O, Joosten A, Suehiro K, et al. A novel mobile phone application for pulse pressure variation monitoring based on feature extraction technology: a method comparison study in a simulated environment. Anesth Analg 2016;123:105–13.

41. Holmes AA, Konig G, Ting V, et al. Clinical evaluation of a novel system for monitoring surgical hemoglobin loss. Anesth Analg 2014;119:588–94.

42. Konig G, Waters JH, Javidroozi M, et al. Real-time evaluation of an image analysis system for monitoring surgical hemoglobin loss. J Clin Monit Comput 2018;32:303–10.

43. Michard F, Gan TJ, Kehlet H. Digital innovations and emerging technologies for enhanced recovery programmes. Br J Anaesth 2017;119:31–9.

44. Michard F, Sessler DI. Ward monitoring 3.0. Br J Anaesth 2018;121:999–1001.

45. Michard F, Bellomo R, Taenzer A. The rise of ward monitoring: opportunities and challenges for critical care specialists. Intensive Care Med 2019;45:671–3.

46. Michard F, Saugel B, Vallet B. Rethinking the post-COVID-19 pandemic hospital: more ICU beds or smart monitoring on the wards? Intensive Care Med 2020;46:1792–3.

47. Luna IE, Peterson B, Kehlet H, et al. Individualized assessment of post-arthroplasty recovery by actigraphy: a methodology study. J Clin Monit Comput 2017;31:1283–7.

48. Cook DJ, Thompson JE, Prinsen SK, et al. Functional recovery in the elderly after major surgery: assessment of mobility recovery using wireless technology. Ann Thorac Surg 2013;96:1057–61.

49. Mobbs RJ, Phan K, Maharaj M, et al. Physical activity measured with accelerometer and self-rated disability in lumbar spine surgery: A prospective study. Glob Spine J 2016;6:459–64.

50. Michard F, Range G, Biais M. Smartphones to assess cardiac function: novelty blindness or fresh perspectives? Crit Care Med 2017;45:e1199–201.

51. Michard F, Teboul JL. Predictive analytics: Beyond the buzz. Ann Intensive Care 2019;9:46.

Machine Learning, Deep Learning, and Closed Loop Devices—Anesthesia Delivery

Theodora Wingert, MD[a,b],*, Christine Lee, PhD[c,d],
Maxime Cannesson, MD, PhD[a,b]

KEYWORDS

- Machine learning • Neural networks • Deep learning • Closed loop devices
- Artificial intelligence

KEY POINTS

- The application of artificial intelligence in anesthesiology with machine learning, neural networks, and closed loop devices has been advancing in frequency, scope, and sophistication.
- This article summarizes some basic tenets of machine learning (supervised, unsupervised, and reinforcement learning), techniques in artificial intelligence (classical machine learning, neural networks, deep learning, and bayesian methods), and applications of these modalities in clinical anesthesiology.
- This article reviews some history and background of closed loop devices, basic tenets of design and engineering of these devices, and their clinical applications.
- Artificial intelligence has the potential to have an impact on the practice of anesthesiology in aspects ranging from perioperative support to critical care delivery to outpatient pain management.

Financial Disclosures: None.
Conflicts of interest: M. Cannesson is a consultant for Edwards Lifesciences and Masimo Corp and has funded research from Edwards Lifesciences and Masimo. He also is the founder of Sironis, owns patents, and receives royalties for closed loop hemodynamic management that have been licensed to Edwards Lifesciences. His department receives funding from the National Institutes of Health (NIH) (R01GM117622; R01 NR013012; U54HL119893; 1R01HL144692). C. Lee is an employee of Edwards Lifesciences.
Clinical trial number: Not Applicable.

[a] University of California Los Angeles, David Geffen School of Medicine, Los Angeles, CA, USA;
[b] Department of Anesthesiology and Perioperative Medicine, Ronald Reagan UCLA Medical Center, 757 Westwood Plaza, Suite 3325, Los Angeles, CA 90095-7403, USA; [c] Edwards Lifesciences, Irvine, CA, USA; [d] Critical Care R&D, 1 Edwards Way, Irvine, CA 92614, USA
* Corresponding author. Department of Anesthesiology and Perioperative Medicine, Ronald Reagan UCLA Medical Center, 757 Westwood Plaza, Suite 3325, Los Angeles, CA 90095-7403.
E-mail address: twingert@mednet.ucla.edu

Anesthesiology Clin 39 (2021) 565–581
https://doi.org/10.1016/j.anclin.2021.03.012
1932-2275/21/© 2021 Elsevier Inc. All rights reserved.

anesthesiology.theclinics.com

BACKGROUND

With the gargantuan volume of data captured during surgeries and procedures, critical care, and pain management, the field of anesthesiology is uniquely suited to the effective application of closed loop technologies, machine learning, and neural networks. In any given aspect of anesthesia practice, be it sedation, the critical care setting, or outpatient pain management, thousands of data points are at the anesthesiologist's disposal in making decisions. Years of experience help with interpreting these, but no matter what is done to optimize clinical decision making, the human brain is subject to bias, distraction, and fatigue. Computational improvements in the recent past have made development of practical tools to augment human intelligence finally feasible. In the past several years, these areas have expanded immensely in both interest and clinical applications.

Historically, anesthesiologists have been early pioneers of closed loop devices. As early as the 1950s, Bickford[1] and others developed an automated delivery of volatile anesthetic based on electroencephalogram (EEG). Subsequent efforts expanded to sophisticated closed loop systems for achieving optimal end-tidal volatile concentration, neuromuscular blockade, and mean arterial pressure.[2–4] The classic open loop control system in anesthesiology, target-controlled infusion devices, in which a hypothetical plasma or effect-site concentration is targeted based on estimations from a population model of drug distribution and effect, bourgeoned outside the United States, from an emerging technology in the 1990s to a mature one today.[5] Particularly in the United States, however, concerns with regulatory issues, safety, and liability and a lack of convincing demonstration of significant clinical impact on patient outcomes have been significant impasses for both open loop and closed loop devices.[6–15]

Concomitant to progress with closed loop innovations have been significant advances in computational techniques and technology, which have made machine learning and other modalities within artificial intelligence (AI) markedly more accessible in recent years. Early efforts at clinical applications within anesthesiology were focused primarily on EEG analysis and depth of anesthesia monitoring but since have expanded considerably.[16–18] Applications of machine learning and other methods within AI span a vast array of purposes but typically fall into 3 common overall goals[19,20]:

1. To analyze large amounts of data in order to search for novel patterns or groups among variables (also known as data mining)
2. To leverage highly complex data sets, such as medical images, EEG waveforms, or multiple hemodynamic signals, over time
3. To generate models or algorithms to predict an event or continuous variable, such as degree of sedation, respiratory depression, or response to nociception

This article provides an overview of the basic tenets of closed loop devices, machine learning, and neural networks. This summary is intended for all audiences within anesthesiology and is by no means exhaustive. Particular emphasis is given to the clinical applications for these technologies. Although the authors have taken efforts to provide as much structure as possible in this text, there inevitably is overlap between these modalities.

WHAT ARE CLOSED LOOP SYSTEMS?

Closed loop control devices are fully automated systems in which a sensor(s) provides feedback to an algorithm that determines the action to take in order to achieve a desired target (**Fig. 1**). In most cases, the sensor(s) measures and provides feedback

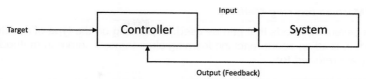

Fig. 1. Basic elements of a closed loop system. A target value range (eg, a mean systolic blood pressure range) is supplied to the controller. These settings then are compared with the output or feedback data (eg, patient blood pressure). The difference between the actual and target values then is processed and action is taken to adjust the input or manipulated variable such that the actual values reach the target range.

to the algorithm repeatedly, and the algorithm repeatedly directs corrective actions, thus creating a closed loop. Also known as automated control systems, closed loop systems act to maintain a given variable at a desired set point via 3 key elements: a sensor, a controller, and an actuator.[15] The sensor or measurement device senses the target parameter and generates a feedback signal that characterizes the status of the controlled variable. The controller queries the disparity between the feedback signal and the desired set point. Then, through a controlled algorithm, the controller generates an output signal for what corrective event should occur. The actuator then converts that signal to actual physical intervention.

The algorithms underlying the closed loop system can be simplistic (eg, if stroke volume variation goes above a certain set threshold, then a bolus is administered) or may utilize AI. In practice, most closed loop systems utilize reinforcement learning, a type of machine learning discussed in more detail later.

Examples of closed loop systems are ubiquitous in daily life—thermostats, clothing dryers, voltage stabilizers, and numerous elements of vehicle navigation, such as cruise control and autopilot systems. In the example of the thermostat, there exists a temperature sensor, a heater or air conditioner, and a unit that allows the user to set a desired temperature; and the heater or air conditioner turns on and off as needed to achieve that temperature based on the measured temperature of the room. These systems have immense potential within medicine. Due to the complexity and variability of inputs, however, not to mention the enormous ramifications of error, the technologies have yet to be rolled out in day-to-day clinical medicine for most practicing anesthesiologists.

WHAT IS ARTIFICIAL INTELLIGENCE?

Just as algorithms underlie closed loop systems, algorithms are at the heart of machine learning and neural networks. The term, *algorithm*, refers to a systematic procedure or method of solving a problem or accomplishing some end. Put simply, machine learning and neural networks are just methodologies within AI, in which computer systems are created to help perform tasks that normally require human intelligence. With that, some basics of AI are delved into.

Types of Outcomes

One way AI within medicine can be classified is by the types of outcomes that are predicted. Classification involves organizing data into categories or discrete groups. Examples of these are models that aim to predict a binary outcome like mortality after surgery.[21] Regression, on the other hand, utilizes modeling to predict continuous variables, such as predicting procedural or recovery times for the purposes of optimizing resource utilization.[22,23]

Types of Machine Learning Methods

There are several methods that can be used, depending on the type of question and data used. In reading about machine learning algorithms, 3 common methodologies frequently are referred to:

1. Supervised learning
2. Unsupervised learning
3. Reinforcement learning

Supervised learning involves creation of an algorithm that is "trained" to predict a defined entity or outcome. Unsupervised learning, by contrast, does not involve introduction of a priori hypotheses; thus, algorithms then are used to identify patterns, structure, or clusters within a data set. In reinforcement learning, an algorithm is trained to perform an action (eg, deliver an anesthetic to a patient) and to receive feedback and learn from its own errors and successes.

Types of Machine Learning Techniques

Although these descriptive terms help in understanding and assessing AI algorithms, it also is important to delve a bit into the types of techniques commonly used to analyze complex or large data sets. Because supervised learning currently is the most common type of machine learning utilized in medicine, this article describes some of the most common supervised learning machine learning algorithms, including neural networks and bayesian techniques. The techniques described are a small subset of what currently exists, and the choice of a machine learning technique is based on several factors, such as experience, data input, interpretability, and so forth.

One of the most popular types of models applied in medicine is logistic regression. Although it is not considered a complex machine learning technique like neural networks, it is important to understand the distinction in order to understand the potential benefits and pitfalls. Logistic regression is considered to be a more traditional and simpler modeling technique, which contrasts in several ways to some of the more state-of-the art AI models. In logistic regression, the structure is simple, the hypothesized effect of an individual variable is straightforward, and the input variables (or features) do not interact with one other. Other machine learning models, like those described later, can allow for relationships between the features and learning of new features as well as learning between features and outcomes.

Another popular model is the decision tree, which utilizes tree models (akin to a rules-based decision flowchart) with branch-points or nodes to establish a target output based on inputs (**Fig. 2**). Each node within a decision tree has an assigned value, with the final node representing an outcome as well as the probability of arriving at that outcome based on the preceding decision tree path.[24] Random forests then are an extension, in a way, of decision trees (see **Fig. 2**). Although a decision tree consists of a single sequential decision tree, a random forest model allows for multiple trees, creating an ensemble model. Each individual decision tree incorporates a random subset of features; the individual trees then are combined to generate a final output.

Bayesian techniques use a known previous probability distribution of an event along with a probability distribution in a given data set.[25] This modality allows for both modeling of uncertainty and updating or learning repeatedly as new data are made available.[26] Similar to classical supervised decision tree learning, there are several assumptions that underlie any results produced.

Neural networks allow for an exponentially higher degree of connections and logic. In a typical neural network, each network is composed of an input layer of neurons,

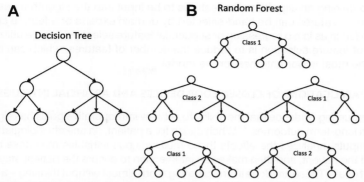

Fig. 2. A simplified decision tree (*A*) and random forest (*B*). A single decision tree is simply a series of sequential questions. A random forest consists of a large number of individual decision trees. Each decision tree is trained on, or utilizes, a random subset of features, or bagged data. These individual decision tree outputs then are aggregated to produce a single model.

which are composed of features that describe the data, as well as a hidden layer of neurons that perform mathematical transformations on input features and an output layer that produces an outcome (**Fig. 3**). Multiple connections between neurons exist and can be weighted differently depending on input-output maps.[24]

Developing a Machine Learning Model

When describing the development of a machine learning algorithm, it also is common to see the phrases, *training data* and *test data*. The training data are used to train the machine learning algorithm to analyze and learn the associations between the inputs and the output of interest. The test data are used to assess the performance of the trained machine learning algorithm on a set of data it has never seen before. For example, 70% to 80% of a data set can be allotted for training, with the remaining 20% to 30% reserved for testing.[24]

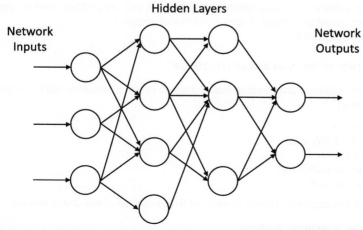

Fig. 3. Basic structure of a neural network. The input layer incorporates features supplied by the user. The hidden layer converts inputs into features useable by the network. The output layer then converts the hidden layer results into an interpretable output.

Prior to training an algorithm, the features to be input into the algorithm need to be decided on. Features can be hand-selected by domain experts or a feature selection algorithm (such as lasso regression or sequential feature selection) can be utilized. The purpose of feature selection is to reduce the number of features, which can be limitless, to the most important ones for the model.

CLINICAL APPLICATIONS OF CLOSED LOOP DEVICES AND ARTIFICIAL INTELLIGENCE

There is mounting evidence that the ability to achieve intraoperative goals has significant effects on long-term outcomes.[27] When caring for a patient, an anesthesiologist takes in multiple inputs, analyzes the effects these multitudinous variables may have on each other and the patient, and then makes an intervention to ensure the patient stays within a range of goals. These are done in an operating room almost without thinking—adjusting ventilator settings, anesthetic gas delivery, titrating infusions, and so forth. Due to the multitude of inputs, individual practice variations, potential distractors, coverage models, and a frequently high-stakes milieu, however, there are numerous ways in which automated intelligent devices can assist in providing optimized care.[15]

There are numerous examples of improved outcomes with reduced interprovider variation and protocol-driven pathways. Kurz and colleagues[28] was one of the first randomized clinical trials demonstrating worse outcomes in patients who did not receive extra measures to ensure normothermia intraoperatively. Numerous randomized studies also now show resounding concrete evidence that proactive use of hemodynamic monitoring along with therapies to control hemodynamics significantly reduced mortality and surgical complications.[29] And there are numerous studies showing excessive depth of anesthesia associated with mortality and other worse outcomes.[27,30–34] Enhanced recovery after surgery pathways, in which multiple aspects of care are targeted for optimization and protocolized, now seemingly are ubiquitous.[35]

Speaking in general terms, closed loop devices and AI techniques within anesthesiology are enlisted to achieve a few common goals in order to improve patient care:

1. Keep patients within some kind of physiologic target range.
2. Reduce variability within an individual patient.
3. Reduce variability of care given to one patient versus another, that is, encounter variation, provider variation, and institutional variation.
4. Improve outcomes.

CLOSED LOOP DEVICES IN ANESTHESIOLOGY

Most current applications of closed loop devices in anesthesiology fall into a handful of clinical arenas[15]:

1. Anesthetics
2. Intravenous (IV) fluid
3. Vasopressors
4. Mechanical ventilation
5. Glucose control

Some of the relevant studies in each of these clinical areas are reviewed.

Closed Loop Anesthetic Systems

The application of closed loop devices to anesthetic agents and depth of anesthesia is to many the apogee of anesthesia research and innovation. Closed loop systems in anesthesia first were pioneered in the 1980s and since have progressed much nearer to more widespread application.[6,7] These systems have shown immense promise in terms of reduction in clinicians' workload and improved control of drug delivery.[14]

There currently are approximately 20 studies in this area. Most have studied adults during the intraoperative period and IV agents (most commonly propofol and remifentanil), and most utilized bispectral index (BIS) as the target variable for anesthetic depth. A range of cases has been studied, including cardiac, general, gynecologic, vascular, thoracic, and spinal surgeries and procedures.[8,12,14,36–41] A meta-analysis by Brogi and colleagues[15] of 15 studies showed automated systems increased the percentage of time the outcome variable (depth of anesthesia) was maintained in the desired range by 17.4%. A subset of these studies also examined the proportion of time that the controlled variable was above or below the targeted set point, with meta-analysis showing 12.3% more undershooting or overshooting in the manual groups compared with the closed loop groups.[8,11,12,14,36,37,39,41–47]

The subset of studies isolated to using BIS and total IV anesthesia showed in meta-analyses that the closed loop anesthetic delivery systems were associated with significant lower doses of propofol at induction of anesthesia and significantly shorter recovery time.[48]

Goal-Directed Fluid Therapy Closed Loop Systems

Although there are several in vivo and in silico studies, currently there have been 2 randomized control trials in humans.[49–51] The smaller of the 2 studies examined 46 moderate-risk to high-risk abdominal surgical patients with an arterial catheter–based cardiac output monitoring system with colloid fluid boluses in response to the closed loop control.[50] Although no difference was found in this study, the groups were small with notable differences in baseline characteristics. In the larger study, Joosten and colleagues[51] studied 104 patients undergoing elective major abdominal surgery. Stroke volume and stroke volume variation were monitored via arterial catheter–based system, and crystalloid or colloid boluses were administered in response to the algorithm.[51] Patients in the closed loop group had significantly shorter length of stay compared with historical controls and reduced incidence of both major and minor postoperative complications.

Closed Loop Vasopressor Devices

Closed loop vasopressor devices have immense promise to improve the ability to maintain optimal therapeutic control of hemodynamics. There have been 2 large randomized controlled studies in this area, both undertaken in the setting of cesarean section with spinal anesthesia.[52,53] Kee and colleagues[52] examined blood pressure and heart rate of 214 patients with a computer-controlled phenylephrine delivery system using both intermittent boluses and continuous infusion. They found blood pressure control to be more precise when computer-controlled phenylephrine was delivered using intermittent boluses rather than continuous infusion. Sng and colleagues[53] evaluated 216 patients' noninvasive blood pressure and utilized computer-controlled phenylephrine for maintenance of blood pressure also during spinal anesthesia for cesarean delivery. In pooled analysis of the 2 studies, the automated systems were found to increase the number of measurements within the target range in comparison to manual control.[15]

There also are a handful of feasibility studies in this area with major promise. Joosten and colleagues[54] demonstrated efficacy in a pig model with an induced hypotension model using nitroglycerine and automated controller–titrated norepinephrine. This study showed efficacy in correcting hypotension to keep the mean arterial pressure within 5 mm Hg of the target for 98% of the time. These same investigators also under-took a feasibility study in 20 human subjects undergoing elective moderate-risk and high-risk surgery.[55] They showed that the closed loop vasopressor control system maintained mean arterial pressure within 5 mm Hg of the target for 91.6% of the intra-operative period and effectively minimized hypotension to 2.6% of the intraoperative period.

Closed Loop Mechanical Ventilation

Nine trials have investigated the accuracy of closed loop ventilation systems in com-parison with manual control of ventilation.[56–63] Mechanical ventilation theoretically should be well suited for the application of closed loop systems; however, there are various inputs and outputs clinicians utilize. Thus, it is not surprising that these studies have a fair degree of heterogeneity within variables utilized as inputs and desired out-comes. Of the current studies, approximately half used oxygen saturation as measured by pulse oximetry as the controlled variable, with an automated fraction of inspired oxygen adjustment. The other studies used tidal volume, respiratory rate, and end-tidal CO_2 ranges in order to examine the feasibility of closed loop pres-sure support ventilation systems to maintain an acceptable ventilation zone.

Subgroup analysis within a recent meta-analysis showed greater maintenance of the controlled variable within the target range in the automated systems versus the control group by approximately 8%.[15] The authors expect in the coming years to see additional progress in this area.

Closed Loop Insulin Administration

More than 10 studies have examined closed loop insulin delivery system for glucose control. This area has made massive strides with both programmable home insulin subcutaneous insulin delivery devices and high-fidelity nearly continuous glucometry. This area also in some ways is much more straightforward than mechanical ventilation, owing to the fact that the controlled therapy (insulin) and target (blood glucose level) are both single, agreed-upon entities.

In patients with type 1 diabetes mellitus, a recent meta-analysis of 8 studies using closed loop insulin delivery systems with pump insulin therapy showed that automated systems were associated with a 21.2% greater time with maintenance in the desired range.[15] Subgroup analyses within the same meta-analysis, demonstrated that compared with the control group, the automated systems also decreased the over-shoots and undershoots, with the automated systems showing a 6.5% reduction in the percentage of time above or below the target range.[15] Meta-analysis of studies in the intensive care setting showed similar benefits; however, these results were not statistically significant.[15]

MACHINE LEARNING IN ANESTHESIOLOGY
Depth of Anesthesia

Anesthetic depth has become a particularly valuable clinical target, with several recent studies suggesting poorer outcomes associated with low BIS or excessive depth of anesthesia.[11,63] A wealth of studies have investigated machine learning and neural networks in the context of depth of anesthesia monitoring.[16–18,64,65] Arguably, the increased utilization and prevalence of BIS have seemed to have spurred methodo-logic efforts and sophistication of anesthetic control systems.[66]

Several studies also have proposed and evaluated alternative AI algorithms for depth of anesthesia versus existing measures, including BIS or the response entropy index. Although BIS is a commonly used modality for measuring depth of anesthesia, by no means is it the only modality available and it is possible that better measures of depth are achievable. Others have utilized auditory evoked potentials and heart rate variability.[67,68] Mirsadeghi and colleagues[64] utilized a method called locally linear embedding, which maps high-dimensional features into a 2-dimensional output space to input direct features from EEG signals. They showed a 88.4% accuracy compared with 84.2% by BIS of identifying awake versus anesthetized patients. Another study by Shalbaf and colleagues[65] applied EEG features within a neural network model to discriminate different states of anesthetic depth and demonstrated 93% accuracy compared with the BIS index's 87% accuracy.

Another exciting target in depth of anesthesia monitoring is identification and potential prediction of awareness events. One study by Ranta and colleagues[68] examined cases of a cohort who had reported intraoperative awareness while under general anesthesia and deployed neural networks using blood pressure, heart rate, and end-tidal carbon dioxide as input features. Although the prediction probability was 66%, the specificity achieved 98%, even with utilization of no EEG features.

Control of Anesthesia

The potential impact of controlled anesthetic delivery systems is vast. Although much emphasis often is placed on depth of anesthesia monitoring in anesthetic control, many forward-thinkers propose systems of complete anesthetic control. A complete system for closed loop control of anesthesia would, in an ideal world, monitor and control hypnosis, nociception, neuromuscular blockade, hemodynamics, ventilation, temperature, and metabolic targets.[69]

Although many aspects of such a system may not require AI, there are many potential places for useful application of such modalities. Not all closed loop systems require AI at all; for example, closed loop temperature control is unlikely to require AI. These methodologies, however, have been applied to helpful use not only in depth of anesthesia systems, discussed previously, but also in systems for maintaining neuromuscular blockade goal as well as systems for controlling or weaning ventilation.[70–75]

Event and Risk Prediction

This area is ripe for application of AI modalities and many studies already exist in this area. Models exist for myriad events in the intraoperative, postoperative, and critical care periods. Examples include postinduction hypotension, hypnotic effect of induction dose of propofol, rate of recovery from neuromuscular blockade, American Society of Anesthesiologists (ASA) status, difficult laryngoscopy, identifying respiratory depression during conscious sedation, and assistance in decision making for the optimal method of anesthesia in pediatric surgery.[76–84] Critical care studies have used machine learning to predict morbidity, ventilator weaning, clinical deterioration, mortality readmission, and detection of sepsis.[85–91]

In the arena of perioperative risks, investigators Hill and colleagues[92] recently described a random forest model that predicts postoperative in-hospital mortality based solely on automatically obtained preoperative features with an area under the curve of 0.932. This model was found to markedly outperform other predictors of mortality, such as the Preoperative Score to Predict Postoperative Mortality, Charlson Comorbidity Index, and ASA physical status. Additionally, deep neural networks have been applied to large data sets in order to predict other common markers of poor postoperative outcomes, such as mortality, readmission, acute kidney injury, and reintubation.[21,93]

Ultrasound Guidance

Studies in ultrasound guidance utilizing AI primarily have utilized neural network techniques. Examples include application of neural networks to distinguish femoral artery versus vein and automated identification of vertebral lamina.[94,95] Several studies exist with cardiac echocardiograms as well.[96] Even in cases of differentiation that seems easy or no better than expert clinical judgment, such simple discriminating abilities potentially could be vastly important and change how to teach trainees learning new imaging modalities.

Pain Management

AI also has significant potential to improve how we understand and treat pain. Examples include development of a nociception-level index based on machine learning analysis of photoplethysmograms and skin conductance waveforms, prediction of opioid dosing, and identification of patients who may benefit from preoperative consultation with a hospital's acute pain service.[97–99] AI also has been deployed to great success in large data studies with the aim of personalization of medicine.[100] This holds potential to optimize drug selection, dosing, and adverse reactions as well as identifying patients at risk for prolonged opioid use and substance use disorders.

Operating Room Logistics

Just as AI has infiltrated business and management, it also has begun to be applied to operating room and hospital logistics. Examples include prediction of the duration of surgical procedures and optimization of bed use.[22,101–103] Machine learning models have been applied successfully to estimating the duration of robotic-assisted surgery.[22] Surgical robotic units are a costly and limited resource; thus, booking robotic cases more accurately represents an example with significant potential business value.

CHALLENGES AND FUTURE DIRECTIONS OF CLOSED LOOP DEVICES AND ARTIFICIAL INTELLIGENCE

Currently, the field of anesthesiology appears to be on an exciting cusp of practical application of AI and closed loop systems. The strides that have been made in computational techniques and hardware, as well as the formation and availability of rich clinical databases, have laid hugely important groundwork. Many experimental systems have been proposed for closed loop control of anesthesia and practical applications of AI in anesthesiology, and the sophistication and intelligent algorithm design and practicalities are improving at lightning speed. Although none of the experimental closed loop systems is commercially available to clinicians at this time, several systems have undergone substantial study and show significant promise, such as the closed loop anesthesia delivery system and Infusion Toolbox 95. To further push for closed loop innovation, significant engagement with regulatory bodies, control, systems, and software engineering will be necessary in the coming future.

With closed loop systems as well as machine learning and neural networks, the next steps seem to be application and demonstration of clear clinical impact and improvement in outcomes. Although numerous studies have shown impressive ability to analyze and predict clinical attributes and outcomes, convincing demonstrations of improved clinically significant outcomes have yet to be seen. Only after clear clinical impact is demonstrated can the cost and other hurdles required of implementation be justified. With the speed of advancement in the past several years, however, studies with demonstration of direct improvement in clinical outcomes are expected to emerge in the near future.

Anesthesiology as a field is genuinely uniquely suited to reap potential benefits and improvements that AI can offer. Anesthesiologists in the operating room are bombarded with digital data points from monitors and anesthesia machines, from within the electronic medical records, and from anesthesia information management systems. This makes incorporation of all these data points all the more challenging in addition to being subject to bias and fatigue. The beauty of AI methodologies is the algorithms' ability to eliminate potential biases and engage in self-learning rather than needing to be fed the features decided on by expert opinion.

At the same time, these seemingly endless digitized data sources enable having access to rich databases from which how to care for patients can be learned and improved. Similar to the revolution in computing abilities and technology, a revolution in these technologies within anesthesiology is expected in the coming years.

CLINICS CARE POINTS

- Given the large amount of data anesthesiologists are required to interpret and prioritize, many closed loop systems and AI modalities have significant potential to reduce unwanted variability in patient care as well as deleterious effects of biases and human error.

- Closed loop systems can be applied to a variety of clinical aspects of the practice of anesthesiology: administration of anesthetics, IV fluids, and vasopressors as well as mechanical ventilation and glucose control.

- AI algorithms have been applied to several clinical arenas within anesthesiology: assessment of anesthetic depth, control of anesthesia, prediction of perioperative events and risks, ultrasound guidance, pain management, and operating room logistics.

REFERENCES

1. Bickford RG. Automatic electroencephalographic control of general anesthesia. Electroencephalog Clin Neurophysiol 1950;2:93–6.
2. Zbinden AM, Frei F, Westenskow DR, et al. Control of end-tidal halothane concentration: Part b: Verification in dogs. Br J Anaesth 1986;58(5):563–71.
3. Brown BH, Perks R, Anthony M, et al. Closed-loop control of muscle relaxation during surgery. Clin Phys Physiol Meas 1980;1(3):203–10.
4. Monk CR, Millard RK, Hutton P, et al. Automatic arterial pressure regulation using isoflurane: Comparison with manual control. Br J Anaesth 1989;63(1):22–30.
5. Absalom AR, Glen JB, Zwart GJC, et al. Target-controlled infusion: a mature technology. Anesth Analg 2016;122(1):70–8.
6. Schwilden H, Stoeckel H, Schüttler J. Closed-loop feedback control of propofol anaesthesia by quantitative eeg analysis in humans. Br J Anaesth 1989;62(3): 290–6.
7. Schwilden H, Schüttler J, Stoeckel H. Closed-loop feedback control of methohexital anesthesia by quantitative EEG analysis in humans. Anesthesiology 1987;67(3):341–7.
8. Puri GD, Kumar B, Aveek J. Closed-loop anaesthesia delivery system (CLADS™) using bispectral index: A performance assessment study. Anaesth Intensive Care 2007;35(3):357–62.
9. Kenny GNC, Mantzaridis H. Closed-loop control of propofol anaesthesia. Br J Anaesth 1999;83(2):223–8.

10. Mortier E, Struys M, De Smet T, et al. Closed-loop controlled administration of propofol using bispectral analysis. Anaesthesia 1998;53(8):749–54.

11. Liu N, Chazot T, Trillat B, et al. Feasibility of closed-loop titration of propofol guided by the Bispectral Index for general anaesthesia induction: a prospective randomized study. Eur J Anaesthesiol 2006;23(6):465–9.

12. Hemmerling TM, Arbeid E, Wehbe M, et al. Evaluation of a novel closed-loop total intravenous anaesthesia drug delivery system: A randomized controlled trial. Br J Anaesth 2013;110(6):1031–9.

13. Hemmerling TM. Automated anesthesia. Curr Opin Anaesthesiol 2009;22(6): 757–63.

14. Dussaussoy C, Peres M, Jaoul V, et al. Automated titration of propofol and remifentanil decreases the anesthesiologist's workload during vascular or thoracic surgery: A randomized prospective study. J Clin Monit Comput 2014;28(1): 35–40.

15. Brogi E, Cyr S, Kazan R, et al. Clinical performance and safety of closed-loop systems: A systematic review and meta-analysis of randomized controlled trials. Anesth Analg 2017;124(2):446–55.

16. Veselis RA, Reinsel R, Wronski M. Analytical methods to differentiate similar electroencephalographic spectra: neural network and discriminant analysis. J Clin Monit 1993;9(4):257–67.

17. Veselis RA, Reinsel R, Sommer S, et al. Use of neural network analysis to classify electroencephalographic patterns against depth of midazolam sedation in intensive care unit patients. J Clin Monit 1991;7(3):259–67.

18. Ortolani O, Conti A, Di Filippo A, et al. EEG signal processing in anaesthesia. Use of a neural network technique for monitoring depth of anaesthesia. Br J Anaesth 2002;88(5):644–8.

19. Gambus PL, Jaramillo S. Machine learning in anaesthesia: reactive, proactive... predictive! Br J Anaesth 2019;123(4):401–3.

20. Connor CW. Artificial Intelligence and Machine Learning in Anesthesiology. Anesthesiology 2019;131(6):1346–59.

21. Hofer IS, Lee C, Gabel E, et al. Development and validation of a deep neural network model to predict postoperative mortality, acute kidney injury, and reintubation using a single feature set. Npj Digit Med 2020;3(1):1–10.

22. Zhao B, Waterman RS, Urman RD, et al. A Machine Learning Approach to Predicting Case Duration for Robot-Assisted Surgery. J Med Syst 2019;43(2). https://doi.org/10.1007/s10916-018-1151-y.

23. Kim WO, Kil HK, Kang JW, et al. Prediction on lengths of stay in the Postanesthesia Care Unit following general anesthesia: Preliminary study of the neural network and logistic regression modelling. J Korean Med Sci 2000;15(1):25–30.

24. Hashimoto DA, Witkowski E, Gao L, et al. Artificial intelligence in anesthesiology: Current techniques, clinical applications, and limitations. Anesthesiology 2020;(2):379–94.

25. Bland JM, Altman DG. Bayesians and frequentists. BMJ 1998;317(7166): 1151–60.

26. Ghahramani Z. Probabilistic machine learning and artificial intelligence. Nature 2015;521(7553):452–9.

27. Monk TG, Saini V, Weldon BC, et al. Anesthetic management and one-year mortality after noncardiac surgery. Anesth Analg 2005;100(1):4–10.

28. Kurz A, Sessler DI, Lenhardt R. Perioperative normothermia to reduce the incidence of surgical-wound infection and shorten hospitalization. Study of Wound Infection and Temperature Group. N Engl J Med 1996;334(19):1209–15.

29. Hamilton MA, Cecconi M, Rhodes A. A systematic review and meta-analysis on the use of preemptive hemodynamic intervention to improve postoperative outcomes in moderate and high-risk surgical patients. Anesth Analg 2011;112(6): 1392–402.

30. Sessler DI, Sigl JC, Kelley SD, et al. Hospital stay and mortality are increased in patients having a "triple low" of low blood pressure, low bispectral index, and low minimum alveolar concentration of volatile anesthesia. Anesthesiology 2012;116(6):1195–203.

31. Watson PL, Shintani AK, Tyson R, et al. Presence of electroencephalogram burst suppression in sedated, critically ill patients is associated with increased mortality. Crit Care Med 2008;36(12):3171–7.

32. Leslie K, Myles PS, Forbes A, et al. The effect of bispectral index monitoring on long-term survival in the B-aware trial. Anesth Analg 2010;110(3):816–22.

33. Lindholm M-L, Träff S, Granath F, et al. Mortality within 2 years after surgery in relation to low intraoperative bispectral index values and preexisting malignant disease. Anesth Analg 2009;108(2):508–12.

34. Kertai MD, Pal N, Palanca BJA, et al. Association of perioperative risk factors and cumulative duration of low bispectral index with intermediate-term mortality after cardiac surgery in the B-Unaware Trial. Anesthesiology 2010;112(5): 1116–27.

35. Ljungqvist O, Scott M, Fearon KC. Enhanced recovery after surgery a review. JAMA Surg 2017;152(3):292–8.

36. De Smet T, Struys MMRF, Neckebroek MM, et al. The accuracy and clinical feasibility of a new bayesian-based closed-loop control system for propofol administration using the bispectral index as a controlled variable. Anesth Analg 2008;107(4):1200–10.

37. Hemmerling TM, Charabati S, Zaouter C, et al. A randomized controlled trial demonstrates that a novel closed-loop propofol system performs better hypnosis control than manual administration. Can J Anaesth 2010;57(8):725–35.

38. Liu N, Chazot T, Genty A, et al. Titration of propofol for anesthetic induction and maintenance guided by the bispectral index: closed-loop versus manual control: a prospective, randomized, multicenter study. Anesthesiology 2006; 104(4):686–95.

39. Liu N, Chazot T, Hamada S, et al. Closed-loop coadministration of propofol and remifentanil guided by bispectral index: a randomized multicenter study. Anesth Analg 2011;112(3):546–57.

40. Liu N, Le Guen M, Benabbes-Lambert F, et al. Feasibility of closed-loop titration of propofol and remifentanil guided by the spectral m-entropy monitor. Anesthesiology 2012;116(2):286–95.

41. Struys MM, De Smet T, Versichelen LF, et al. Comparison of closed-loop controlled administration of propofol using Bispectral Index as the controlled variable versus "standard practice" controlled administration. Anesthesiology 2001;95(1):6–17.

42. Le Guen M, Liu N, Bourgeois E, et al. Automated sedation outperforms manual administration of propofol and remifentanil in critically ill patients with deep sedation: a randomized phase II trial. Intensive Care Med 2013;39(3):454–62.

43. Locher S, Stadler KS, Boehlen T, et al. A new closed-loop control system for isoflurane using bispectral index outperforms manual control. Anesthesiology 2004;101(3):591–602.

44. Madhavan JS, Puri GD, Mathew PJ. Closed-loop isoflurane administration with bispectral index in open heart surgery: randomized controlled trial with manual control. Acta Anaesthesiol Taiwan 2011;49(4):130–5.

45. Solanki A, Puri GD, Mathew PJ. Bispectral index-controlled postoperative sedation in cardiac surgery patients: a comparative trial between closed loop and manual administration of propofol. Eur J Anaesthesiol 2010;27(8):708–13.

46. Biswas I, Mathew PJ, Singh RS, et al. Evaluation of closed-loop anesthesia delivery for propofol anesthesia in pediatric cardiac surgery. Paediatr Anaesth 2013;23(12):1145–52.

47. Agarwal J, Puri GD, Mathew PJ. Comparison of closed loop vs. manual administration of propofol using the Bispectral index in cardiac surgery. Acta Anaesthesiol Scand 2009;53(3):390–7.

48. Pasin L, Nardelli P, Pintaudi M, et al. Closed-loop delivery systems versus manually controlled administration of total IV Anesthesia: A meta-analysis of randomized clinical trials. Anesth Analg 2017;124(2):456–64.

49. Rinehart J, Lee C, Canales C, et al. Closed-loop fluid administration compared to anesthesiologist management for hemodynamic optimization and resuscitation during surgery: An in vivo study. Anesth Analg 2013;117(5):1119–29.

50. Lilot M, Bellon A, Gueugnon M, et al. Comparison of cardiac output optimization with an automated closed-loop goal-directed fluid therapy versus non standardized manual fluid administration during elective abdominal surgery: first prospective randomized controlled trial. J Clin Monit Comput 2018;32(6):993–1003.

51. Joosten A, Coeckelenbergh S, Delaporte A, et al. Implementation of closed-loop-assisted intra-operative goal-directed fluid therapy during major abdominal surgery: A case-control study with propensity matching. Eur J Anaesthesiol 2018;35(9):650–8.

52. Ngan Kee WD, Tam YH, Khaw KS, et al. Closed-loop feedback computer-controlled phenylephrine for maintenance of blood pressure during spinal anesthesia for cesarean delivery: A randomized trial comparing automated boluses versus infusion. Anesth Analg 2017;125(1):117–23.

53. Sng BL, Tan HS, Sia ATH. Closed-loop double-vasopressor automated system vs manual bolus vasopressor to treat hypotension during spinal anaesthesia for caesarean section: A randomised controlled trial. Anaesthesia 2014;69(1): 37–45.

54. Joosten A, Delaporte A, Alexander B, et al. Automated titration of vasopressor infusion using a closed-loop controller: in vivo feasibility study using a Swine Model. Anesthesiology 2019;130(3):394–403.

55. Joosten A, Alexander B, Duranteau J, et al. Feasibility of closed-loop titration of norepinephrine infusion in patients undergoing moderate- and high-risk surgery. Br J Anaesth 2019;123(4):430–8.

56. Claure N, Bancalari E, D'Ugard C, et al. Multicenter crossover study of automated control of inspired oxygen in ventilated preterm infants. Pediatrics 2011;127(1):e76–83.

57. Claure N, Gerhardt T, Everett R, et al. Closed-loop controlled inspired oxygen concentration for mechanically ventilated very low birth weight infants with frequent episodes of hypoxemia. Pediatrics 2001;107(5):1120–4.

58. Dojat M, Harf A, Touchard D, et al. Clinical evaluation of a computer-controlled pressure support mode. Am J Respir Crit Care Med 2000;161(4 Pt 1):1161–6.

59. Johannigman JA, Branson R, Lecroy D, et al. Autonomous control of inspired oxygen concentration during mechanical ventilation of the critically injured trauma patient. J Trauma 2009;66(2):386–92.

60. Hallenberger A, Poets CF, Horn W, et al, CLAC Study Group. Closed-loop automatic oxygen control (CLAC) in preterm infants: a randomized controlled trial. Pediatrics 2014;133(2):e379–85.

61. Schädler D, Engel C, Elke G, et al. Automatic control of pressure support for ventilator weaning in surgical intensive care patients. Am J Respir Crit Care Med 2012;185(6):637–44.

62. Urschitz MS, Horn W, Seyfang A, et al. Automatic control of the inspired oxygen fraction in preterm infants: a randomized crossover trial. Am J Respir Crit Care Med 2004;170(10):1095–100.

63. Lellouche F, Bouchard P-A, Simard S, et al. Evaluation of fully automated ventilation: a randomized controlled study in post-cardiac surgery patients. Intensive Care Med 2013;39(3):463–71.

64. Mirsadeghi M, Behnam H, Shalbaf R, et al. Characterizing awake and anesthetized states using a dimensionality reduction method. J Med Syst 2016;40(1):13.

65. Shalbaf A, Saffar M, Sleigh JW, et al. Monitoring the depth of anesthesia using a new adaptive neurofuzzy system. IEEE J Biomed Heal Informatics 2018;22(3):671–7.

66. Zaouter C, Hemmerling TM, Lanchon R, et al. The feasibility of a completely automated total IV anesthesia drug delivery system for cardiac surgery. Anesth Analg 2016;123(4):885–93.

67. Nagaraj SB, Biswal S, Boyle EJ, et al. Patient-Specific Classification of ICU sedation levels from heart rate variability. Crit Care Med 2017;45(7):e683–90.

68. Ranta SOV, Hynynen M, Räsänen J. Application of artificial neural networks as an indicator of awareness with recall during general anaesthesia. J Clin Monit Comput 2002;17(1):53–60.

69. Dumont GA, Ansermino JM. Closed-loop control of anesthesia: A primer for anesthesiologists. Anesth Analg 2013;117(5):1130–8.

70. Shieh JS, Kao MH, Liu CC. Genetic fuzzy modelling and control of bispectral index (BIS) for general intravenous anaesthesia. Med Eng Phys 2006;28(2):134–48.

71. Motamed C, Devys JM, Debaene B, et al. Influence of real-time Bayesian forecasting of pharmacokinetic parameters on the precision of a rocuronium target-controlled infusion. Eur J Clin Pharmacol 2012;68(7):1025–31.

72. Martinoni EP, Pfister CA, Stadler KS, et al. Model-based control of mechanical ventilation: Design and clinical validation. Br J Anaesth 2004;92(6):800–7.

73. Schäublin J, Derighetti M, Feigenwinter P, et al. Fuzzy logic control of mechanical ventilation during anaesthesia. Br J Anaesth 1996;77(5):636–41.

74. Schädler D, Mersmann S, Frerichs I, et al. A knowledge- and model-based system for automated weaning from mechanical ventilation: technical description and first clinical application. J Clin Monit Comput 2014;28(5):487–98.

75. Lendl M, Schwarz UH, Romeiser HJ, et al. Nonlinear model-based predictive control of non-depolarizing muscle relaxants using neural networks. J Clin Monit Comput 1999;15(5):271–8.

76. Hatib F, Jian Z, Buddi S, et al. Machine-learning algorithm to predict hypotension based on high-fidelity arterial pressure waveform analysis. Anesthesiology 2018;129(4):663–74.

77. Lin C-S, Chiu J-S, Hsieh M-H, et al. Predicting hypotensive episodes during spinal anesthesia with the application of artificial neural networks. Comput Methods Programs Biomed 2008;92(2):193–7.

78. Lin C-S, Chang C-C, Chiu J-S, et al. Application of an artificial neural network to predict postinduction hypotension during general anesthesia. Med Decis Making 2011;31(2):308–14.
79. Lin C-S, Li Y-C, Mok MS, et al. Neural network modeling to predict the hypnotic effect of propofol bolus induction. Proc AMIA Symp 2002;450–3. Available at: http://www.ncbi.nlm.nih.gov/pubmed/12463864.
80. Santanen OAP, Svartling N, Haasio J, et al. Neural nets and prediction of the recovery rate from neuromuscular block. Eur J Anaesthesiol 2003;20(2):87–92.
81. Zhang L, Fabbri D, Lasko TA, et al. A System for Automated Determination of Perioperative Patient Acuity. J Med Syst 2018;42(7):123.
82. Moustafa MA, El-Metainy S, Mahar K, et al. Defining difficult laryngoscopy findings by using multiple parameters: A machine learning approach. Egypt J Anaesth 2017;33(2):153–8.
83. Berkenstadt H, Ben-Menachem E, Herman A, et al. An evaluation of the Integrated Pulmonary Index (IPI) for the detection of respiratory events in sedated patients undergoing colonoscopy. J Clin Monit Comput 2012;26(3):177–81.
84. Hancerliogullari G, Hancerliogullari KO, Koksalmis E. The use of multi-criteria decision making models in evaluating anesthesia method options in circumcision surgery. BMC Med Inform Decis Mak 2017;17(1):14.
85. Gao L, Smielewski P, Czosnyka M, et al. Cerebrovascular Signal Complexity Six Hours after Intensive Care Unit Admission Correlates with Outcome after Severe Traumatic Brain Injury. J Neurotrauma 2016;33(22):2011–8.
86. Zappitelli M, Bernier PL, Saczkowski RS, et al. A small post-operative rise in serum creatinine predicts acute kidney injury in children undergoing cardiac surgery. Kidney Int 2009;76(8):885–92.
87. Bonds BW, Yang S, Hu PF, et al. Predicting secondary insults after severe traumatic brain injury. J Trauma Acute Care Surg 2015;79(1):85–90 [discussion: 90].
88. Jalali A, Bender D, Rehman M, et al. Advanced analytics for outcome prediction in intensive care units. Conf Proc Annu Int Conf IEEE Eng Med Biol Soc IEEE Eng Med Biol Soc Annu Conf 2016;2016:2520–4.
89. Clermont G, Angus DC, DiRusso SM, et al. Predicting hospital mortality for patients in the intensive care unit: a comparison of artificial neural networks with logistic regression models. Crit Care Med 2001;29(2):291–6.
90. Desautels T, Das R, Calvert J, et al. Prediction of early unplanned intensive care unit readmission in a UK tertiary care hospital: a cross-sectional machine learning approach. BMJ Open 2017;7(9):e017199.
91. Desautels T, Calvert J, Hoffman J, et al. Prediction of sepsis in the intensive care unit with minimal electronic health record data: a machine learning approach. JMIR Med Informatics 2016;4(3):e28.
92. Hill BL, Brown R, Gabel E, et al. An automated machine learning-based model predicts postoperative mortality using readily-extractable preoperative electronic health record data. Br J Anaesth 2019;123(6):877–86.
93. Mišić VV, Gabel E, Hofer I, et al. Machine Learning Prediction of Postoperative Emergency Department Hospital Readmission. Anesthesiology 2020;(5):968–80.
94. Pesteie M, Lessoway V, Abolmaesumi P, et al. Automatic Localization of the Needle Target for Ultrasound-Guided Epidural Injections. IEEE Trans Med Imaging 2018;37(1):81–92.
95. Hetherington J, Lessoway V, Gunka V, et al. SLIDE: automatic spine level identification system using a deep convolutional neural network. Int J Comput Assist Radiol Surg 2017;12(7):1189–98.

96. Ghorbani A, Ouyang D, Abid A, et al. Deep learning interpretation of echocardiograms. Npj Digit Med 2020;3(1):1–10.

97. Ben-Israel N, Kliger M, Zuckerman G, et al. Monitoring the nociception level: a multi-parameter approach. J Clin Monit Comput 2013;27(6):659–68.

98. Olesen AE, Grønlund D, Gram M, et al. Prediction of opioid dose in cancer pain patients using genetic profiling: not yet an option with support vector machine learning. BMC Res Notes 2018;11(1):78.

99. Tighe PJ, Lucas SD, Edwards DA, et al. Use of machine-learning classifiers to predict requests for preoperative acute pain service consultation. Pain Med 2012;13(10):1347–57.

100. Williams AM, Liu Y, Regner KR, et al. Artificial intelligence, physiological genomics, and precision medicine. Physiol Genomics 2018;50(4):237–43.

101. Combes C, Meskens N, Rivat C, et al. Using a KDD process to forecast the duration of surgery. Int J Prod Econ 2008;112(1):279–93.

102. Devi SP, Rao KS, Sangeetha SS. Prediction of surgery times and scheduling of operation theaters in ophthalmology department. J Med Syst 2012;36(2):415–30.

103. Houliston BR, Parry DT, Merry AF. TADAA: Towards Automated Detection of Anaesthetic Activity. Methods Inf Med 2011;50(5):464–71.

Telemedicine for Anesthesiologists

Kathryn Harter Bridges, MD*, Julie Ryan McSwain, MD

KEYWORDS

- Telemedicine • Preoperative care • Postoperative care • Remote consultation
- Surgical intensive care • Smartphone

KEY POINTS

- Preoperative telemedicine evaluation is associated with high satisfaction rates, increased patient cost savings and convenience, and equivalent day-of-surgery procedure cancellation rates compared with in-person evaluation.
- Preoperative teleconsultation may be performed via a direct-to-consumer approach with patient smartphone or tablet or a facilitated visit using a brick-and-mortar teleconsultation center.
- The intraoperative use of telemedicine for either educational purposes or direct patient care remains sparsely reported but requires highly reliable data transmission and communication.
- Virtual intensive care units can provide high levels of care to postoperative patients when traditional intensive care unit beds are in short supply.
- Compliance with federal and state regulations, medical licensing, equipment purchasing, data encryption, and informed consent must be addressed when initiating a telemedicine program.

INTRODUCTION

According to the World Health Organization, telemedicine is defined as the provision of health care services via the use of communication technology for the diagnosis and treatment of diseases.[1] Telemedicine technology is currently used across numerous medical specialties, including primary care, emergency services, critical care medicine, radiology, psychiatry, and anesthesiology. Virtual preoperative evaluation and remote intraoperative and postoperative care represent exciting areas of potential growth, expanding the provision of critical care services in times of need. The coronavirus disease 2019 (COVID-19) pandemic has reinforced the need for telehealth program expansion to allow delivery of care in the face of mandated distancing and

Department of Anesthesia and Perioperative Medicine, Medical University of South Carolina, 25 Courtenay Drive, Suite 4200, MSC 240, Charleston, SC 29425, USA
* Corresponding author.
E-mail address: bridgek@musc.edu

Anesthesiology Clin 39 (2021) 583–596
https://doi.org/10.1016/j.anclin.2021.04.006
1932-2275/21/© 2021 Elsevier Inc. All rights reserved.

anesthesiology.theclinics.com

staff shortages. Anesthesiologists may see an increase in telemedicine opportunities in the preoperative, intraoperative, and postoperative periods that can further the advancement of the specialty.

PREOPERATIVE CARE

One of the first reported efforts to overcome distance barriers for health care purposes was telemetry research performed by the National Aeronautics and Space Administration in its manned space-flight program. This program showed that physiologic functions for astronauts in space could be monitored successfully by physicians on Earth.[2,3] In 1964, advances in closed-circuit television and video telecommunications allowed the establishment of the first interactive video link between the Nebraska Psychiatric Institute in Omaha and the Norfolk State Hospital, located 112 miles away.[2] Further technological developments paired with increased federal funding led to telemedicine growth over the subsequent decades, especially in psychiatry, emergency medicine, and radiology. The first reported use of telemedicine in anesthesiology occurred in 2004, in which 10 patients underwent preoperative evaluation using a nurse-operated video monitor.[4] Both the patients and anesthesiologists reported high satisfaction with the experience, and similar satisfaction and examination concordance rates were noted in multiple later studies.[5–7] These early studies were performed in a manner now labeled as facilitated visits, in which patients used a brick-and-mortar teleconsultation site with video and examination equipment operated by a trained staff member with data transmitted in real time to a physician in a separate facility.[8]

Potential benefits of remote preoperative evaluation include cost savings to patients, convenience, and reduced day-of-surgery cancellation rates. Introduction of remote preoperative evaluation within the Department of Veterans Affairs (VA) health care system was met with positive feedback, as 87.5% of patients thought that the use of telemedicine saved them time and money.[9] Similarly, Dick and colleagues[5] reported an average savings of approximately $1300 in lodging and travel costs when patients living more than 1288 km (800 miles) from the tertiary care center were provided the option of teleconsultation. Further, the VA health care system, after initiating preoperative telemedicine evaluation, noted an average yearly savings of $18,000 in patient travel reimbursement.[10] Benefits from telehealth preoperative evaluation are not limited to those patients who live rurally. Patients living in metropolitan areas and subject to traffic concerns have also experienced direct and opportunity cost savings when offered virtual evaluation.[11] Remote consultation may further reduce costs by reducing the need for patients to take time off work and/or arrange alternative childcare. Because it is known that distance may contribute to patients failing to attend an in-person preoperative clinic visit, overall compliance with preoperative evaluation may be improved with the availability of a remote option.[12]

Failure to undergo a preoperative anesthesia evaluation may result in day-of-surgery cancellation, which negatively affects hospitals and patients. Inadequate preoperative work-up is to blame for up to 25% of surgery cancellations.[13] Preoperative clinics have been proven to decrease the risk of cancellations and delays.[14–18] Thus, they may reduce the financial impact on hospital systems, as cancellation costs range from $1400 to $7500 per procedure in the private sector.[19] Telemedicine assessment has a similar efficacy to physical preoperative clinics in terms of impact on cancellation rates, with multiple studies reporting limited or no cancellations for incomplete preoperative evaluation.[6,9,20,21] Tam and colleagues[22] reported a day-of-surgery cancellation rate of 1.3%, consistent with the international average, in patients who underwent tele-health evaluation. More recently, Kamdar and colleagues[11] showed no difference in cancellation rates between patients who underwent telehealth preoperative evaluation (2.95% cancellation rate) versus in-person evaluation (3.23% cancellation rate). For hospitals, the cost of implementing telemedicine technology ranges from $1700 to $7000 and depends on the platform used. Hospitals with high cancellation rates or those with large numbers of patients who live remotely may see cost reduction following implementation of telemedicine services.

Appropriate patient selection is an important consideration for remote preoperative evaluation. The use of virtual evaluation has been studied in numerous patient populations, including those living in rural areas and, more recently, metropolitan areas.[4–7,11] Before oral and maxillofacial surgery, incarcerated patients with complicated travel needs underwent successful telemedicine preoperative evaluation with no noted complications, suggesting that the prison population in particular may benefit from remote evaluation.[20] Patients who live remotely and are scheduled for surgery within a short time frame and those in metropolitan areas with long commute times may find teleconsultation beneficial because of time constraints. Given the aging population in the United States, the need for preoperative evaluation of these patients will continue to expand. Teleconsultation may be of particular benefit in elderly patients in whom travel is challenging, including those who are bedbound, use wheelchairs, or rely on medical transport. Very few studies have identified what, if any, patient comorbidities exclude patients from potential telemedicine evaluation. The requirement for a physical examination of the heart and lungs may be a deciding factor in patient qualification for remote services, depending on the type of telemedicine equipment available. Although the ability to conduct visits with patients in their own homes via personal smartphone or tablet adds convenience, to complete a full physical evaluation, including vital signs and cardiopulmonary examination, patients must travel to a local teleconsultation center that contains the appropriate equipment as well as a health care provider who can assist in using the equipment. Whether patients with significant comorbidities are well suited to preoperative evaluation via personal smartphone or home computer, also known as direct-to-consumer visits, has been questioned. Kamdar and colleagues[11] showed that patients deemed American Society of Anesthesiologists physical status classification 3 and 4 can successfully undergo teleconsultation preoperatively with no noted difference in procedure cancellation rates.

INTRAOPERATIVE CARE

The successful intraoperative use of telemedicine in direct patient care has been described by case reports published over the past 2 decades. In 2004, Cone and colleagues[23] described the use of telemonitoring between an anesthesiologist in the state of Virginia (United States) to an operating room in Ecuador for a patient undergoing cholecystectomy. The patient had both an unexpected challenging airway with direct laryngoscopy as well as a simultaneous change in heart rhythm, which resulted in a shared decision to emerge the patient from the general anesthetic and perform an awake nasal intubation. Given the success of this collaboration, the investigators went on to publish a follow-up report whereby they used telemedicine for 7 other procedures during 2 separate surgical missions.[24] The investigators used real-time standard patient monitoring, audio transmission of heart and lung sounds via an electronic stethoscope, and visual transmission of the airway with fiberoptic cameras. In 2009, Fiadjoe and colleagues[25] reported the use of remote monitoring during liver transplant in which a Philadelphia-based team was able to successfully use telemedicine to assist with 2 separate liver transplants in India. Similarly, Hemmerling and colleagues[26] assessed the feasibility of transcontinental anesthesia between Canada and Italy for 20 adult patients undergoing elective thyroid surgery. Patients in Italy underwent total intravenous anesthesia via a closed-loop automated drug delivery system that was controlled remotely by anesthesiologists in Montreal, Canada, via a standard Internet connection. The investigators were successful in maintaining excellent or good control over the performance of the hypnotic infusion approximately 69% of the time as defined by maintaining a bispectral index value within 10% to 20% of the target goal of 45. These early case reports not only detail the use of transcontinental teleanesthesia but also describe the concept of telementoring, whereby teams can collaborate and provide educational instruction in real time using a range of audiovisual equipment.[24]

Extending beyond a standard Internet connection for vital signs monitoring, Miyashita and colleagues[27] reported reliable communication between mainland Japan and Sado Island, a private island 300 km off the coast of Japan, via use of a virtual private network and FaceTime (Apple Inc, Cupertino, CA) application. Teleanesthesia was instituted between these 2 sites as a means to overcome a shortage of qualified anesthetists on Sado Island in scenarios where 2 patients required simultaneous intraoperative care. Although the anesthetist at the local hospital was able to care for 1 patient directly, a remote anesthetist on mainland Japan directed the intraoperative care of the second patient via a nurse who physically received and executed anesthetic commands, including the management of vasopressor and anesthetic medications. In total, this pilot study provided parallel anesthesia for 25 patients with only 7 reported FaceTime disconnections lasting a total of 10 minutes, all of which occurred at times when no anesthetic commands were given and thus had no negative impact on operative care.

Because patient conditions can change rapidly within the intraoperative setting, losing data transmission and communication could result in catastrophic patient outcomes with significant liability issues. Although previously described pilot studies and case reports highlight the feasibility of instituting teleanesthesia using a variety of audiovideo tools, they are small in sample size and often include only healthy patients undergoing minor procedures. It is therefore difficult to draw conclusions on the overall safety of teleanesthesia for intraoperative care based on the available literature. For telemedicine to be safely used in direct patient care during the intraoperative period, equipment would need to consistently transmit all patient data, including, at minimum, electrocardiography, pulse oximetry, noninvasive blood pressure readings, and endtidal carbon dioxide concentration in real time. Procedures that involve prolonged operative time, large blood loss, or sustained periods of intraoperative instability may prove difficult to handle reliably via teleanesthesia. Another concern may be the unfamiliarity of the anesthesiologist with the remote staff who are providing direct patient care. Differences in skill sets, communication styles, and practice may give anesthesiologists pause because complications can occur in even the simplest of procedures. Therefore, it may be reasonable to ensure a baseline level of staff competency with common intraoperative procedures before instituting an intraoperative teleanesthesia program.

It is known that telemedicine can be used for educational purposes, primarily for instruction in procedural techniques. Miyashita and colleagues[28] describe the use of free real-time video conferencing tools to remotely educate and assist anesthesiologists in conducting ultrasonography-guided peripheral nerve blocks. Although the investigators primarily assessed the feasibility of different devices in providing the best real-time visual feedback, the possibility exists for future studies to investigate the use of telemedicine to remotely guide anesthesia providers in performing new procedures.

In addition, the intraoperative use of telemedicine could be extended to disaster situations, including mass casualty events, natural disasters, or infectious outbreaks, which can overwhelm normal staffing models and care pathways. These situations often necessitate the delivery of emergent care to large groups of people in 1 geographic region at a time, resulting in significant limitations to staffing resources. Looking to the future and building on successful programs of the past, applications of intraoperative telemedicine could expand to include monitoring in space and in the most remote areas of Earth.

POSTOPERATIVE CARE

Telemedicine has been extensively used for postoperative clinic visits as well as monitoring surgical patients immediately postprocedure in the hospital and following discharge.[29–32] Collins and colleagues[33] created a virtual intensive care unit (ICU) for patients in the postanesthesia care unit who needed ICU-level care but for whom ICU beds were not currently available. Approximately 72% of patients monitored via virtual care were able to transfer directly to the floor. This ability eliminated the need for physical ICU bed space while maintaining a safe solution for patients requiring a high level of care. Telemedicine for ICU patients also allows critical care physicians to care for patients at locations that may not have dedicated 24-hour critical care specialists. At our institution, the Medical University of South Carolina (MUSC), adult intensivists routinely provide round-the-clock ICU care to 10 different hospitals within the state of South Carolina.

Remote monitoring of medical data is a rapidly developing area of medical technology that has utility for anesthesiologists involved in the postoperative care of patients.[34] A recent pilot study described a mobile application to record in-hospital adherence to 15 different enhanced recovery program processes and monitor 6 patient outcomes in patients undergoing colorectal surgery.[35] Approximately 89% of the patients stated that the application was helpful in their recovery, and 76% stated that it increased motivation to recover.

Remote monitoring technology has the potential to affect care delivered by anesthesiologists who participate in Perioperative Surgical Home models as well as Enhanced Recovery Pathways.[36] Remote monitoring of patient data via wireless medical-grade biosensors is also being used in the care of postsurgical patients. At present, postoperative vital signs are taken intermittently, and deteriorations between measurements may be missed. In contrast, wearable biosensors monitor patient vital signs continuously. When combined with real-time analysis, this could lead to earlier notification of patient deterioration and decreased complication rates.[37,38] Biosensor technology may also have the ability to decrease activation of rapid response teams and failure to rescue events by alerting ward teams to an immediate change in patient condition.[38] However, it is not yet clear which patient populations these devices would best serve. Further, high-quality research needs to be conducted to determine whether such wearable devices can decrease complication rates in postsurgical patients. In addition, reliability, sustainability, and cost-effectiveness need to be critically evaluated before such wearable devices become mainstream. Development of virtual ICUs may present a potential solution when there is a shortage of critical care beds. However, there also needs to be further research into which surgical populations may best benefit from postoperative telemonitoring as well as evaluating the cost-benefit ratio of using this type of postoperative care compared with traditional approaches, both from a space and staffing perspective.

EQUIPMENT

Telemedicine equipment needs vary depending on the functionality desired, especially as it relates to physical examination capability. Formal video towers are highly capable, associated with high day-of-surgery examination concordance, and available in a wide price range.[6] These towers combine audiovisual communication technology, including a video screen and high-quality microphones and speakers for 2 way communication, with integrated physical examination tools (eg, digital stethoscopes, otoscopes, and movable cameras) to allow for a complete airway and cardiopulmonary examination[8] (**Fig. 1**). A dedicated staff member at the remote site moves the camera to allow examination of the head and neck, lower extremities, and any other relevant area. Video towers are available via multiple different vendors[39] and may offer more in-depth examination tools, including digital spirometers, 12-lead electrocardiogram testing, and ultrasonography probes for nerve, cardiac, or vascular imaging (**Fig. 2**).

As an alternative to full telemedicine video tower technology, various personal and business-oriented software programs exist to facilitate videoconferencing with patients via personal smartphone or home computer, including Skype (Skype Technologies, Palo Alto, CA), GoToMeeting (LogMeIn Inc, Boston, MA), Zoom (Zoom Video Communications, San Jose, CA), Doxy.me (Doxy.me LLC, Rochester, NY), Vidyo (Vidyo, Inc, Hackensack, NJ), and numerous others. Software programs should include a high degree of security encryption to ensure compliance with the Health Insurance Portability and Accountability Act of 1996 (HIPAA).[39] Ultimately the software choice may depend on desired electronic medical record (EMR) integration. For example, Zoom software may be used alongside the Epic-based EMR, whereas Vidyo can be used directly within Epic.[11] **Table 1** compares the equipment needs for remote preoperative evaluation via home tablet versus a teleconsultation center.

HEALTH INSURANCE PORTABILITY AND ACCOUNTABILITY ACT COMPLIANCE

With regard to telemedicine, essential requirements for HIPAA compliance include login controls, data encryption, and auditing ability.[40] Ensuring compliance with federal privacy laws can seem like an insurmountable hurdle, and noncompliance is a

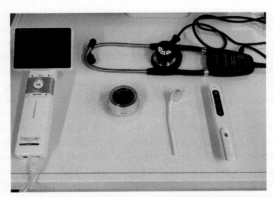

Fig. 1. Telehealth towers may be equipped with numerous physical examination tools. As pictured from left to right, these tools include a movable camera, ophthalmoscope attachment, dental mirror, movable light for airway examination, and electronic stethoscope (*top* of image).

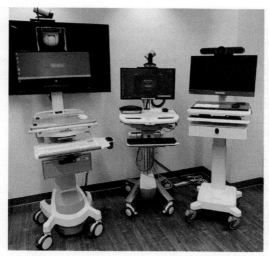

Fig. 2. Telehealth towers are offered from a range of vendors with various functionality and price points.

serious offense that can include heavy monetary fines with civil and criminal charges. In addition, medical providers must adhere to HIPAA's Omnibus Final Rule of 2013, which expanded and more rigorously defined the responsibilities of third party business associates to encompass all those who have access to patient data, such as software companies, hardware technicians, and training support staff.[41] In order to maintain compliance with HIPAA regulations and ensure data security, third parties involved in data storage must have a business associate agreement in place with the health care provider to provide liability protection in case of a data breach. However, no device is HIPAA compliant on its own, because compliance also encompasses the software used by the device to communicate with other technologies.[40]

The potential for data misuse cannot be understated because data collection, storage, access, and use from commercial products is under-regulated and not standardized within the United States.[42] For example, commonly used commercial communication platforms such as Skype, as well as Google-based platforms, are problematic because they store communication information on their own servers[43] and were not originally designed to meet the high standards of patient protection set forth by HIPAA. As such, choosing equipment and platforms to establish a HIPAA-compliant telemedicine program usually requires consultation with security and institutional compliance experts. Current events and reports regarding data use, storage, and sharing or selling between third parties among some of the largest tech companies in the world have made many citizens wary of sharing health data over mobile platforms, a hurdle that must be overcome in the expansion of telehealth.[42]

MEDICAL LICENSURE AND BILLING

Other legal concerns with regard to telemedicine include individual state medical licensing laws, teleprescription, and billing for virtual services. Medical licensure laws require that, whether conducting an in-person or remote evaluation, the physician is licensed in the state where the patient is physically located. This requirement imposes potential limitations on the performance of teleconsultation across state

Table 1
Comparison of telemedicine evaluation via personal smartphone or home computer versus facilitated telemedicine visit at a remote teleconsultation site

	Personal Smartphone or Computer	Facilitated Telemedicine Visit
Able to discuss medical history and anesthesia plan	Yes	Yes
Airway examination capability	Yes	Yes
Cardiopulmonary examination capability	No	Yes
Face-to-face interaction	Yes	Yes
Medical staff needed to operate equipment	No	Yes
Administrative support needed to identify and schedule patients	Yes	Yes
Basic testing capability (electrocardiogram, spirometry)	No	Yes
Patient participation from home	Yes	No
Minimum equipment required for patient	Two-way video and audio-capable device (smartphone, tablet, laptop, or home computer) Internet access	None
Minimum equipment required for institution	Video-capable device (laptop or computer) EMR access for charting Speakers or audio headset Internet access	For physician: Video-capable device (laptop or computer) EMR access for charting Speakers or audio headset Internet access At remote center: Video tower Electronic stethoscope Movable camera Internet access

lines. However, there is an Interstate Medical Licensure Compact (IMLC) that has been gaining acceptance. The IMLC is an agreement between 29 states, District of Columbia, and Territory of Guam that provides a voluntary expedited pathway to licensure of qualified physicians with the goal of increasing access to health care, especially in rural or underserved areas.[44] Although licensure through the Federation of State Medical Boards may be quicker under this agreement, it still requires physicians to pay licensure fees for all states in which they will practice. In contrast, VA hospitals enacted a national licensure in 2018 that enables VA practitioners to treat veterans no matter where the veteran or doctor is located.[45] Many states have developed reciprocity agreements in the midst of the COVID-19 pandemic to allow providers to care for patients across state lines and authorize telehealth services as accepted modes of care.[46] However, whether these temporary waivers extend beyond the pandemic crisis is unknown. In addition, several states are mandating commercial insurance coverage for telehealth services during the COVID-19 crisis.

In general, payment bundling does not change regardless of manner of evaluation, whether in-person or via a telemedicine visit. For example, at MUSC, preoperative clinic visits with an anesthesiologist are bundle billed with the anesthetic. However, our preoperative clinic also uses hospitalists who see patients as consults and therefore bill consultations, whether in-person or via telehealth, as a separate charge. Teleprescribing is less of a concern in most anesthesia-run preoperative clinics because rarely do anesthesiologists prescribe home medications before surgery.

INFORMED CONSENT

In the context of teleanesthesia, informed consent requires that patients be informed of how their treatment may deviate from conventional treatment, including the risks and benefits as well as limitations of teleconsultation. Patients should also be informed on who is participating in their care as well as the staff member's skill set and expertise. For example, the individuals making medical decisions for the care of the patient may be in a different physical location than those individuals carrying out those decisions and performing needed procedures. In addition, patients should be informed on how transmitted medical information will be used in their care (educational vs diagnostic) and the policies in place to store such medical information with the understanding that there exists the possibility of unauthorized access.[47] Regulation regarding informed consent varies between states, with some states requiring written consent and others allowing verbal consent. Using a consent form that includes names and credentials of all involved health care providers and a description of all telehealth services performed may be the best protection from a legal standpoint.[48] Current state laws and reimbursement policies with regard to telehealth can be found at the Center for Connected Health Policy at www.cchpca.org.

THE COVID-19 PANDEMIC

The Coronavirus Aid, Relief, and Economic Security (CARES) Act of 2020 lifted many of the restrictions placed on telehealth services and greatly expanded access to and billing for telehealth services. In addition, health care providers and patients across the world have shown rapid acceptance and flexibility in using both new and existing telehealth services given the health care climate during the COVID-19 pandemic. Although telemedicine use during the pandemic is perceived to be satisfactory to both patients and providers,[49,50] it is unclear whether most patients and health care providers will choose to continue with such robust use once the pandemic ends. Zhu and colleagues[50] reported that only a minority of surgical patients would continue to use telemedicine after the pandemic ends, with many stating that virtual visits may be better suited for long-term follow-up rather than immediate perioperative care. Patients reported a desire to have vital signs taken and a physical examination performed, as many tactile examinations are not possible during a telemedicine visit.[50]

In an effort to limit the spread of COVID-19 and comply with regional lockdown measures, many preoperative clinics have either limited or eliminated in-person preoperative clinic visits at various time points during the pandemic. Many institutions across the globe have instead quickly leveraged existing telehealth platforms or implemented new technology to conduct virtual preoperative visits. Although these visits, when performed from the comfort of a patient's home via personal tablet, may preclude a detailed physical examination or ability to perform on-site diagnostic testing, most patient information, as well as certain physical traits such as the airway, can be examined reliably. Virtual preoperative assessments may also help identify patients who are in need of timely surgery, especially when restrictions caused by regional COVID prevalence may limit the type and amount of elective surgery performed.[51] Some preoperative clinics may be uniquely situated to provide centralized assistance in both preoperative screening and testing for the novel coronavirus (severe acute respiratory syndrome–coronavirus-2 [SARS-CoV-2]) in the surgical patient population. Two recent publications describe institutional preoperative clinic pathways to instituting SARS-CoV-2 PCR testing, symptom screening, and infection prevention education in addition to routine preoperative care for presurgical patients.[52,53] Both pathways resulted in marked improvement in the percentage of patients with appropriately timed COVID-19 test results before surgery.[52,53] In addition, virtual preoperative clinic visits may help to alleviate some of the financial burden on health care systems caused by COVID-19 by continuing to provide billable patient care.[51]

The COVID-19 pandemic has strained inpatient health care resources across the globe. In particular, ICUs have suffered, with large volumes of critically ill patients admitted in short periods of time, making planning and forecasting resource needs extremely difficult, especially during the initial outbreak.[54] Large waves of admissions within days to weeks strain both medical equipment resources such as personal protective equipment and ventilators as well as ICU staffing resources, because these patients require time-intensive monitoring and care.[55,56] Many institutions across the world have leveraged telecritical care (TCC) as a method to deal with staffing inequities and expand ICU care. TCC delivered via synchronous 2-way audiovisual communication has evolved with prior global pandemics, including H1N1 influenza and SARS.[57] However, unique issues with regard to the COVID-19 pandemic include an unknown extent and speed of contagion that may challenge the effectiveness of existing TCC guidelines within institutions. Houston Medical Center broadened their existing virtual ICU (vICU) platform to meet the needs of a COVID-19 surge. Conservation of personal protective equipment, protection of medical staff consulting and working in COVID-19 units, and virtual visitation by patients' family members were all noted benefits of using a tiered vICU staffing model.[58] Singh and colleagues[59] also detail their institution's approach to leveraging an existing TCC system to meet the demands of COVID-19. Use of TCC allowed providers to minimize personal protective equipment use by decreasing the need for in-person care with patients in isolation and assist in monitoring and communication during high-risk procedures, including intubation, which allowed minimal staff entering or exiting rooms during aerosolizing procedures. However, increasing the scale of their existing TCC program involved the purchase of 130 additional mobile telehealth carts, a significant capital investment.[59] Smaller institutions may not have the resources or funds to increase infrastructure in such a fashion. One institution described the use of commercially available teleconferencing software and the installation of microphone-enabled high-definition webcams beside every computer to expand virtual capabilities during the pandemic, thus allowing continuous real-time communication with staff working in quarantined zones without the need for large-scale capital investment.[60]

Tiered virtual staffing models and telementoring can extend ICU care to those areas that may not traditionally have capacity to care for critically ill patients. This ability may provide ready access to specialty trained critical care physicians for patients who are quickly decompensating, and limit transfers between facilities, thus reducing risk of transmission.[61] The Society of Critical Care Medicine in collaboration with the Advanced Technology Research Center are investigating the establishment of a National Emergency Tele-Critical Care Network, which may further vICU care for future national and global emergencies.[61]

SUMMARY

Telemedicine has expanded rapidly over the past decade, and growth will continue as technology advances. Remote preoperative evaluation has proven benefits for patients and has been successfully used to allow resumption of needed care during the COVID-19 pandemic. As licensing compacts broaden to facilitate remote care, providers may see an expansion in their ability to care for patients across state lines. The use of telemedicine in anesthesiology, although new, offers great potential; however, care must be taken to ensure data security and HIPAA compliance. Institutions developing or expanding telehealth programs should perform cost-benefit analysis to guide the scope of development and determine equipment purchasing needs. The COVID-19 pandemic has led to the sharing of knowledge regarding virtual patient evaluation, and such collaboration must continue to allow advancement of telemedicine practice.

CLINICS CARE POINTS

- Remote preoperative evaluation can be performed via either patient-owned smartphone/tablet or a brick-and-mortar teleconsultation site and is associated with high patient and provider satisfaction rates, day-of-surgery examination concordance, and patient cost savings with no difference in surgical procedure cancellation rates compared with a physical preoperative clinic visit.

- Preoperative teleconsultation requires compliance with HIPAA laws and state medical licensure boards as well as potential equipment and software purchasing to ensure adequate data encryption.

- Intraoperative teleanesthesia has been described by several case reports with transcontinental success noted; however, potential pitfalls include lack of supervising anesthesiologist familiarity with staff providing direct patient care and questions regarding safety and legal liability in the event of data communication disruption.

- Postoperative telemedicine uses include both virtual ICUs to expand critical care services in rural areas or in times of bed shortages and as a means to conduct postoperative evaluation at home via patient's personal electronic device, both of which have been proven successful.

- The COVID-19 pandemic has expanded the reach of telemedicine, with several institutions reporting increased volume of patients undergoing telepreoperative evaluation and others noting growth of TCC capacity; however, capital investment may be required to facilitate virtual ICU growth.

DISCLOSURE

The authors have nothing to disclose.

REFERENCES

1. WHO. A health telematics policy in support of WHO's Health-For-All strategy for global health development: report of the WHO group consultation on health telematics, 11–16 December, Geneva, 1997. Geneva (Switzerland): World Health Organization; 1998.
2. Zundel KM. Telemedicine: history, applications, and impact on librarianship. Bull Med Libr Assoc 1996;84(1):71–9.
3. Bashshur R, Lovett J. Assessment of telemedicine: results of the initial experience. Aviat Space Environ Med 1977;48(1):65–70.

4. Wong DT, Kamming D, Salenieks ME, et al. Preadmission anesthesia consultation using telemedicine technology: a pilot study. Anesthesiology 2004;100(6): 1605–7.

5. Dick PT, Filler R, Pavan A. Participant satisfaction and comfort with multidisciplinary pediatric telemedicine consultations. J Pediatr Surg 1999;34(1):137–41 [discussion: 141–2].

6. Applegate RL 2nd, Gildea B, Patchin R, et al. Telemedicine pre-anesthesia evaluation: a randomized pilot trial. Telemed J E Health 2013;19(3):211–6.

7. Roberts S, Spain B, Hicks C, et al. Telemedicine in the Northern Territory: an assessment of patient perceptions in the preoperative anaesthetic clinic. Aust J Rural Health 2015;23(3):136–41.

8. Shih J, Portnoy J. Tips for Seeing Patients via Telemedicine. Curr Allergy Asthma Rep 2018;18(10):50.

9. Zetterman CV, Sweitzer BJ, Webb B, et al. Validation of a virtual preoperative evaluation clinic: a pilot study. Stud Health Technol Inform 2011;163:737–9.

10. Russo J, McCool R, Davies L. VA telemedicine: an analysis of cost and time savings. telemedicine and e-Health. Telemed J E Health 2016;22(3):209–15.

11. Kamdar NV, Huverserian A, Jalilian L, et al. Development, implementation, and evaluation of a telemedicine preoperative evaluation initiative at a major Academic Medical Center. Anesth Analg 2020;131(6):1647–56.

12. Seidel JE, Beck CA, Pocobelli G, et al. Location of residence associated with the likelihood of patient visit to the preoperative assessment clinic. BMC Health Serv Res 2006;6:13.

13. Yu K, Xie X, Luo L, et al. Contributing factors of elective surgical case cancellation: a retrospective cross-sectional study at a single-site hospital. BMC Surg 2017;17(1):100.

14. Argo JL, Vick CC, Graham LA, et al. Elective surgical case cancellation in the Veterans Health Administration system: identifying areas for improvement. Am J Surg 2009;198(5):600–6.

15. Ferschl MB, Tung A, Sweitzer B, et al. Preoperative clinic visits reduce operating room cancellations and delays. Anesthesiology 2005;103(4):855–9.

16. Seim AR, Fagerhaug T, Ryen SM, et al. Causes of cancellations on the day of surgery at two major university hospitals. Surg Innov 2009;16(2):173–80.

17. van Klei WA, Moons KG, Rutten CL, et al. The effect of outpatient preoperative evaluation of hospital inpatients on cancellation of surgery and length of hospital stay. Anesth Analg 2002;94(3):644–9 [table of contents].

18. Knox M, Myers E, Hurley M. The impact of pre-operative assessment clinics on elective surgical case cancellations. Surgeon 2009;7(2):76–8.

19. Campbell C MA, Russo S, Abdur-Rahman N,Pierre N, Rosinia F, Bent S. The Financial Burden of Cancelled Surgeries: Implications for Performance Improvement. Paper presented at: American Society of Anesthesiologists' Practice Management Conference. Houston (TX), January 28-30, 2011.

20. Rollert MK, Strauss RA, Abubaker AO, et al. Telemedicine consultations in oral and maxillofacial surgery. J Oral Maxillofac Surg 1999;57(2):136–8.

21. Mullen-Fortino M, Rising KL, Duckworth J, et al. Presurgical assessment using telemedicine technology: impact on efficiency, effectiveness, and patient experience of care. Telemed J E Health 2018;25(2):137–42.

22. Tam A, Leung A, O'Callaghan C, et al. Role of telehealth in perioperative medicine for regional and rural patients in Queensland. Intern Med J 2017;47(8):933–7.

23. Cone SW, Gehr L, Hummel R, et al. Case report of remote anesthetic monitoring using telemedicine. Anesth Analg 2004;98(2):386–8, table of contents.

24. Cone SW, Gehr L, Hummel R, et al. Remote anesthetic monitoring using satellite telecommunications and the Internet. Anesth Analg 2006;102(5):1463–7.

25. Fiadjoe J, Gurnaney H, Muralidhar K, et al. Telemedicine consultation and monitoring for pediatric liver transplant. Anesth Analg 2009;108(4):1212–4.

26. Hemmerling TM, Arbeid E, Wehbe M, et al. Evaluation of a novel closed-loop total intravenous anaesthesia drug delivery system: a randomized controlled trial. Br J Anaesth 2013;110(6):1031–9.

27. Miyashita T, Mizuno Y, Sugawara Y, et al. A pilot study of tele-anaesthesia by virtual private network between an island hospital and a mainland hospital in Japan. J Telemed Telecare 2015;21(2):73–9.

28. Miyashita T, Iketani Y, Nagamine Y, et al. FaceTime((R)) for teaching ultrasound-guided anesthetic procedures in remote place. J Clin Monit Comput 2014;28(2):211–5.

29. Nikolian VC, Williams AM, Jacobs BN, et al. Pilot Study to Evaluate the Safety, Feasibility, and Financial Implications of a Postoperative Telemedicine Program. Ann Surg 2018;268(4):700–7.

30. Gunter RL, Chouinard S, Fernandes-Taylor S, et al. Current Use of Telemedicine for Post-Discharge Surgical Care: A Systematic Review. J Am Coll Surg 2016;222(5):915–27.

31. Vyas KS, Hambrick HR, Shakir A, et al. A Systematic Review of the Use of Telemedicine in Plastic and Reconstructive Surgery and Dermatology. Ann Plast Surg 2017;78(6):736–68.

32. McGillicuddy JW, Gregoski MJ, Weiland AK, et al. Mobile health medication adherence and blood pressure control in renal transplant recipients: a proof-of-concept randomized controlled trial. JMIR Res Protoc 2013;2(2):e32.

33. Collins TA, Robertson MP, Sicoutris CP, et al. Telemedicine coverage for post-operative ICU patients. J Telemed Telecare 2017;23(2):360–4.

34. Safavi KC, Driscoll W, Wiener-Kronish JP. Remote surveillance technologies: realizing the aim of right patient, right data, right time. Anesth Analg 2018;129(3):726–34.

35. Pecorelli N, Fiore JF Jr, Kaneva P, et al. An app for patient education and self-audit within an enhanced recovery program for bowel surgery: a pilot study assessing validity and usability. Surg Endosc 2018;32(5):2263–73.

36. Merchea A, Larson DW. Enhanced recovery after surgery and future directions. Surg Clin North Am 2018;98(6):1287–92.

37. Joshi M, Ashrafian H, Aufegger L, et al. Wearable sensors to improve detection of patient deterioration. Expert Rev Med Devices 2019;16(2):145–54.

38. Boer C, Touw HR, Loer SA. Postanesthesia care by remote monitoring of vital signs in surgical wards. Curr Opin Anaesthesiol 2018;31(6):716–22.

39. Meyer BC, Clarke CA, Troke TM, et al. Essential telemedicine elements (tele-ments) for connecting the academic health center and remote community providers to enhance patient care. Acad Med 2012;87(8):1032–40.

40. Baker J, Stanley A. Telemedicine technology: a review of services, equipment, and other aspects. Curr Allergy Asthma Rep 2018;18(11):60.

41. Levy M. The new world of interaction recording for medical practices. J Med Pract Manage 2016;31(4):245–50.

42. Schairer CE, Rubanovich CK, Bloss CS. How could commercial terms of use and privacy policies undermine informed consent in the age of mobile health? AMA J Ethics 2018;20(9):E864–72.

43. HIPAA Guidelines on Telemedicine. HIPAA Journal. Available at: https://www.hipaajournal.com/hipaa-guidelines-on-telemedicine/. Accessed January 14, 2019.
44. Interstate medical licensure compact. Available at: https://www.imlcc.org/a-faster-pathway-to-physician-licensure/. Accessed October 1, 2020.
45. Affairs DoV, editor. Authority of health care providers to practice telehealth, vol. 38. Federal Register; 2018. p. 8. CFR Part 17.
46. Federation of state medical boards: U.S. States and territories modifying requirements for telehealth in response to COVID-19. Available at: https://www.fsmb.org/siteassets/advocacy/pdf/states-waiving-licensure-requirements-for-telehealth-in-response-to-covid-19.pdf. Accessed October 1, 2020.
47. Dreezen I. Telemedicine and informed consent. Med L 2004;23(3):541–9.
48. Reisenwitz C. 2 big telemedicine malpractice risks - and how to protect yourself 2017. Available at: https://blog.capterra.com/2-big-telemedicine-malpractice-risks-and-how-to-protect-yourself/. Accessed January 14, 2019.
49. Holtz BE. Patients perceptions of telemedicine visits before and after the coronavirus disease 2019 pandemic. Telemed J E Health 2020;27(1):107–12.
50. Zhu C, Williamson J, Lin A, et al. Implications for telemedicine for surgery patients after COVID-19: survey of patient and provider experiences. Am Surg 2020;86(8):907–15.
51. Mihalj M, Carrel T, Gregoric ID, et al. Telemedicine for preoperative assessment during a COVID-19 pandemic: Recommendations for clinical care. Best Pract Res Clin Anaesthesiol 2020;34(2):345–51.
52. Pai SL, Irizarry-Alvarado JM, Pitruzzello NE, et al. Responding to the COVID-19 pandemic: a new surgical patient flow utilizing the preoperative evaluation clinic. Am J Med Qual 2020;35(6):444–9.
53. McSwain JR, Bridges KH, Wilson SH, et al. Positive or Negative? Implementation Processes and Pitfalls of Preoperative SARS-CoV-2 Testing at a Single Academic Institution. Perioper Care Oper Room Manag 2020;21:100132.
54. Grasselli G, Pesenti A, Cecconi M. Critical Care Utilization for the COVID-19 outbreak in lombardy, italy: early experience and forecast during an emergency response. JAMA 2020;323(16):1545–6.
55. Ranney ML, Griffeth V, Jha AK. Critical Supply Shortages - The Need for Ventilators and Personal Protective Equipment during the Covid-19 Pandemic. N Engl J Med 2020;382(18):e41.
56. Xie J, Tong Z, Guan X, et al. Critical care crisis and some recommendations during the COVID-19 epidemic in China. Intensive Care Med 2020;46(5):837–40.
57. Lilly CM, Zubrow MT, Kempner KM, et al. Critical care telemedicine: evolution and state of the art. Crit Care Med 2014;42(11):2429–36.
58. Dhala A, Sasangohar F, Kash B, et al. Rapid Implementation and Innovative Applications of a Virtual Intensive Care Unit During the COVID-19 Pandemic: Case Study. J Med Internet Res 2020;22(9):e20143.
59. Singh J, Green MB, Lindblom S, et al. Telecritical care clinical and operational strategies in response to COVID-19. Telemed J E Health 2020;27(3):261–8.
60. Thakuria L, Igra A, Cervera-Jackson R, et al. Rapid deployment of virtual ICU support when resources are compromised. J Crit Care 2020;59:55–6.
61. Scott BK, Miller GT, Fonda SJ, et al. Advanced Digital Health Technologies for COVID-19 and future emergencies. Telemed J E Health 2020;26(10):1226–33.